SHORT TEXTB
ANESTHESIA

Disclaimer

Medicine is an ever and rapidly changing science. The author has tried his best to obtain the information from the sources which he has believed to be the most reliable and in accordance with the latest guidelines and recommendations. However, there is always a possibility of error and change in guidelines. Therefore, author and publisher disclaim all the responsibilities arising from any act of commission or omission, because of the information used from the contents of this book.

SHORT TEXTBOOK OF
ANESTHESIA

Sixth Edition

Ajay Yadav
MD (Anesthesiology)
Senior Consultant and Head
Department of Anesthesia and Critical Care
W Pratiksha Hospital
Gurugram, Haryana, India

JAYPEE *The Health Sciences Publisher*
New Delhi | London | Panama

Jaypee Brothers Medical Publishers (P) Ltd.

Headquarters
Jaypee Brothers Medical Publishers (P) Ltd
4838/24, Ansari Road, Daryaganj
New Delhi 110 002, India
Phone: +91-11-43574357
Fax: +91-11-43574314
E-mail: jaypee@jaypeebrothers.com

Overseas Offices

J.P. Medical Ltd
83, Victoria Street, London
SW1H 0HW (UK)
Phone: +44 20 3170 8910
Fax: +44 (0)20 3008 6180
E-mail: info@jpmedpub.com

Jaypee-Highlights Medical Publishers Inc
City of Knowledge, Bld. 235, 2nd Floor, Clayton
Panama City, Panama
Phone: +1 507-301-0496
Fax: +1 507-301-0499
E-mail: cservice@jphmedical.com

Jaypee Brothers Medical Publishers (P) Ltd
17/1-B, Babar Road, Block-B, Shaymali
Mohammadpur, Dhaka-1207
Bangladesh
Mobile: +08801912003485
E-mail: jaypeedhaka@gmail.com

Jaypee Brothers Medical Publishers (P) Ltd
Bhotahity, Kathmandu
Nepal
Phone: +977-9741283608
E-mail: kathmandu@jaypeebrothers.com

Website: www.jaypeebrothers.com
Website: www.jaypeedigital.com

© 2018, Jaypee Brothers Medical Publishers

Short Textbook of Anesthesia

Sixth Edition: **2018**

ISBN: 978-93-5270-464-4

Printed at: Paras Offset Pvt. Ltd., New Delhi

Dedicated to

My father Late Shri HS Yadav
Freedom Fighter, Indian National Army
and
All those great countrymen who
sacrificed their lives to make India
free and build a great nation

A Very Simple Thought to Kill Piracy

How much are we justified in getting the photocopy of original books?

What psychology do we have that we do not mind spending any amount of money on entertainment, electronic gadgets, fashion, food or fiction books, but for professional books, we feel burdened in spending even a little amount which may be just a cost of popcorn at the multiplex or a burger meal at a fast food point. Do not we think that it is the same profession by which we are earning for entertainment, electronic gadgets, fashion, food or fiction books?

By doing this, are not we insulting our profession or in fact ourselves?

You being the most educated class of society, just think over it and decide.

Preface to the Sixth Edition

As we know that medicine is ever changing, anesthesia has seen rapid changes in the last few years. In this edition, I have tried my best to incorporate the most recent advances in drugs, equipment and techniques; Cardiopulmonary resuscitation (CPR) guidelines are based on American Heart Association (AHA) 2015 guidelines. All the chapters have been thoroughly revised and updated with addition of few new chapters; there have been significant changes in almost all chapters.

This edition has been divided into nine sections providing a basic knowledge of physiology and pharmacology related to anesthesia, anesthesia machine and equipment, various anesthetic drugs and techniques in normal subjects and patients suffering from medical ailments and subspecialty management. I hope that chapters on intensive care management and cardiopulmonary resuscitation will be very useful to students.

To make the revision easier at the last time where a student does not get enough time to read the whole subject, the most important points are presented in italics, and moreover, key points are given at the end of each chapter. Wherever possible, a summary of topics has been presented in tabulated form. However, I will sincerely advise the students to go through the whole text at least once.

Although every effort has been made to minimize the scope of error, but still no one is perfect in this world. So, minor grammatical errors may be overlooked, but any major error or controversy may immediately be brought to the notice of author/publisher either through e-mail address or in writing. My e-mail address is dryadavajay@rediffmail.com. We will be highly obliged and try to rectify the mistake or clear up the controversy as soon as possible.

I hope that this edition of the book would be of immense value in providing the basic knowledge of anesthesia to undergraduate students. I am sure that this book would not only help in solving the anesthesia questions, but also questions related to intensive care therapy, applied physiology and emergency medicine.

I thank M/s Jaypee Brothers Medical Publishers (P) Ltd., New Delhi, India, for their efforts in bringing out this book in this elegant shape.

Ajay Yadav

Preface to the First Edition

Anesthesia is often the overlooked subject during undergraduation; however, the requirement of basic knowledge of anesthesia at undergraduate level has become necessary because of multiple reasons. Firstly, because of the increasing scope of this specialty which is not only restricted to operation theaters, but also to intensive care units, pain management and emergency medicine. Secondly, and also very importantly, the questions of anesthesiology asked in different postgraduate (PG) entrance examinations are not only increasing in number, but also getting tougher and can only be answered if the student is having reasonable knowledge of the subject.

To fulfill these requirements, I decided to write *Short Textbook of Anesthesia*.

In this book, I put my efforts to provide a comprehensive text keeping more focus on topics which are frequently asked in various pre-PG examinations.

One more point I kept in mind while writing this book was to take care of the controversies commonly encountered during preparation of pre-PG examination because of different values and criteria mentioned in different books. For example, the color of oxygen cylinder in India and in most of the countries is black, while in USA, it is green. A blood transfusion criterion in India is volume loss more than 20%, while in western countries, it is 25–30%. In my book, values and criteria which are applicable in India have been mentioned and wherever found necessary difference to western countries has also been mentioned. I would like to advise the students to abide by the Indian standards, at least in anesthesiology.

Any suggestions, criticisms and controversies which can really help in improving this book are most welcome.

I wish best of luck to all the students appearing for the various pre-PG examinations.

Ajay Yadav

Acknowledgments

First of all I would like to thank my teachers at PGIMS, Rohtak, Haryana, India, who enabled me to do my undergraduation.

I wish to express my sincere thanks to my first teachers Dr Neelam and Dr Meenakshi, SMS Medical College, Jaipur, Rajasthan, India, from whom I learned the ABC of anesthesia.

I would be failing in my duty if I do not express my gratitude to my eminent guide, Dr Vijender Sharma, under whom I not only did my thesis, but also learnt a lot about life. I have yet to come across a person gentler than him; whatever goodness I have, I owed it to him.

I would also like to thank my seniors, Dr Madhu Jain, Dr Madhu Dixit, Dr S Kumar, and my colleagues, at Hindu Rao Hospital, New Delhi, India, whose indispensable help led me to start this venture.

I feel pleasure in conveying my sincere thanks to Mr Nishant Bajaj, CEO and Dr Ragni Agrawal, Medical Director, W Pratiksha Hospital, Gurugram, Haryana, India, for providing such an excellent and encouraging academic atmosphere in the hospital.

I am very thankful to my department colleagues, at the W Pratiksha Hospital, the discussions with whom have really helped me in keeping update with recent advances.

I would like to pay my very special thanks to my wife Promila, who has been a constant source of inspiration for me every moment. I would also like to pay my thanks to my sons, Vasu and Eklavya, friends and family members, who always stood like pillars for me.

I would be failing in my duty if I do not express my thanks to all undergraduate students who have really inspired me to write this book.

And last but not least, I would like to thank M/s Jaypee Brothers Medical Publishers (P) Ltd., New Delhi, India, for their technical help and kind support without which this venture would have not been possible.

Contents

SECTION 6 Regional Anesthesia

SECTION 7 Anesthesia for Coexisting Diseases

SECTION 8 Subspecialty Anesthetic Management

SECTION 9 Cardiorespiratory Care

Plate 1

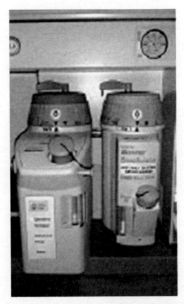

Fig. 2.12: Desflurane (with blue dial knob) and sevoflurane (with yellow dial knob) vaporizer

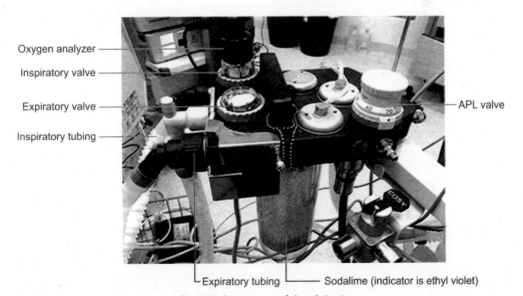

Fig. 2.19: Components of closed circuit

Plate 2

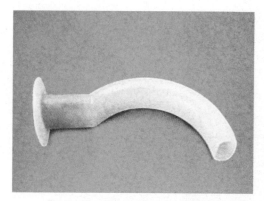

Fig. 3.1: Guedel's oropharyngeal airway

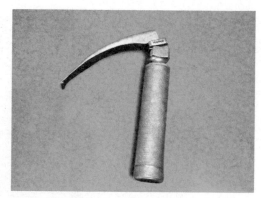

Fig. 3.5: Macintosh laryngoscope

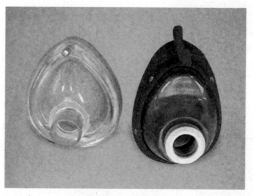

Fig. 3.2: Facemask

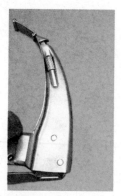

Fig. 3.6: McCoy laryngoscope

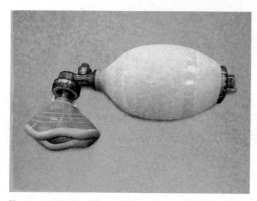

Fig. 3.4: AMBU bag (Note there is an option for attaching reservoir bag and oxygen supply)

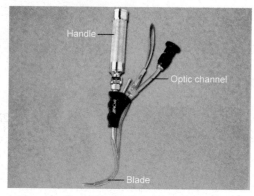

Fig. 3.7: Bullard laryngoscope

Plate 3

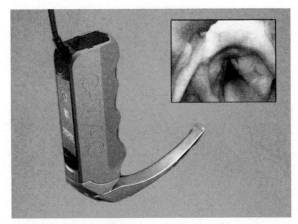

Fig. 3.8: C-MAC laryngoscope and picture of glottis seen on screen

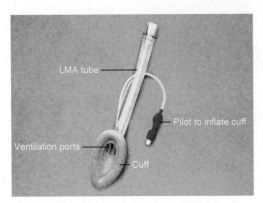

Fig. 3.10: Laryngeal mask airway (Classic)

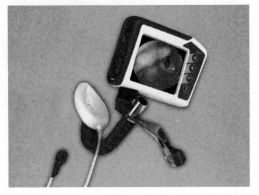

Fig. 3.15: LMA C-Trach

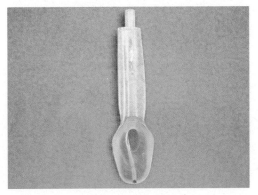

Fig. 3.14: I-Gel

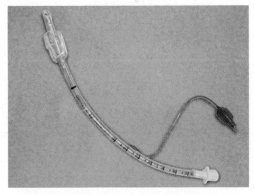

Fig. 3.17A: Cuffed endotracheal tube (PVC type)

Plate 4

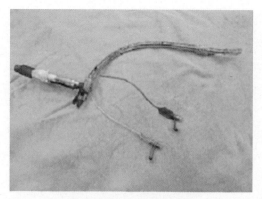

Fig. 3.19: Double lumen tube
(Note 2 cuffs, 2 pilot system and 2 ventilation ports)

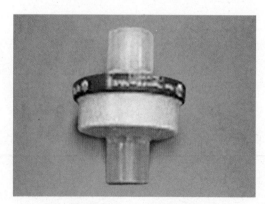

Fig. 3.20: Heat and moisture exchanger

Fundamental Concepts

CHAPTER 1

Applied Anatomy, Physiology and Physics

RESPIRATORY PHYSIOLOGY

Anatomy of Airways

Larynx (Fig. 1.1)

It is the organ of voice extending from root of tongue to trachea and lies opposite C3 to C6.

Distance between teeth and vocal cords is 12–15 cm and distance between vocal cords and carina is 10–15 cm.

It consists of 3 paired cartilages namely arytenoid, corniculate and cuneiform and three unpaired cartilages, namely thyroid, cricoid and epiglottis.

The glottis is the narrowest part in adults while *subglottis (at the level of cricoid) is the narrowest part in children up to the age of 6 years.* As subglottis is the narrowest part, the cuff of endotracheal tube can cause subglottic edema and stenosis, therefore the traditional approach had been not to use cuffed tube in children, however this approach is not followed in current day practice.

Nerve supply: All muscles of the larynx are supplied by recurrent laryngeal nerve except cricothyroid which is supplied by external branch of superior laryngeal nerve.

Sensory supply: Up to vocal cords by internal branch of superior laryngeal nerve and below vocal cords by recurrent laryngeal nerve.

Arterial supply: By laryngeal branches of superior and inferior thyroid arteries.

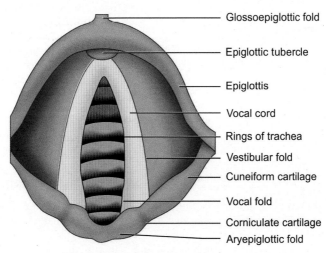

Glossoepiglottic fold

Epiglottic tubercle

Epiglottis

Vocal cord

Rings of trachea

Vestibular fold

Cuneiform cartilage

Vocal fold

Corniculate cartilage

Aryepiglottic fold

Fig. 1.1: Laryngoscopic view of larynx

Paralysis of Nerves of Larynx

- Paralysis of recurrent laryngeal nerve of one side has no serious consequences as it is compensated by other side. There is only hoarseness of voice.
- In *bilateral partial paralysis of recurrent laryngeal nerve,* the abductors (posterior cricoarytenoids) will go first (Semon's Law) causing the cords to be held in adduction producing respiratory stridor.
- In *complete paralysis of recurrent laryngeal nerve,* the cords are still held in adducted position due to tensing action of cricothyroid which is supplied by superior laryngeal nerve, causing severe respiratory distress, stridor, aphonia and complete obstruction. A tracheostomy is usually required for the management.
- In *complete paralysis of both recurrent and superior laryngeal nerves,* the cords are held in mid-position (*cadaveric position*).
- *Cords are also in cadaveric position during anesthesia with muscle relaxants.*

Trachea

- Length of the trachea is 10–12 cm.
- It starts from cricoid ring (C6) and ends at carina (T5). Anteriorly carina corresponds to second costal cartilage at the junction of manubrium with sternal body *(angle of Louis).*
- It consists of 16–20 incomplete rings.
- The diameter of trachea is 1.2 cm.

Bronchial Tree (Fig. 1.2)

At carina trachea divides into right and left main bronchus. Distance of carina from upper incisors is 28–30 cm.

Further right main bronchus divides into right upper, middle and lower lobe bronchus and left main bronchus into left upper and lower lobe bronchus.

- Due to shorter, wider and less acute angle *chances of endotracheal tube to be positioned on right side (endobronchial intubation) are more* **(Table 1.1).**
- In children the angle of both right and left bronchus is same, i.e. *55° up to the age of 3 years.*

Right upper lobe bronchus divides into apical, posterior and anterior segment bronchi.

Right middle lobe bronchus divides into lateral and medial segment bronchi.

Right lower lobe bronchus divides into apical, medial basal, anterior basal, lateral basal and posterior basal segment bronchi.

Left upper lobe bronchus divides into apical, anterior and posterior segment bronchi. Left upper lobe bronchus also gives rise to lingular bronchus, which is further subdivided into superior and inferior segment bronchi.

Left lower lobe bronchus divides into apical, anterior basal, posterior basal and lateral basal segment bronchi.

Segmental bronchi along with lung paren-chyma constitutes *bronchopulmonary segments* which are 10 in number on right side, viz.

Upper lobe: Apical, posterior and anterior.

Middle lobe: Lateral and medial.

Lower lobe: Apical (superior), medial basal (cardiac), anterior basal, lateral basal and posterior basal.

On the left side bronchopulmonary segments are 9 in number, viz.

Upper lobe: Apical, posterior and anterior.

Lingular lobe: Superior lingular and inferior lingular.

Lower lobe: Apical, inferior basal, lateral basal and posterior basal.

These segmental bronchi further divide and re-divide till terminal bronchioles. Further these terminal bronchioles lose their cartilage to form *respiratory bronchiole* which with alveolar duct and alveolar sac forms the *respiratory unit. It is at this alveolar capillary membrane where gaseous exchange takes place.* The thickness of alveolar capillary membrane is 0.3 mm.

Total number of alveoli is 300 million with surface area of 70 m^2.

Alveolar epithelium has type I and type II cells. Type II cells secrete surfactant.

FOREIGN BODY ASPIRATION

Due to shorter, wider and less acute angle of right bronchus foreign body aspiration is more common on right side.

- In *supine position most commonly involved segment is apical segment of right lower lobe.*

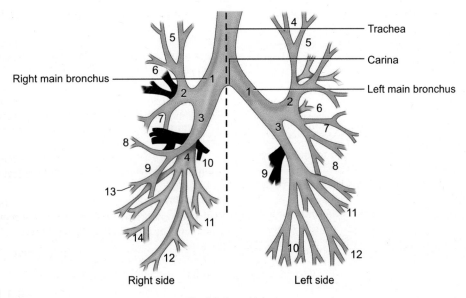

Fig. 1.2: Bronchial tree

Right side	Left side
1. Right main bronchus	1. Left main bronchus
2. Right upper lobe bronchus	2. Left upper lobe bronchus
3. Right middle lobe bronchus	3. Left lower lobe bronchus
4. Right lower lobe bronchus	4. Apical upper lobe bronchus
5. Apical segment bronchus	5. Posterior upper lobe bronchus
6. Posterior segment bronchus	6. Anterior upper lobe bronchus
7. Anterior segment bronchus	7. Superior bronchus
8. Lateral segment bronchus	8. Inferior bronchus
9. Medial segment bronchus	9. Apical bronchus
10. Apical segment bronchus	10. Anterior basal bronchus
11. Medial basal bronchus	11. Lateral basal bronchus
12. Anterior basal bronchus	12. Posterior basal bronchus
13. Lateral basal bronchus	
14. Posterior basal bronchus	

■ **Table 1.1:** Comparison of the anatomy of the right and left bronchus

Right bronchus	Left bronchus
Shorter (length 2.5 cm)	Longer (length 5 cm)
Wider	Narrower
The angle with vertical is 25°	The angle is 45°
—	Aorta arches over the left main bronchus

- In lateral position, most commonly involved segment is posterior segment of upper lobe (right upper lobe in right lateral and left upper lobe in left lateral).

- In standing/sitting aspiration, most commonly aspiration occurs in posterior basal segment of right lower lobe.

Mucosa: Ciliated epithelium up to terminal bronchioles after which non-ciliated epithelium.

Ciliary activity is inhibited by all inhalational agents except ether.

Arterial supply: Bronchial artery up to terminal bronchioles and beyond terminal bronchioles by pulmonary artery.

Nerve supply: Parasympathetic by vagus (causes bronchoconstriction).

Sympathetic by T2 to T5 (causes broncho-dilatation).

REGULATION OF RESPIRATION

Mediated by:
- Pneumotaxic center in upper pons.
- Apneustic center in lower pons.
- Ventral group of neurons in medulla (expiratory group).
- Dorsal group of neurons in medulla (inspiratory group).

Normally pneumotaxic center has inhibitory effect on apneustic center which otherwise produces apneustic breathing or inspiratory spasm.

Normal respiration is maintained by expiratory and inspiratory neurons of medulla.

During inspiration stretch receptors in lung parenchyma, which are supplied by vagus get stimulated leading to inhibition of inspiratory group of neurons, and hence stopping the inspiration.

Expiration is normally passive and expiratory group of neurons comes into play only during active expiration.

These central respiratory centers are most sensitive to changes in CSF pH, which in turn is influenced by pCO_2 (partial pressure of carbon dioxide in blood).

Increase in pCO_2 stimulates the respiration while decrease in pCO_2 inhibits respiration. Other factors effecting respiratory centers are:
- Body temperature
- Hypoxia
- Exercise
- Pain
- Hypothalamus
- Cortex.

Peripheral chemoreceptors: These are present in carotid body and aortic arch. *Carotid body receptors are very sensitive to hypoxia.*

All inhalational agents (except nitrous oxide and minimum with ether) have depressant effect on ventilatory response to increased CO_2 and hypoxia.

MUSCLES OF RESPIRATION

Inspiration

Diaphragm is the most important muscle of inspiration (moves 1.5 cm in quiet respiration and 6–10 cm in deep breathing).

External intercostals, pectoralis minor and scalene also assist in normal inspiration.

Pectoralis major, latissimus dorsi and sternomastoids are needed during deep inspiration.

Respiration in males is abdominothoracic while in children and females, it is thoracoabdominal.

Expiration

Expiration is normally passive. Forced expiration is mediated by internal intercostals and abdominal muscles.

During anesthesia with inhalational agents expiration is active, mediated by abdominal muscles.

AIRWAY RESISTANCE

For air to flow in lungs a pressure gradient must develop to overcome the airway resistance. This pressure gradient depends on airway caliber and pattern of airflow.

At laminar flows (which occurs below the main bronchi where velocity is less), resistance is proportional to flow rates but at turbulent flow (seen in trachea and main bronchi) resistance is square of flow rates. In other words, it can be said that *maximum airway resistance to airflow occurs in trachea and then main bronchus and minimum in terminal bronchi.*

VENTILATION/PERFUSION (V/Q)

Both ventilation and perfusion is more at bases as compared to apex but perfusion at base is comparatively higher decreasing V/Q ratio towards base (from 2.1 at apex to 0.3 at base, average 0.8).

This ventilation perfusion mismatch is responsible for producing *alveolar dead space* (i.e. alveoli are only ventilated but not perfused, wasting the oxygen in alveoli).

This V/Q mismatch creates alveolar to arterial oxygen difference [(A–a) pO_2 difference] which is normally 3–5 mm Hg.

This A-a difference is increased in lung pathologies affecting alveoli such as pulmonary edema, acute respiratory distress syndrome (ARDS) and interstitial lung disease.

DEAD SPACE

Total dead space (also called as physiological dead space) = Anatomical dead space + Alveolar dead space.

Anatomical Dead Space

It is constituted by air which is not participating in diffusion. Therefore it is constituted by air present in nose, trachea and bronchial tree (up to terminal bronchioles). Normally, it is 30% of tidal volume or 2 mL/kg or 150 mL.

Anatomical dead space is increased in:
- Old age
- Neck extension
- Jaw protrusion
- Bronchodilators
- Increasing lung volume
- Atropine (causes bronchodilatation)
- Anesthesia mask, circuits
- *Intermittent positive pressure ventilation (IPPV) and positive end-expiratory pressure (PEEP).*

Anatomical dead space is decreased by:
- *Intubation* (nasal cavity is bypassed and diameter of tube is less than airway diameter)
- *Tracheostomy* (upper airways and nasal cavity bypassed)
- Hyperventilation (decreasing lung volume)
- Neck flexion
- Bronchoconstrictors.

Alveolar Dead Space

It is constituted by alveoli which are only ventilated but not perfused. It is 60–80 mL in standing position and zero in lying position (in lying position perfusion is equal in all parts of lung). It is increased by:
- Lung pathologies affecting diffusion at alveolar capillary membrane such as interstitial lung disease, pulmonary embolism, pulmonary edema and ARDS.
- General anesthesia.
- IPPV.
- PEEP.
- Hypotension.

Anesthesia and Dead Space
- All anesthesia circuits, masks, humidifiers increase the anatomical dead space.
- Endotracheal tubes, tracheostomy decreases the anatomical dead space by bypassing the upper airways.
- All inhalational agents increase both anatomical and alveolar dead space. Anatomical dead space is increased because all these agents are bronchodilators. Alveolar dead space is increased because of hypotension (decreased perfusion) produced by these agents.
- Positions during anesthesia, especially lateral position causes more ventilation in upper lung (non-dependent) and more blood flow in lower lung (dependent lung), thereby increasing the V/Q mismatch, and hence alveolar dead space. Other positions such as Trendelenburg, lithotomy also causes the V/Q mismatch.
- Anesthesia ventilation techniques such as IPPV, PEEP increase both anatomical and alveolar dead space. Anatomical dead space is increased by increasing lung volume and alveolar dead space is increased because of hypotension produced by IPPV and PEEP (Increase in intrathoracic pressure produced by IPPV/PEEP decreases the venous return, cardiac output and hence hypotension).

OXYGEN AND CARBON DIOXIDE IN BLOOD

Oxygen

Normal oxygen uptake is 250 mL/min.

Oxygen is mainly carried in blood attached to hemoglobin (1 g of Hb carries 1.34 mL of oxygen). Very less amount, 0.003 mL/dL/mm Hg is carried as dissolved fraction. Oxygen content of arterial blood is 20 mL/dL and that of venous blood is 15 mL/dL.

Oxygen Dissociation Curve (Fig. 1.3)

Normally, Hb is 97% saturated at normal partial pressure (pO_2) of oxygen, which is 95–98 mm Hg.

At 60 mm Hg, saturation is still 90%. After this point, there is sudden drop in oxygen saturation leading to significant desaturation of Hb (*cyanosis appears when pO_2 fall below 50–60 mm Hg*).

P_{50} is the partial pressure at which oxygen saturation is 50%. The partial pressure of oxygen for 50% saturation is 26 mm Hg. P_{50} is not effected by anesthetics.

Bohr effect: Alkalosis shifts O_2 dissociation curve to left and acidosis to right.

Oxygen flux: It is the amount of oxygen leaving left ventricle/minute.

It is *1,000 mL/min.*

Shift of oxygen dissociation curve is seen with:

To left	To right
Alkalosis	Acidosis
Low pCO_2	High pCO_2
Decreased 2,3 DPG	Increased 2,3 DPG
Carbon monoxide poisoning	Hyperthermia
Abnormal hemoglobins like methemoglobin, fetal hemoglobin, etc.	Inhalational anesthetics
Hypophosphatemia	
Hypothermia	

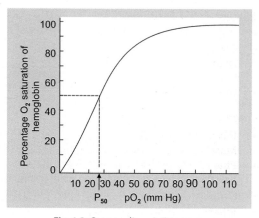

Fig. 1.3: Oxygen dissociation curve

Carbon Dioxide

Transported in blood as:
- Bicarbonate (90%).
- Dissolved (0.0308 mmol/L/mm Hg): 5% of total.
- As carbamino compounds.

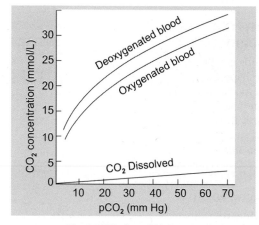

Fig. 1.4: CO_2 dissociation curve

CO_2 Dissociation Curve (Fig. 1.4)

It is relationship between pCO_2 and CO_2 content.

Deoxygenated blood has more CO_2 content at a given pCO_2, this is called as Haldane effect.

ABNORMALITIES OF CHEST MOVEMENTS

Paradoxical Respiration

Seen in flail chest.

Treatment: IPPV.

Tracheal Tug

This is downward movement of trachea during deep inspiration. It is seen in:
- Deep anesthesia (by inhalational agents).
- Partially curarized patient.

- Upper airway obstruction (this is the main reason of tracheal tug at the end of anesthesia as airway can get obstructed by secretions).

Mechanism: During deep anesthesia and partially curarized patient diaphragm is not supported by costal margins. Also larynx is not supported by neck muscles so strong contraction of central part of diaphragm pulls the trachea downwards.

Sigh

It is deep inspiratory hold.

Hiccup

Intermittent clonic spasm of diaphragm of reflex origin.

Causes

- Light anesthesia.
- Gastric and bowel distension.
- Diaphragm irritation by touching diaphragm in upper abdominal surgeries.
- Uremia.

Treatment

- Increase the depth of anesthesia.
- Muscle relaxants.
- Pharyngeal stimulation by nasal catheter, Valsalva maneuver, CO_2 inhalation.
- Drugs such as amyl nitrate.
- Ether.
- For intractable hiccups, phrenic nerve block may be required.

HYPOXIC PULMONARY VASOCONSTRICTION

This is a protective mechanism. Whenever there is hypoxia, there occurs vasoconstriction in these hypoxic areas leading to shunting of blood to well-perfused area, decreasing the V/Q mismatch. *All inhalational agents blunt this hypoxic pulmonary vasoconstriction (HPV) response thereby increasing the shunt fraction (maximum with halothane).*

PULMONARY FUNCTION TESTS

Lung Volumes (Fig. 1.5)

Tidal volume: Volume of gas inspired or expired in each breath during normal quiet respiration.
It is 400–500 mL (10 mL/kg).

Inspiratory reserve volume: It is the maximum volume of gas which a person can inhale from end inspiratory position.
It is 2400–2600 mL.

Inspiratory capacity: It is the maximum volume which can be inhaled from end expiratory position i.e. it is inspiratory reserve volume + tidal volume.
It is 2500 (IRV) + 500 (TV) = 3,000 mL

Expiratory reserve volume: Maximum volume of gas that can be exhaled after normal expiration.
It is 1200–1500 mL.

Vital capacity: It is the maximum amount of gas that can be exhaled after maximum inhalation, i.e. it is IRV + TV + ERV.
It is 4200–4500 mL (75–80 mL/kg).

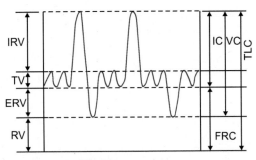

Fig. 1.5: Lung volumes

TV = Tidal volume
IRV = Inspiratory reserve volume
IC = Inspiratory capacity
ERV = Expiratory reserve volume
RV = Residual volume
FRC = Functional residual capacity
VC = Vital capacity
TLC = Total lung capacity
All these lung volumes are approximately 5% less in females (except residual volume).

Residual volume: It is volume of gas still present in lungs after maximal expiration.
It is 1200–1500 mL.

Maximum breathing capacity: Maximum volume of air that can be breathed/minute. It is 120–170 L/min (normally it is measured for 15 seconds and expressed as L/min).

Minute volume: It is tidal volume × respiratory rate.
It is 500 × 12 = 6000 mL/min.

Total lung volume: IRV + TV + ERV + RV.
It is 5500–6000 mL.

Functional residual capacity (FRC): It is the volume of gas in lungs after end expiration. It is ERV + RV. It is 2400–2600 mL.
During general anesthesia FRC decreases by 15–20%.

Simple Bedside Test

- *Breath-holding time:* It is very simple and useful bedside test. Normal is > *25 seconds.* Patients with breath-holding time of 15–25 seconds are considered borderline cases and breath holding time < 15 seconds indicate severe pulmonary dysfunction.
- *Match test:* Person is asked to blow-off match stick from a distance of 15 cm. A person with

normal pulmonary reserve will blow off the match-stick from this distance.

- *Tracheal auscultation:* If breath sounds are audible for more than 6 seconds it denotes significant airway obstruction.
- Able to blow a balloon.
- Spirometry by pocket size microspirometers can now be performed on bed side.

Spirometry

It is the instrument used to measure following lung volumes:

- Tidal volume
- Inspiratory reserve volume
- Inspiratory capacity
- Expiratory reserve volume
- Vital capacity.

It cannot measure residual volume, therefore any lung volume which requires measurement of residual volume, i.e. functional residual capacity and total lung volume cannot be measured by spirometry.

Forced Spirometry
(Timed Expiratory Spirogram)

Forced vital capacity (FVC): Expiration is performed as hard as possible. It is 4200–4500 mL (75–80 mL/kg)

Forced expiratory volume (FeV): It is the volume of gas expired in 1 second (FeV$_1$), 2 seconds (FeV$_2$), 3 seconds (FeV$_3$) measured from the start of expiration after full inspiration (forced vital capacity). Normal person can exhale 83–85% of FVC in 1 second (so *FeV$_1$ is 83–85%*), 93% in 2 seconds (*FeV$_2$ is 93%*) and 97% in 3 seconds (*FeV$_3$ is 97%*).

FeV$_1$/FVC ratio is important as this ratio is decreased in obstructive lung diseases. It is expressed as percentage.

Peak expiratory flow rate: Normal 500–600 L/min.

Forced mid-expiratory flow rate: Measures flow rate during 25–75% of exhalation.

Flow Volume Loops

These are more sensitive and informative in detecting pulmonary diseases than conventional spirometry. Modern microprocessor controlled recording spirometers automatically generate these flow volume loops.

Body Plethysmography, Helium Dilution, Nitrogen Washout

These techniques are employed for measuring functional residual capacity, residual volume and total lung capacity.

Helium dilution technique is also used to measure closing capacity, which is the volume at which airway closes. *Normally it is 1 litre less than functional residual capacity.* If functional residual capacity falls below closing capacity there will be significant hypoventilation and V/Q abnormalities.

Body plethysmograph is also used to measure airway resistance (normal = 2.5 cm H_2O/L/second).

Lung Compliance

It is volume change per unit of pressure.

Lung compliance : 0.2 L/cm H_2O
Chest wall compliance : 0.2 L/cm H_2O
Total compliance : 0.1 L/cm H_2O (lung and chest wall compliance act in opposite direction).

Blood Gas Analysis

Described in Chapter 40, page no. 293.

Pleural Pressures

Normal intrapleural pressure is –3 to –5 cm H_2O.

During inspiration, it becomes more negative up to –7 cm H_2O.

During expiration, it is +1 to +2 cm H_2O.

Fitness for Surgery and Pulmonary Functions

- Patients with FVC < 20 mL/kg and FeV$_1$ <15 mL/kg require appropriate preoperative preparation before surgery such as chest physiotherapy, antibiotics, bronchodilators, etc.
- Patient with FeV$_1$< 10 mL/kg and history of dyspnea at rest or on minimal activity should be subjected to only life-saving operations.

Three most important criteria to indicate severe respiratory compromise are:

1. Dyspnea at rest or on minimal activity.
2. FeV$_1$ < 15 mL/kg (normal 65 mL/kg).
3. pO_2 < 60 mm Hg (or oxygen saturation < 90%) on room air.

PHYSICS RELATED TO ANESTHESIA

Boyle's Law

At a constant temperature, volume of gas is inversely proportional to the pressure.

Charle's Law

At a constant pressure, volume of gas is directly proportional to temperature.

Graham's Law

The rate of diffusion of gas is inversely proportional to square root of their molecular weight.

An ideal gas should follow all the above said laws.

Partial Pressure of Gas

It is the pressure exerted by each gas in a gaseous mixture.

Vapor

Vapor is the gaseous state of liquid.

Avogadro Number

The number of molecules contained in one gram molecular weight of any compound. It is 6.23×10^{23}.

Critical Temperature

It is the temperature below which a gas can be stored in liquid form.

Flow of Gases

Flow may be laminar or turbulent.

Laminar

Laminar flow is produced when the gas pass through straight tube. Flow is smooth. *Laminar flow is more dependent on viscosity.*

At laminar flow, *Hagen–Poiseuille law* is applicable which states that flow rate is directly proportional to pressure gradient and fourth power of radius of tube and inversely proportional to viscosity and length.

$$Q \propto \frac{\pi (P_1 - P_2) r^4}{8 \eta l}$$

Q = Flow rate
$P_2 - P_2$ = Pressure gradient (P_1 and P_2 are pressure at each end of tube)
η = Viscosity
l = Length.

Turbulent

Turbulent flow is produced, if flow rate is very high or if gas passes through bends, constrictions. Flow is rough. Reynolds number must exceed to 2,000 for turbulence. *Turbulent flow is more dependent on density.*

VENTURI PRINCIPLE

When a fluid or gas passes through a tube of varying diameter, the pressure exerted by fluid (lateral pressure) is minimum where velocity is maximum (pressure energy drops where kinetic energy increases: *Bernoulli's law*).

This principle is very much utilized in anesthesia particularly with Venturi masks. By increasing flow rate (velocity) through narrow constriction sub atmospheric pressure can be created in vicinity enthralling air to mix in fixed proportion (through pores in mask) with oxygen. Jet ventilation and suction apparatus also works on this principle.

POYNTING EFFECT

Mixing of liquid nitrous oxide at low pressure with oxygen at high pressure (in Entonox) leads to formation of gas of nitrous oxide. Therefore, oxygen and nitrous oxide both are present in gaseous state in Entonox cylinder.

KEY POINTS

- Subglottis is the narrowest part in children up to the age of 6 years however, this does not act as deterrent to use cuffed tubes in children.
- During general anesthesia with muscle relaxants the cords are held in cadaveric position.

Contd…

Contd...

- Due to shorter, wider and less acute angle chances of endobronchial intubation are more on right side.
- Aspiration in supine position most commonly involves apical segment of right lower lobe.
- Maximum airway resistance to airflow occurs in trachea and then main bronchus and minimum in terminal bronchi.
- Endotracheal tubes and tracheostomy decrease the anatomical dead space by bypassing the upper airways.
- During general anesthesia alveolar dead space is increased.
- P_{50} i.e. partial pressure at which oxygen saturation is 50% is not affected by anesthetics.
- All inhalational agents blunt hypoxic pulmonary vasoconstriction (HPV) response thereby increasing the shunt fraction.
- Closing capacity is normally 1 L less than functional residual capacity.
- Venturi principle is often utilized in anesthesia particularly with Venturi masks.

Equipment in Anesthesia

CHAPTER 2

Anesthesia Delivery Systems (Anesthesia Machine and Circuits)

ANESTHESIA MACHINE

First anesthesia machine was invented by Edmund Gaskin Boyle in 1917 (that's why anesthesia machine used to be called as Boyle's machine). The Boyle's machine is *continuous flow machine* used for administration of anesthesia.

Over the years, anesthesia machine has evolved from Boyle's basic **(Fig. 2.1)** to Boyle's major **(Fig. 2.2)** to anesthesia work stations **(Fig. 2.3)**. Anesthesia work stations are not only the machines but are the compact systems having *all essential monitors* (capnograph, pulse oximeter, oxygen analyzer, spirometer, airway pressure monitor), *all essential alarms*, ventilator, storage drawers for equipment, suction port, auxiliary oxygen source, provision for closed and semiclosed circuits, scavenging system and electric plugs integrated as a single unit.

As different parts of anesthesia machine works on different pressures, it is divided into three parts—high pressure system, intermediate pressure system and low pressure system:

HIGH PRESSURE SYSTEM

It extends from yoke assembly to high pressure regulator (1st stage pressure reducing valve). It includes yoke assembly (Cylinders and yoke), high pressure regulator and oxygen flush.

Cylinders

Cylinders are made up of *molybdenum steel* because molybdenum steel can withstand high pressures. Some of the newer cylinders also contains chromium alloy to decrease their weight. As steel is not compatible with MRI, special

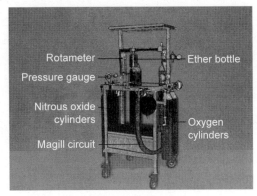

Fig. 2.1: Boyle's basic

aluminum cylinders (and aluminum machine) are used in MRI suites.

Oxygen Cylinder (Fig. 2.4)

The color of oxygen cylinder is black body with white shoulders (top) and pressure is 2,000 pounds per square inch (psi) or 137 kg/cm² [1 kg/cm² = 14.7 psi]. Smallest size available is AA and the largest is H. *The cylinder mounted on anesthesia machine is type E.*

As oxygen is consumed cylinder pressure falls in proportion to its content, i.e. if the pressure gauge is showing 1,000 psi that means oxygen cylinder is half full.

Acceptable purity is 99%. The cylinder should have the following details: Name of the owner, serial number, capacity of cylinder, symbol of gas, tare weight (weight of empty cylinder) and date of hydraulic test. Cylinders should be tested every 5 years.

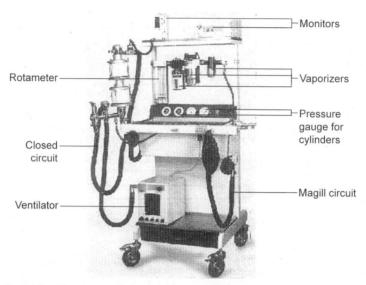

Fig. 2.2: Boyle's major anesthesia machine (cylinders are fitted on the back side therefore cannot be visualized in diagram)

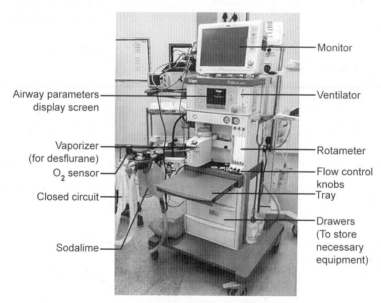

Fig. 2.3: Anesthesia work station

Liquid oxygen: Any gas can be stored in liquid form below its critical temperature. The critical temperature of oxygen is –119°C, therefore oxygen reservoirs storing oxygen in liquid form has to maintain a temperature below –119°C, which make them quite expensive.

As 1 mL of liquid oxygen gives 840 mL of gas, the advantage of liquid oxygen is that it can be stored in large volumes in small containers making them very useful for remote locations like wars or disasters.

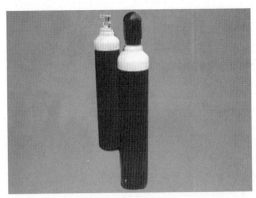

Fig. 2.4: Oxygen cylinder

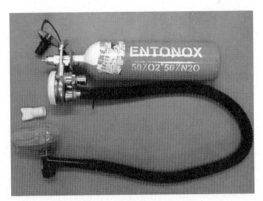

Fig. 2.6: Entonox cylinder

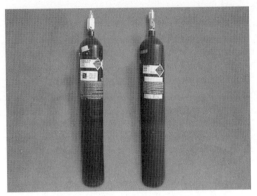

Fig. 2.5: Nitrous oxide cylinders

Nitrous Oxide Cylinder (Fig. 2.5)

Nitrous oxide is stored in blue color cylinders at a pressure of 760 psi.

As the critical temperature of nitrous oxide is 36.5°C, it is filled in liquid form. Vaporization of liquid produces gas leading to heat loss which sometimes may produce frost on cylinder. Small amount of liquid present in cylinder may still vaporize to produce gas leading the pressure gauge to show the pressure of full cylinder therefore, *contents of cylinder are measured by weight, not by the pressure gauge.*

Entonox Cylinder (Fig. 2.6)

Entonox, the mixture of 50% oxygen and 50% nitrous oxide, is mainly used to produce analgesia during labor. *It is stored in blue color cylinders*

(representing nitrous oxide) *with white shoulders* (representing oxygen) *at a pressure of 2000 psi.*

Heliox Cylinder

Heliox, the mixture of 79% helium and 21% oxygen, is mainly used in upper airway obstruction. *It is stored in black color cylinders* (representing oxygen) *with brown and white shoulders* (brown representing helium) at a pressure of 2000 psi.

Air Cylinder

Air is stored in grey color cylinders (representing CO_2) with black and white shoulders (representing oxygen) at a pressure of 2000 psi.

Cyclopropane and carbon dioxide, which are no more used in anesthesia, used to be stored respectively in orange color cylinders at a pressure of 75 psi and grey color cylinders at a pressure of 750 psi. They were stored in liquid form.

Filling Ratio (Also Called as Filling Density)

It is the percentage of weight of gas in container to weight of water it can hold at 60°F. This is to prevent overfilling. It is 68% for nitrous oxide and oxygen (in liquefied state).

Cylinder Valves

Cylinder valves are fitted at the top of cylinder. Different type of cylinder valves are available like flush type (most commonly used), bull nosed, etc. To start and close gas, these valves are rotated anticlockwise and clockwise, respectively. (For summary of gas cylinders see **Table 2.1**).

■ **Table 2.1:** Summary of gas cylinders

Gas	Type*	Filled as	Color**	Pressure	Capacity
Oxygen	E	Gas	Black body White shoulders	2000 psi	660 L
	H	Gas	Black body White shoulders	2,000 psi	6900 L
Nitrous oxide	E	Liquid	Blue	760 psi	1,590 L
	H	Liquid	Blue	760 psi	15,800 L
Air	E	Gas	Grey body Black and white shoulders	2000 psi	625 L
Heliox	E and H	Gas	Black body Brown and white shoulders	2000 psi	—
Entonox	E and H	Liquid and gas	Blue body White shoulders	2,000 psi	—
Carbon dioxide	E	Liquid	Grey	750 psi	1,590 L
Cyclopropane	E	Liquid	Orange	75 psi	—

*Commonly used type
**Different countries use different color coding for cylinders. The colors mentioned here are as per Indian Standard adopted by the Indian Standards Institution on 24th November 1966, after the draft finalized by the Gas Cylinders Sectional Committee (Clause 2.1, 2.2 and 2.3)

Pressure Gauge

It is used to measure the cylinder pressure. Most commonly used is Bourdon type.

Yoke Assembly

Yoke is that part of the machine where cylinders get fitted. It consists of index pins, a gas seal (Bodok seal) to prevent leak between cylinder and yoke and a filter **(Fig. 2.7)**.

Pin Index System (Table 2.2)

It is the safety mechanism to prevent wrong fitting of cylinders at other's position. It consists of 2 pins, 4 mm and 6 mm long on yoke of the anesthesia machine. The pins are so positioned that the cylinder with the holes at corresponding distance can only be fitted at that position.

Making of Pin Index System

A 9/16 inch circumference semicircle is made and 6 equidistant points are made on arc (additional 7th point, if entonox is to be used) **(Fig. 2.8)**.

The pins at the yoke of oxygen are at 2 and 5 position. Oxygen cylinders have holes at the same position making only oxygen cylinder possible to be placed at this position. Similarly, yoke of nitrous oxide has pins positioned at 3, 5 position; nitrous oxide cylinder has holes at same position making

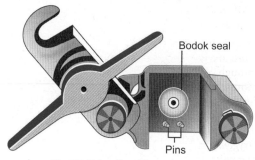

Fig. 2.7: Yoke of anesthesia machine

■ **Table 2.2:** Pin index position for gases on yoke of anesthesia machine

Gas	Pin position
Oxygen	2, 5
Nitrous oxide	3, 5
Cyclopropane	3, 6
Air	1, 5
Nitrogen	1, 4
Entonox	7
Carbon dioxide (< 7.5%)	2, 6
Heliox	2, 4

only nitrous oxide cylinder possible to be placed at this position.

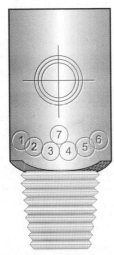

Fig. 2.8: Cylinder valves showing position of holes (these holes correspond to same pins at yoke of machine)

Central Supply of Oxygen and Nitrous Oxide

In large hospitals where consumption of gases is more, oxygen, nitrous oxide and air are supplied through central supply pipelines. In central supply rooms, oxygen and nitrous oxide are stored in a set of 4–8 large (type H) cylinders connected to a common manifold (many hospitals use liquid oxygen tanks instead of cylinders). In India, *Oxygen, medical air and nitrous oxide are supplied at a pressure of 60 psi through central supply.*

There is color coding for central supply pipelines; white for oxygen, blue for nitrous oxide and black for air. Majority of the hospitals having central supply of gases also have central suction-mediated through yellow color pipes.

Like pin index system which prevent wrong fitting of cylinders to machine *Diameter index safety system (DISS)* prevent wrong fitting of central supply pipes to machine. As the name suggests the diameter of oxygen, nitrous oxide, air and suction pipes are different so that couplers of oxygen, nitrous oxide, air and suction can only receive their pipes.

Oxygen Flush (Emergency Oxygen Flush)

It is a bypass system which bypasses the intermediate and low pressure system and oxygen directly reaches at machine outlet. *It delivers 35 liters of oxygen per minute at a pressure of 45–60 psi.*

High Pressure Regulator

High pressure regulator is also known as 1st stage pressure reducing valve. It converts high pressure in cylinder to constant working pressure suitable for anesthesia machine. It reduces the pressure to 45–60 psi.

INTERMEDIATE PRESSURE SYSTEM

It extends from 2nd stage pressure reducing valve to flow control knobs. It includes:
- 2nd stage pressure reducing valve which further reduces the pressure to 15–35 psi.
- *Oxygen failure alarms:* Machine starts alarming, if the pressure of oxygen falls below a preset pressure.
- *Fail safe valve:* This is an important safety device which in case of decreased oxygen pressure either cut-off or proportionately decreases the flow of nitrous oxide and other gases (that is why also called as oxygen supply failure protection devices), thus preventing the delivery of hypoxic mixture.

LOW PRESSURE SYSTEM

Downstream to flow control knob constitutes low pressure system. It includes rotameter, vaporizers and check valve.

Rotameter

One of the most important component of low pressure system is rotameter which contains flowmeter tubes specific for each gas and flow control knob **(Figs 2.9 and 2.10)**.

The flow to each tube is adjusted by rotating the flow control knob clockwise and anticlockwise. As a safety measure (to prevent opening of wrong knob), these flow control knobs are color-coded (blue for nitrous oxide, white for oxygen and black for air), chemical formula of gas is embedded on each knob and oxygen knob is made physically different from other knobs (it is more fluted, more prominent and large in diameter).

Flowmeter tubes are glass tubes which are transparent and have *variable orifice, (tapered—narrow at base and wider at apex)* with markings on each tube indicating flow. These tubes are also called as *Thorpe's tube.* Although the tubes are

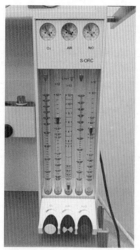

Fig. 2.9: Rotameter with two flowmeters
Note that newer machines have double flowmeter tubes for oxygen and nitrous oxide. A fine flow tube for low flow rates (200 mL to 1 L) and coarse tube for high flow rates (1–10 L).

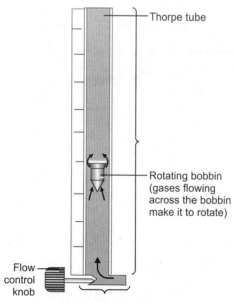

Fig. 2.10: Flowmeter

transparent but still it is not possible to see the gas flowing through it therefore, to ensure continuous flow of gases each tube contains aluminum float-called as bobbin. The gas stream passing all around the bobbin keeps it rotating continuously ensuring continuous flow of gases. *Upper end of bobbin determines the flow rate.* For example, in **Figure 2.9** nitrous oxide is flowing at flow rate of 3 L/min. and oxygen at 5 L/min. The pressure around the bobbin remains constant throughout therefore these flowmeters tubes are considered as *constant pressure* tubes. The flow at low flow rates is laminar therefore *viscosity determines the flow while density becomes an important determinant at high flow rates.*

The whole unit with flowmeter tubes and flow control knobs is called as *rotameter* (named so because of rotating bobbin).

Safety Features of Rotameter

- *Position of flowmeter tubes* (**Fig. 2.11**): Most vulnerable point of leakage is the junction of flow meter tube and common manifold at the top of machine. If oxygen tube is upstream it can leak at 6 positions (**1, 2, 3, 4, 5, 6 of Fig. 2.11**), while if it is most downstream, then possibility of leakage is only at 2 points (**5, 6 of Fig. 2.11**). Therefore, *oxygen tube should be most downstream, i.e. oxygen should be the last gas to enter the rotameter.*
- *Oxygen-nitrous ratio controller/oxygen nitrous proportioning system:* Oxygen and nitrous oxide knobs are interconnected by a pulley in such a manner that rotation of nitrous oxide knob will automatically start oxygen flow making it impossible to deliver singular flow of nitrous oxide. *This ensures a minimum FiO_2 (delivered concentration of oxygen) of 25% which is mandatory to prevent hypoxia.*
- Florescent back panel of rotameter so that it can be visualized in dark.
- Rotameters are hand-calibrated to minimize errors.
- They are antistatic to prevent sticking of Bobbin to flowmeter tube.

Other types of flowmeter:
- *Heidbrink flowmeter:* Used in past, it consists of metal-tapered tube with inverted black float. The upper end projects in glass tube.
- *Connell flowmeter:* Again used in past, it contains a round float (bobbin). Reading was taken from the center of float.

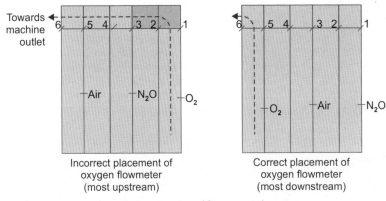

Fig. 2.11: Position of flowmeter tubes

Vaporizers (Fig. 2.12)

Vaporizers are the devices which are used to deliver inhalational agents. Inhalational agents are in liquid form in vaporizer. As the inhalational agents are volatile, fresh gases passing over the agent vaporizes them and their vapors get incorporated in fresh gases to be delivered to the patient.

The vaporizer material should have *high specific heat and high thermal conductivity*. As Copper possesses these properties, vaporizers are made up of copper.

In the last few decades, there has been continuous development in vaporizers. Old vaporizers of the past-like ether bottle, trielene bottle and Goldman vaporizer has been replaced by newer vaporizers such as Tec. 5, Tec. 6 (heated and pressurized vaporizer, specifically designed for desflurane) or Tec. 7.

Aladin cassette vaporizer is the latest vaporizer which can be used to deliver all inhalational agents. It just requires insertion of color-coded cassette of each agent, rest everything is automatically adjusted by vaporizer.

The *characteristics* of new vaporizers are:

- Temperature compensated (vaporizer output not affected by changes in temperature which occurs due to vaporization of inhalational agent).
- *Variable bypass*: By rotating the dial knob, it can be decided how much fresh gas will pass through vaporizer and how much to be bypassed (therefore called as splitting ratio). This decides the concentration of anesthetic

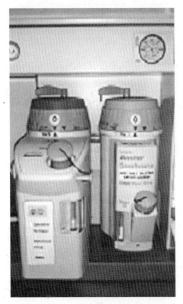

Fig. 2.12: Desflurane (with blue dial knob) and sevoflurane (with yellow dial knob) vaporizer *(For color version, see Plate 1)*

agent to be delivered, i.e. at 5% concentration most of the gas will pass through vaporizer and at 0.1% most of gas will be bypassed.

- Flow over, i.e. gas flow passes over the agent. Other type is bubble through in which gas passes through the agent.
- Not affected by pumping effect (back pressure).
- Outside the circuit (i.e. not in breathing circuit).

■ **Table 2.3:** Physical properties of inhalational agents

Agent	Boiling point	Vapor pressure (mm Hg)
Sevoflurane	58°C	160
Halothane	50°C	243
Isoflurane	49°C	240
Desflurane	23.5°C	680

- *Agent specific*: Although all vaporizers used nowadays are agent specific. However, the agents with similar vapor pressure can be used interchangeably. For example, halothane and isoflurane with almost identical vapor pressure can be used interchangeably with accurate delivery **(Table 2.3)**.

Sequence of Vaporizers

One machine contains more than one vaporizer at a time. *The agent with lower boiling point should be placed first,* i.e. near to rotameter otherwise condensed particles will be recovered from the second vaporizer **(Table 2.3)**.

Safety Features in Vaporizers

- Newer vaporizers are agent specific. They have special key filling system specific for each agent.
- There are color code markings mentioned on vaporizers; the dial knob and filling system are also of the same color. *Color code* is: *Red* for halothane, *Purple* for isoflurane, *Yellow* for sevoflurane and *Blue* for desflurane.
- Interlock devices which prevent more than one vaporizer to be turned on at same time
- *One-way check valve:* It is placed just before machine outlet to prevent backflow effect of positive pressure ventilation.

OTHER PARTS OF ANESTHESIA MACHINE

Anesthesia Ventilators

Ventilators in the newer anesthesia work stations have almost the same features as in ICU ventilators, i.e. they can work in volume as well as pressure mode. *Majority of the newer machines prefers ascending bellows over descending bellows* because leaks are better detected in ascending bellows (they will not ascend, if there is leak while descending bellows will continue to descend in the presence of leakage).

Fresh gas flow compensation and *fresh gas decoupling* are very important safety feature in the ventilators used with new machines. They provide compensation of leakage in fresh gas flow to maintain stable delivery of preset tidal volume.

Scavenging System

It is the system to eliminate exhaled gases to minimize the theater pollution.

Maximum *permissible concentration of nitrous oxide in theater is 25 parts per million (ppm)* and that of halogenated agents less than 2 ppm.

Mechanics of Gas Flow in Anesthesia Machine (Fig. 2.13)

Gases in cylinders are at high pressure. The high (1st stage/primary) pressure regulator reduces the pressure to 45–60 psi. The pressure is further reduced to 15–35 psi by secondary (2nd stage) pressure regulator. Gases from 2nd stage pressure regulator reaches the flowmeters where flow is regulated by rotating the flow control knobs.

These gases mix in a common manifold at the top of flowmeter; from there they pass through a vaporizer containing inhalational agent. The vapors of inhalational agents get mixed in gaseous mixture which is *finally delivered at machine outlet at a pressure of 5 to 8 psi.* The final gaseous mixture delivered from machine outlet is *called as fresh gas flow.* Traditionally this gas flow consists of 66.6% nitrous oxide + 33.3% oxygen + Inhalational agent.

BREATHING CIRCUITS

Breathing circuits connect patient (either through endotracheal tube or mask) to the anesthesia machine. These are divided into open, semiopen, semiclosed and closed systems.

Open System

Inhalational agent is directly poured over patient mouth and nostril by placing a wire like mask (Schimmelbusch mask). Open systems were used in past for delivery of ether and chloroform. In current day practice open systems are obsolete as it is not possible to control the delivered

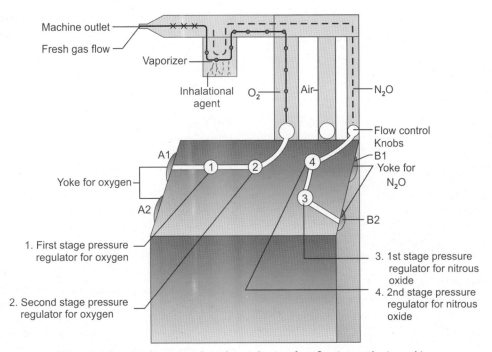

Fig. 2.13: Schematic diagram to show the mechanics of gas flow in anesthesia machine.
A1, A2—yoke of oxygen; B1, B2—yoke for nitrous oxide

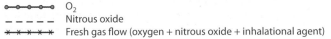 O_2
– – – – – Nitrous oxide
✳✳✳✳✳ Fresh gas flow (oxygen + nitrous oxide + inhalational agent)

concentration. Moreover, patient directly exhales into the atmosphere causing uncontrollable theater pollution.

If a folded towel is placed over Schimmelbusch mask to prevent escape of inhalational agent it constitutes *semiopen system* which is also no more used in modern practice.

Semiclosed Circuits

These circuits were described by *Mapleson therefore called as Mapleson circuits*. These are divided into six types: Type A, B, C, D, E, F (**Fig. 2.14**). (Because of similarity in characteristics some authors have classified them in three groups: A, BC and DEF group).

Type A

It is also called *Magill circuit* (**Fig. 2.15**).

Fresh gases from machine (shown as continuous line in **Fig. 2.15**) reach the patient.

Most of the expired gases from patient (broken lines) are exhaled from pressure relief valve; however, some of the gases go back into the tubing (that is why these circuits are called as semiclosed circuits). These expiratory gases which have gone back in the tubing may be reinhaled by the patient in next breath. This is called as rebreathing (patient rebreathing his/her expired gases). To prevent this rebreathing, there are recommendations for fresh gas flow for each circuit; fresh gas flow should be sufficient enough to push these expiratory gases out in atmosphere through expiratory valve before getting delivered to the patient.

For Magill circuit fresh gas flow should be equal to minute volume to prevent rebreathing in a spontaneously breathing patient.

If this circuit is used for controlled ventilation (no spontaneous breathing, patient is on artificial ventilation) very high flows (3 times of minute volume or > 20 L) is required and in spite of

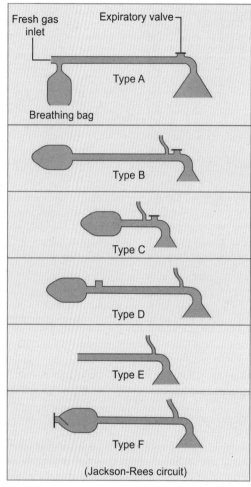

Fig. 2.14: Mapleson circuits

such high flows prevention of rebreathing is still unpredictable therefore *Magill circuit should not be used for controlled ventilation.* It is the *circuit of choice for spontaneous ventilation.*

Pressure Relief Valve

It is also called *adjustable pressure limiting (APL) valve, expiratory valve and rebreathing prevention valve.* Most commonly used is Heidbrink type valve. *The expiratory valve should be as near to the patient to minimize rebreathing* and it should be fully open during spontaneous breathing and partially closed during controlled ventilation.

Reservoir (Breathing) Bag (Fig. 2.16)

These are attached to anesthesia breathing circuits to ventilate the patient. Bags with different capacities are available for various age groups.

Neonates	:	250 mL
Children (up to 3 years)	:	500 mL
Children > 3 years	:	1,000 mL
Adults	:	2,000 mL

The capacity of bag should be more than the patient tidal volume.

Lack System

It is a coaxial (containing one tube in other) modification of Magill circuit with two tubes. Outer tube is inspiratory and inner tube is expiratory.

Type B

Fresh gas flow inlet brought near APL valve. It did not offer any advantage therefore no more used. Functionally, it is almost equally efficient for spontaneous and controlled ventilation.

Type C (Water's Circuit)

Corrugated tubing is shortened. It also did not offer any advantage therefore no more used. Functionally it is almost equally efficient for spontaneous and controlled ventilation.

Type D (Fig. 2.17)

APL valve was brought near the bag. It did not offer any advantage but a modification in Type D was made by scientist Bain, who incorporated an inner tube in Type D circuit making it as coaxial. Fresh gases are delivered through inner tube so that mixing of fresh gases and exhaled gases can be minimized. *Bain circuit is most commonly used semiclosed circuit in anesthesia.*

Bain circuit is the circuit of choice for controlled ventilation. Fresh gas flow for controlled ventilation is: (i) *1.6 times of minute ventilation* at normal respiratory rates (10–12 breath/min) or (ii) *70–100 mL/kg/min* (which is almost equal to minute ventilation), if respiratory rate is increased to 16 breath/min. Many clinicians prefer (ii) method.

Bain circuit can also be used for spontaneous ventilation but fresh gas flow requirement is higher, i.e. *2.5 times of minute volume.*

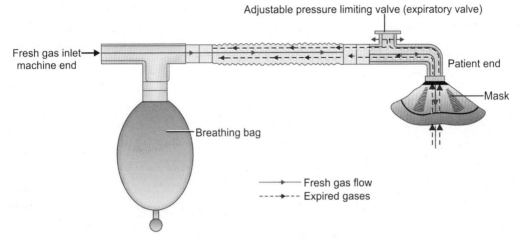

Fig. 2.15: Magill circuit

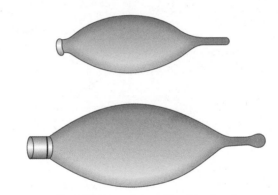

Fig. 2.16: Reservoir bags (Breathing bags)

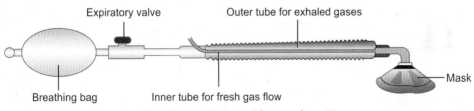

Fig. 2.17: Bain circuit (modification of type D)

Advantages of Bain circuit are:
- Light weight.
- Corrugated tubing is long (1.8 meters), making it useful for head and neck surgeries where anesthetist is away from patient.
- Resistance is less (< 0.7 cm H$_2$O).
- Sterilization is easy.

Disadvantages: Inner tube may become folded or kinked causing obstruction or may get disconnected. To decrease these complications the outer tube is made transparent.

Type E (Fig. 2.14)

It is Ayre's T piece with corrugated tubing. It is a *pediatric circuit*. As it does not have breathing bag it cannot be considered complete circuit. It is basically a circuit only meant for spontaneous respiration, however can be utilized for controlled ventilation by intermittently occluding the end of expiratory limb.

Type F Circuit (Jackson and Rees Circuit) (Fig. 2.14)

Ayre's T piece was made complete by attaching a breathing bag to it by Jackson and Rees. Jackson-Rees circuit, which is considered as Mapleson F, *is the most commonly used pediatric semiclosed circuit to be used in children < 6 years of age or <20 kg.*

Fresh gas flow recommendations are similar to Bains, i.e. 1.6 times of minute volume for controlled ventilation and 2.5 times for spontaneous ventilation.

Type E and type F circuits are made *valveless* to decrease the resistance (mostly F circuits have hole in the tail of bag but valve may be present in some F circuits).

To conclude, semiclosed circuits *in terms of efficiency for spontaneous ventilation: A> DEF > BC and for controlled ventilation: DFE >BC>A.*

Other Semiclosed Circuits

Hafina system: These are modifications of A, B, C and D. Expiratory valve is replaced by suction port and ejector flowmeter. This is to decrease the theater pollution.

Humprey (ADE) system: A single lever changes from one circuit to other.

For summary of semiclosed circuits see **Table 2.4**.

Closed Circuit

In closed circuit (**Fig. 2.18**) expiratory gases pass through the expiratory limb to reach canister containing sodalime. Sodalime absorbs the carbon dioxide from these expired gases and the same gases are reused by the patient. Since no gases are venting out in atmosphere these are considered as closed circuits.

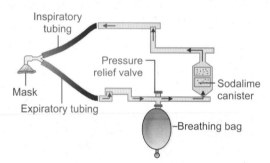

Fig. 2.18: Closed circuit (Circle system)

■ **Table 2.4:** Summary of semiclosed circuits

Circuit	Fresh gas flow		Comments
	Spontaneous	Controlled	
Type A (Also called as Magill circuit)	Equal to minute volume	Very high flow (3 × minute volume)	Circuit of choice for spontaneous ventilation, should not be used for controlled ventilation
Type B	2 × minute volume	2.25 × minute volume	No more used
Type C (Also called as Water's circuit)	2 × minute volume	2.25 × minute volume	No more used
Type D (Bain circuit)	2.5 × minute volume	1.6 × minute volume (or 70–100 mL/kg)	Circuit of choice for controlled ventilation. Most commonly used semiclosed circuit.
Type E (Ayre's T piece)	2.5 × minute volume	3 × minute volume	Pediatric, incomplete circuit
Type F (Jackson-Rees circuit)	2.5 × minute volume	1.5–2 × minute volume	commonly used pediatric circuit

Note: If fresh gas flow for Magill circuit is asked without being mentioned for spontaneous or controlled ventilation, it should be considered equal to minute volume as it is circuit of choice for spontaneous ventilation. Similarly for Bain's circuit, it should be considered 1.6 times of minute volume as it is circuit of choice for controlled ventilation.

As the same gases are being reused, only the oxygen consumed by body need to be replaced requiring very low flows and that is why the anesthesia given with closed circuit is called as *Low flow anesthesia.*

There are two types of closed circuits, *circle system* which is commonly used and *to and fro system* which is no more used.

In human beings, the closed circuit system was first introduced by Water's in 1923.

COMPONENTS OF CLOSED CIRCUIT (FIG. 2.19)

Carbon Dioxide Absorbents

Sodalime

Sodalime is the most commonly used CO_2 absorbent. The reaction between sodalime and CO_2 is exothermic therefore heat and water is produced during the reaction.

Composition of sodalime: Although the composition may vary in different countries or between the companies with in same country, the standard traditional composition of soda lime is:
- Ca (OH)$_2$: 94%
- NaOH : 5% (NaOH acts as catalyst)
- KOH : 1%

- *Color indicator:* Color indicator indicates whether the sodalime is fresh or has been exhausted. Different countries uses different color indicators, however in India, the most commonly used absorbent is *Durasorb which is pink when fresh and becomes white on exhaustion.* Few of the centers have started to use ethyl violet which is white when fresh and becomes purple on exhaustion.
- Silica (to prevent dust formation)

Properties of sodalime granules (*Fig. 2.20*):
- Hardness of granules should be more than 75, otherwise, there may be dust formation which may be inhaled by patient. Sodalime is made hard by adding silica.
- Moisture (14–19%) is needed for carbon dioxide absorption.
- Size of sodalime granules is *4–8 mesh* (or 3–6 mm).
- As reaction takes place on surface of granule, air space should be >50%.
- *100 g of sodalime can absorb 24–26 L of carbon dioxide.*

Barylime

Barylime, which has 80% Ca(OH)$_2$ and 20% Ba(OH)$_2$, has been withdrawn from the market because of the possibility of life-threatening *fire*

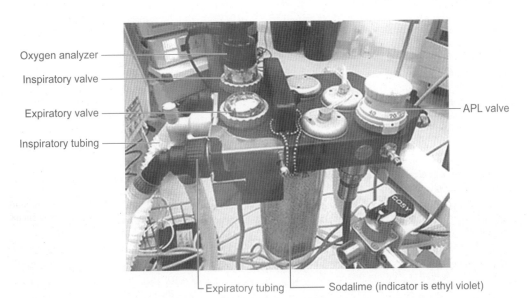

Fig. 2.19: Components of closed circuit *(For color version, see Plate 1)*

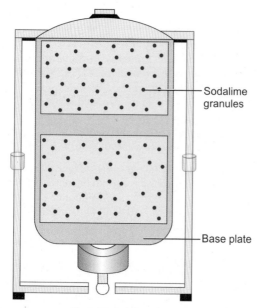

Fig. 2.20: Sodalime canister

and explosions in breathing circuits with sevoflu-rane (In experiments, absorber temperatures has been seen to reach > 200°C).

Reaction of Sodalime/Barylime with Inhalational Agents

- *Sevoflurane by reacting with sodalime and Barylime can produce compound A which is nephrotoxic. The factors which can increase the production of Compound A are:*
  - Low-flow (< 2 L/min.)
  - Higher concentrations of sevoflurane
  - Type of absorbent (Barylime > Sodalime)
  - Higher absorbent temperatures
  - Fresh absorbent
- *Desiccated (dry) sodalime and barylime (Barylime > Sodalime) can produces carbon monoxide with the following inhalational agents in decreasing order- Desflurane > > Isoflurane >> halothane = Sevoflurane. Desiccated sodalime can cause burns of respiratory mucosa with sevoflurane by producing hydrogen fluoride*
- Trielene by reacting with sodalime can produce dichloroacetylene (which is neurotoxic) and phosgene gas (which can cause ARDS).
- Methoxyflurane and halothane can react with the rubber tubing of closed circuit.

Amsorb (Also Called as Calcium Hydroxide Lime)

It is a new carbon dioxide absorbent containing calcium hydroxide and calcium chloride. *Amsorb neither produces compound A nor carbon monoxide with desiccated sodalime and barylime.*

The disadvantage of Amsorb is its high cost and less absorptive capacity (almost half of soda-lime).

Lithium Hydroxide

Like Amsorb lithium-based absorbents do not produce compound A and carbon monoxide. Moreover, they are believed to have more absorbing capacity than soda lime, however, they are more expensive and can cause burns of skin and respiratory tract.

Other Components of Closed Circuit

- Expiratory and inspiratory tubes
- *Expiratory and inspiratory valves:* These valves maintains the unidirectional flow of gases and ensures that expiratory gases does not enter the inspiratory limb and vice versa.
- *Oxygen analyzer:* It is fitted in the inspiratory limb. *It is one of the most important safety measures as it measures the final delivered concentration of oxygen to the patient.* The oxygen analyzers used in most of the modern machines are electrochemical. Oxygen passes through the sensor membrane (galvanic cell or polarographic cell) gets reduced and generates current. The rate at which current is generated is proportional to the partial pressure of oxygen which is converted into percentage by software.
- *Flow sensor:* The use of flow sensors is considered mandatory by American Society of Anesthesiology. It is connected at the end of breathing circuit. It collects a sample from expiratory gases and deliver it to monitor to measure:
  - The concentration of expired carbon dioxide ($ETCO_2$) and inhalational agents
  - To measure expired tidal volume, respiratory rate and airway pressures. New monitor not only measures the volume and pressure but also display the pressure and volume graphs.

■ **Table 2.5:** Comparison between closed and semiclosed systems

Closed system (Circle system)	Semiclosed system (Mapleson system)
Advantages	*Disadvantages*
• Economical (same gases and inhalational agent can be reused)	• Not economical (requires very high gas flows)
• Less theater pollution	• High theater pollution
• Humidity is well preserved (reaction between CO_2 and sodalime produces water)	• Humidity not preserved (water content of dry 100% O_2 is 0 mg/L)
• For conditions in which there is very high production of CO_2 only closed circuit can eliminate such high CO_2 (e.g. malignant hyperthermia)	• Cannot eliminate such high CO_2 levels
Disadvantages	*Advantages*
• Heavy weight due to tubing, canister and accessories	• Light weight
• If sodalime gets exhausted or expiratory valve gets stuck there can be dangerous hypercapnia	• No such risk
• Production of toxic compounds like dichloroacetylene and phosgene gas with trilene and compound A with sevoflurane	• No such possibility
• Desiccated sodalime/Barylime can produce carbon monoxide with desflurane (and other agents) and burns of respiratory tract with sevoflurane	• No such possibility
• Cross-infection from apparatus may occur	• Chances are less
• Breathing resistance and dead space is high	• Less
• As low flows are used so high level of monitoring is essential	• More useful when only basic monitoring is available

Flow sensor is one of the most important safety measure to detect life-threatening complications such as ventilatory failure, extubation, bronchospasm, etc.

Factors affecting carbon dioxide absorption in closed circuit:
- Freshness of sodalime
- *Tidal volume of patient:* Tidal volume should be equal or less than airspace otherwise large tidal volumes will pass through canister without CO_2 being absorbed.
- *High flows:* High flows allow less time for CO_2 absorption.
- *Dead space:* Increased dead space in canister decreases the CO_2 absorption.
- *Inadequate filling of sodalime:* Too loosely filled sodalime allows gas to pass through the gap between sodalime granules and canister wall without absorption, this is called *channeling*. Too tightly filled sodalime decreases air space decreasing CO_2 absorption.
- *Resistance to outflow:* Increasing the resistance to outflow permit gases to remain in contact of sodalime for more time, and thus allowing more CO_2 absorption.

Universal F

It is a single limb closed circuit intended to decrease the cumbersomeness of circle system.

For comparison between closed and semiclosed systems see **Table 2.5**.

CHECKING OF ANESTHESIA MACHINE AND CIRCUITS

Although many of the latest machines provides a series of automatic self-check tests but a manual comprehensive tests must be performed before using anesthesia machine to avoid any mishap. The checking should begin from high pressure system up to breathing circuits.

High Pressure System

- Open oxygen cylinder and ensure that it is at least half full (Pressure> 1000 psi).

- Verify that hoses for central supply are appropriately connected and pressure gauges for central supply should read 50-60 psi (depending on country).

Low Pressure System

Ensure that gases are flowing smoothly in rotameter.

Open singular flow of nitrous oxide to see the integrity of oxygen nitrous oxide proportioning system and fail safe valve. Machine should not allow singular flow of nitrous oxide.

Test to Detect Leaks in Low Flow System

Positive Pressure Test

Open oxygen flow and occlude machine outlet. If there is no leak, then due to back pressure the height of float (bobbin) should drop and should bounce back to normal after releasing occlusion. The limitation of this test is that it cannot be performed in machine which have back pressure valve just before machine outlet (which is installed to prevent back pressure effects of positive pressure ventilation on vaporizer output).

Negative Pressure Test

Off all flows and attach a suction bulb to machine outlet. Keep on squeezing till, it collapses completely. This will generate a negative pressure in machine. If there is leak, then air will be sucked in leading to inflation of bulb otherwise, it will remain collapsed. If its remains collapsed > 10 seconds, it should be considered that there is no leak. Do the same test by opening each vaporizer (there may leakage in vaporizer). As it can be done, even if there is back pressure valve and is *most sensitive of all tests to detect leak (can detect leak as low as 30 mL), therefore called as universal leak test.*

Check for Breathing System

- Check completeness of all attachments.
- Close APL valve and occlude end of breathing circuit (Y piece in case of closed circuit) with finger and flush system with oxygen to attain a pressure of 30 cm H_2O. If same pressure is maintained for > 10 seconds that means there is no leak.

If opening of APL valve releases pressure that means APL valve is intact. Site of leak can be detected by soap bubble solution.

Final Check for Whole System

Attach a breathing bag (called as test lung) at the end of circuit. Start flow at 5 L/min. and start ventilation (with bag or ventilator). *Bag should expand and collapse like a normal lung.*

Checking the Accuracy of Oxygen Analyzer

Since it tells the final delivered concentration of oxygen to the patient therefore *checking its accuracy* is *very vital.* It should show 21% when exposed to air and > 90% when the system is flushed with oxygen.

Set alarms limits, check all monitors and do the ventilator settings before starting the case.

SAFETY FEATURES OF ANESTHESIA DELIVERY SYSTEMS

- Antistatic rubber tyres (to prevent current flow).
- *Pin index system* to prevent wrong cylinder placement and diameter index safety system to prevent wrong fitting of central supply pipelines.
- 1st stage and 2nd stage pressure regulators.
- Fail safe valve (stops or decreases flow of other gases, if oxygen pressure falls).
- *Oxygen failure alarms.*
- Color coding of flow control knobs.
- Different physical appearance of oxygen knob.
- *Oxygen-nitrous proportioning devices.*
- Fluorescent back panel of rotameter (to be visualized in darkness).
- *Oxygen flowmeter tube placed most downstream.*
- Trielene lock for closed circuit (in old machines).
- Pressure relief valve (open when there is excessive pressure in machine).
- Oxygen flush can deliver high flow in emergency.
- One way valve before machine outlet to prevent backpressure effects of positive pressure ventilation.
- *Oxygen analyzer* to detect final delivered concentration of oxygen to patient.
- *Flow sensors* to detect ventilatory failure, disconnections, Extubation, Bronchospasm, etc.

KEY POINTS

- The color of oxygen cylinder is black body with white shoulders (top) and pressure is 2,000 pounds per square inch (psi).
- Nitrous oxide is stored in blue color cylinders at a pressure of 760 psi.
- Entonox is the mixture of 50% oxygen and 50% nitrous oxide.
- Pin index system is to prevent the wrong fitting of cylinders while diameter index safety system is to prevent the wrong fitting of central supply pipe lines.
- Fail safe valve, oxygen-nitrous oxide proportionater and oxygen tube placed most downstream are to decrease the possibility of delivery of hypoxic mixture to patient.
- Upper end of bobbin determines the flow rate in rotameter.
- Aladin cassette vaporizer is the latest vaporizer, which can be used to deliver all inhalational agents.
- Magill circuit is the circuit of choice for spontaneous ventilation. Fresh gas flow should be kept equal to minute volume to prevent rebreathing in a spontaneously breathing patient.
- Bain circuit is the circuit of choice for controlled ventilation. Fresh gas flow for controlled ventilation is 1.6 times of minute ventilation.
- Jackson Rees (Mapleson F) is the most commonly used semiclosed circuit for children.
- Sevoflurane by reacting with sodalime and barylime can produce compound A.
- Desiccated (dry) sodalime and Barylime (Barylime > Sodalime) can produces carbon monoxide with the following inhalational agents in decreasing order: Desflurane > > Isoflurane >> halothane = Sevoflurane.
- Desiccated sodalime can cause burns of respiratory mucosa with sevoflurane by producing hydrogen fluoride.
- Amsorb neither produces compound A nor carbon monoxide with desiccated sodalime and Barylime.

CHAPTER 3

Equipment

EQUIPMENT FOR AIRWAY MANAGEMENT

AIRWAYS

The aim of airway is *to prevent the tongue fall.* Most commonly used is *Guedel airway* **(Fig. 3.1)**. The tip, inserted between tongue and posterior pharyngeal wall prevents tongue falling back on posterior pharyngeal wall, and thus maintaining the patency of airway. Airways are available in many sizes. The appropriate length is the distance between tip of nose and tragus plus 1 cm.

Nasal airways are also available which are inserted through nostril.

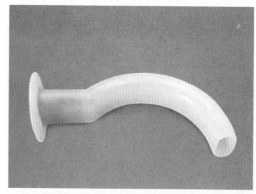

Fig. 3.1: Guedel's oropharyngeal airway
(For color version, see Plate 2)

FACEMASKS (FIG. 3.2)

Facemask is used to ventilate the patient without intubation. They are available in sizes from 0 (smallest) to 6 (largest). Facemask should be made of antistatic rubber. At the bottom of mask, there is air-filled cuff which has soft cushioning effect.

As the plastic masks are transparent allowing visualization of cyanosis and secretions they are preferred over rubber masks.

As mask ventilation carries many disadvantages, it can be used only as a tide over phase till definite airway (intubation) is accomplished. The *disadvantages* of mask ventilation are:
- Dead space volume is increased
- Ventilation with mask is tiring
- A significant amount of air leaks into esophagus and can easily increase the intragastric pressure significant enough (> 28 cm H_2O) to cause *aspiration.*

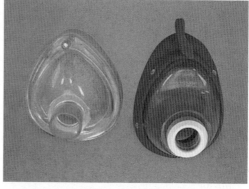

Fig. 3.2: Facemask *(For color version, see Plate 2)*

AMBU BAG RESUSCITATOR (FIGS 3.3 AND 3.4)

AMBU stands for artificial manual breathing unit. It is used to ventilate the patient. The AMBU

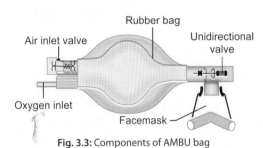

Fig. 3.3: Components of AMBU bag

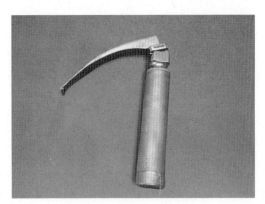

Fig. 3.5: Macintosh laryngoscope
(For color version, see Plate 2)

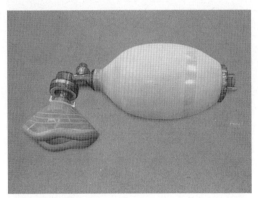

Fig. 3.4: AMBU bag (Note there is an option for attaching reservoir bag and oxygen supply) *(For color version, see Plate 2)*

unit consists of one self-inflating bag made up of rubber or silicone, a non-rebreathing valve and a mask. Non-breathing valve closes the expiratory port when the bag is manually squeezed letting the air inside the bag to pass to facemask. During expiration, bobin of valve comes to normal position letting the expired air to void to atmosphere.

- AMBU bags are available in a capacity of 1,200 mL for adults, 500 mL for children and 250 mL for newborns.
- 100% oxygen can be delivered by AMBU bag by attaching oxygen source and oxygen reservoir.

LARYNGOSCOPES (FIG. 3.5)

Laryngoscope is used for visualizing the glottis to facilitate intubation. Laryngoscopy may be direct where glottis is directly visualized or indirect where glottis is visualized through optic channels. Based on method of laryngoscopy, laryngoscopes has been classified as: (1) Direct rigid laryngoscopes; (2) Indirect (fiberoptic) rigid laryngoscopes; (3) Flexible (fiberoptic) laryngoscopes.

Direct Rigid Laryngoscopes

Direct rigid laryngoscope consists of a handle (containing 2 batteries), a blade with a bulb. They are named on the shape of the blade. Although there are number of laryngoscopes available in the market, however, the most common in use are:

- *Macintosh* **(Fig. 3.5)**: *It is most commonly used.* It has *curved blade* and is available in 4 sizes; smallest for children and largest for adults with long necks.
- *McCoy:* It has got a movable tip, which can be used to maneuver the glottis **(Fig. 3.6)**.
- *Miller:* It has a straight blade with curve at the tip.

Blades for Infants and Newborns

- *Magill:* Magill is *straight blade* used for neonates. Neonatal epiglottis is large, leafy and more anterior, therefore it need to be lifted by straight blade to visualize glottis (Adult's epiglottis just need to be pushed anteriorly, therefore curved blade is used).
- *Oxford infant blade:* Used for infants.

Indirect Rigid Laryngoscopes (Fiberoptic)

In this technique, the glottis is not visualized directly but through the fiberoptic channels. The

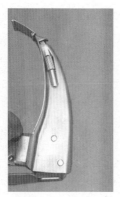

Fig. 3.6: McCoy laryngoscope
(For color version, see Plate 2)

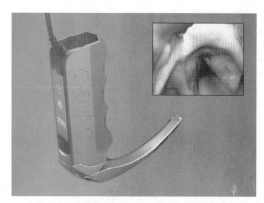

Fig. 3.8: C-MAC laryngoscope and picture of glottis seen
on screen *(For color version, see Plate 3)*

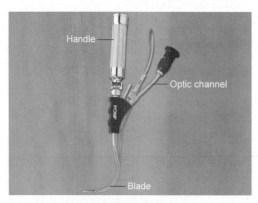

Fig. 3.7: Bullard laryngoscope
(For color version, see Plate 2)

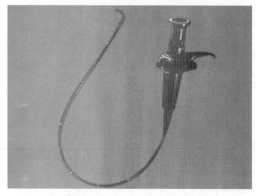

Fig. 3.9: Flexible fiberoptic laryngoscope

classical example of such laryngoscope is *Bullard laryngoscope* **(Fig. 3.7)**. WuScope is another commonly used indirect laryngoscope, which has a channel for guiding endotracheal tube.

Video Laryngoscopes (Fig. 3.8)

Video laryngoscopes (VLs) are just one step ahead, where the video of the real time refracted image of glottis is obtained on a screen. Some of the video laryngoscopes have the option to obtain the image on any laptop or smart phone screen.

Studies have reported intubation success rates of 94–99% for video laryngoscopy as a rescue modality after failed direct laryngoscopy.

Although like direct laryngoscopes, video laryngoscopes are also available in different shapes of blades such as highly curved or distally angulated, however, the *most commonly used and prototype is C-MAC* the design of which is based on the Macintosh blade **(Fig. 3.8)**.

Flexible Laryngoscopes/Bronchoscopes (Fiberoptic) (Fig. 3.9)

Intubation done under the guidance of fiberoptic laryngoscope/bronchoscope is called as flexible scope intubation (FSI). It is considered as *gold standard technique for the management of difficult/ failed intubation.* It is less traumatic, does not require any specific position of neck and can be performed in awake patients. The limitations are cost, technical expertise and time consuming.

Complications of Laryngoscopy

- *Dental injury: Most vulnerable are upper incisors.*
- Damage to soft tissues and nerves.
- Injury to cervical spinal cord in case of aggressive manipulation of pre-existing injury.
- *Hemodynamic alterations:* Tachycardia, hypertension and cardiac arrhythmias.
- Breakage and aspiration of bulb.

SUPRAGLOTTIC AIRWAY DEVICES

As the name suggests these devices are placed above glottis for airway management. These devices serve as a niche between facemask and endotracheal tubes. They are so commonly used in current day practice that we can say that it is an era of supraglottic devices. The most popular and most commonly used supraglottic device used is laryngeal mask airway.

Laryngeal Mask Airways

Laryngeal mask airways (LMA) has been classified as 1st generation and 2nd generation LMA.

First Generation LMA

Classical LMA: Discovered by Archie Brain, therefore also called as *Brain Mask*. It is placed blindly in oropharynx and the cuff is inflated with large volume of air (30 to 40 mL for adult size) **(Fig. 3.10)**. Inflated cuff seals the lateral and posterior pharyngeal walls, and patient can be ventilated through ventilation ports.

LMA are available in 7 different sizes (in some countries 8th size is also available)—the smallest one for neonate and largest for large adults.

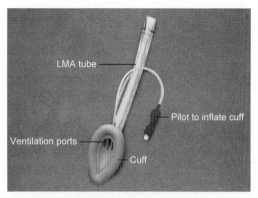

Fig. 3.10: Laryngeal mask airway (Classic)
(For color version, see Plate 3)

Indications

- As an alternative to intubation where difficult intubation is anticipated.
- Securing airway in emergency situations where intubation and mask ventilation becomes impossible.
- As an elective method for minor-to-moderate surgeries where anesthetist electively wants to avoid intubation.
- As a conduit for bronchoscopes, small size tubes and gum elastic bougies.

Advantages

- Easy to insert (even paramedical staff can insert).
- Does not require any laryngoscope and muscle relaxants.
- Does not require any specific position of cervical spine, therefore can be used in cervical injuries.
- Less sympathetic stimulation as compared to intubation
- Complications of intubation can be avoided
- Patient awakening is smooth as compared to intubation
- Reusable (up to 40 times)

Disadvantages/Complications

- As air can leak into the esophagus, *LMA increases the risk of aspiration.* Moreover, if there occurs gastric distension due to leakage of air in esophagus it is not possible to decompress the stomach as there is no place to pass

Size	Indication (is on basis of weight)	Cuff volume
1	Up to 5 kg	4 mL
1.5	5–10 kg	7 mL
2	10–20 kg	10 mL
2.5	20–30 kg	14 mL
3	30–50 kg	20 mL
4	50–70 kg	30 mL
5	> 70 kg (or 70–100 kg)	40 mL
6 (only available in few countries)	> 100 kg	50 mL

suction catheter/Ryles tubes because of the occupation of oropharynx by the cuff of LMA.
- Can cause *laryngospasm* and airway obstruction, if displaces anteriorly.
- Trauma to oral cavity and injury to hypoglossal and lingual nerve, if excessive pressures are being used. The cuff pressure for LMA should be kept between 40–60 cm H_2O
- Sore throat—incidence is 10–20%

Contraindications

- Full stomach patients.
- Hiatus hernia, pregnancy (where chances of aspiration are high).
- Oropharyngeal abscess or mass.

LMA Unique: It is single use disposable LMA

LMA Flexible: The tube of LMA is enforced with a wire making it flexible, i.e. nonkinkable making it useful for head and neck surgeries.

Second Generation LMA

Second generation LMA provides better seal *thereby decreasing the chances of aspiration.*
- *Intubating LMA (also called as LMA Fastrach):* Up to 8 no. endotracheal tube can be guided through it **(Fig. 3.11).**
- *Proseal LMA:* It has larger and posterior cuff, which provides better seal. Moreover, it has drain tube which can be used to deflate the stomach **(Fig. 3.12).**
- *Supreme LMA*: Supreme LMA is like proseal LMA with a bite block to avoid damage to LMA tube, if the patient bites **(Fig. 3.13).**
- *I-Gel:* As the name suggests the cuff is prefilled with gel avoiding the complications of air filled cuff such as cuff leakage, damage and puncture. Like Proseal, I-gel also contains a drain tube, which can be used to deflate the stomach **(Fig. 3.14).**
- *LMA C-Trach:* Like video laryngoscopy, the LMA is attached to screen to visualize the structures **(Fig. 3.15).**

Other Supraglottic Devices

The success of LMA has led to manufacturing of number of similar devices but none could replace LMA. Out of > 10 kind of supraglottic devices, few which are used are:

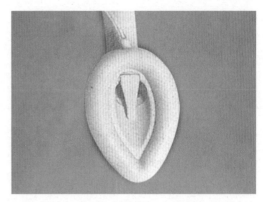

Fig. 3.11: Intubating LMA (Note a single port which allows the passage of endotracheal tube)

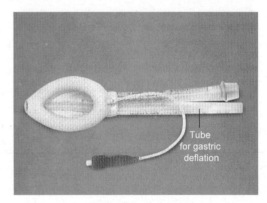

Fig. 3.12: Proseal LMA

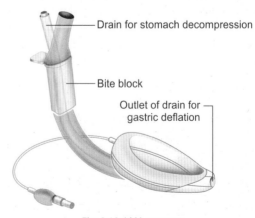

Fig. 3.13: LMA supreme

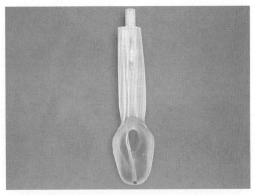

Fig. 3.14: I-Gel *(For color version, see Plate 3)*

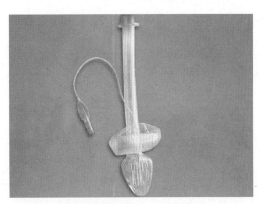

Fig. 3.16: Peripharyngeal airway

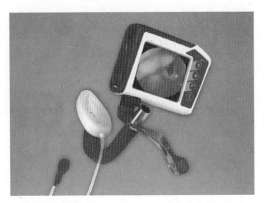

Fig. 3.15: LMA C-Trach *(For color version, see Plate 3)*

Peripharyngeal airway (Cobra-PLMA) *(Fig. 3.16)*: It has high volume oval cuff, which seals the hypopharynx while patient can be ventilated through the ventilation slots at the tip.

Combitube: It is double lumen tube used for providing patent airway in emergency and difficult intubation. It was popular in past but due to high rate of complications, it is hardy used now a day.

INFRAGLOTTIC AIRWAY DEVICES

As the name suggests, they are placed below the glottis. These devices are further classified as definitive and emergency airway management devices. *Definitive airway management devices include endotracheal tube and tracheostomy,* while infraglottic emergency airway includes cricothyroidotomy.

Definitive Airway Management Devices

Endotracheal Tubes

Endotracheal tubes have 2 ends, proximal end (machine end) and distal end (patient end). Patient end is beveled with angle of 45° in oral tubes and 30º in nasal tubes. They are mainly of two types, red rubber and PVC **(Table 3.1)**.

The endotracheal tubes may be uncuffed or cuffed **(Figs 3.17A and B)**.

Technique of Intubation

The patient should lie supine. *There should be extension at atlanto-occipital joint and flexion at cervical spine* **(Fig. 3.18)**. This position is achieved by putting a 6 to 8 cm thick pillow under the occiput. The laryngoscope blade should be inserted from right side of mouth and advanced slowly displacing the tongue to left until epiglottis is visualized. Once the epiglottis is visualized, it is lifted anteriorly to visualize the glottis. Once the glottis is seen the endotracheal tube is passed between the cords.

The cuff is inflated and the cuff should be well below vocal cords in adults. *The position of tube is verified by capnography* and auscultation over chest for air entry. The tube should be well secured at the angle of mouth with adhesive tape or bandage.

Cuff

The aim of inflating the cuff is to prevent aspiration. Usually, 4–8 mL of air is required to fill the cuff. During cuff inflation, ensure cuff pressure to be

■ **Table. 3.1:** Comparison of red rubber and PVC endotracheal tubes.

Red rubber	PVC
• Costlier	• Cheap
• Reusable (Can be autoclaved up to 6 times without damage)	• Disposable
• *Cuff: High pressure and low volume.* Because of this high pressure cuff chances of tracheal injury is more	• *Cuff: Low pressure and high volume.* Because of the low pressure, these tubes produce less tracheal injury
• Radiolucent	• Contains a radiopaque line therefore can be visualized in X-ray
• Nontransparent	• Transparent therefore secretions and mist can be visualized
• No Murphy eye is present	• Contains an additional hole near the tip called as Murphy's eye so that if main lumen gets blocked patient can still be ventilated through Murphy's eye
• Slightly more rigid so does not conform to the anatomy of airways	• Easily conforms to the anatomy of airways
• Less incidence of sore throat	• High incidence of sore throat (because of large cuff)
• It contains preservative lead (which imparts red color to these tubes)	—

less than 30 cm H_2O to prevent tracheal ischemia. Cuff should be filled with saline (instead of air) when tube is used for laser surgeries, surgeries at mines and when hyperbaric oxygen is used. The cuff should be 2–2.5 cm below the vocal cords.

The traditional approach of not using cuffed tubes in children up to 10 years does not hold true in present day practice (for details see Chapter 29, page no. 237).

Endotracheal Tube and Dead Space

As the endotracheal tube by passes the dead space constituted by nasal pathways, *anatomical dead is reduced by almost 50% (70 mL).*

Deciding the Size of Endotracheal Tube

For a normal healthy male usually 8.5 number (means internal diameter 8.5 mm) tube is used, while for normal healthy female usually 7.5 number tube is used. In children, the size of endotracheal tube is as follows:

- Prematures   : 2.5 no.
- 0–6 months   : 3–3.5 no.
- 6 months to 1 year : 3.5–4 no.
- For children 1 year to 6 years, the size is calculated by formula:

$$\frac{\text{Age (in years)}}{3} + 3.5$$

- For children > 6 years:

$$\frac{\text{Age (in years)}}{4} + 4.5$$

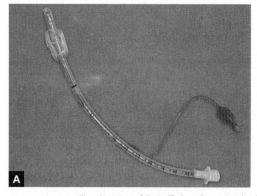
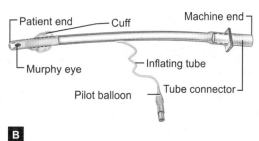

Figs 3.17A and B: Cuffed endotracheal tube (PVC type) *(For color version, see Plate 3)*

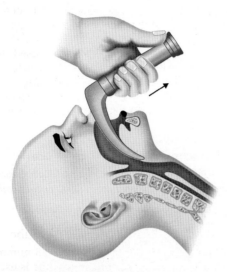

Fig. 3.18: Position for laryngoscopy (extension at atlanto-occipital joint and flexion at cervical spine)

For example, for a 5-year-old child, the tube size required will be:

5/3 + 3.5 = 1.6 + 3.5 = 5.1 (means 5 number tube).

Smallest size of tube available is 2.5 mm and the largest is 10.5 mm.

Deciding the Length of Tube

Optimal length is the length at which air entry is equal on both sides of the chest. Usually, it is 23 cm in adult males and 21 cm in adult females. In other words, *tip of the tube should lie 4–5 cm above the carina* (distance between incisors and carina is 26–28 cm). A rough guide is that length is twice the length from tip of nose to ear lobule.

- In children, the length of oral tube is calculated by formula:

$$\frac{\text{Age (in years)}}{2} + 12 \text{ cm}$$

For calculating length for nasal intubation 3 cm is added to oral length.

Example: For 5-year-old child length will be:

$$= \frac{5}{2} + 12$$

$$= 2.5 + 12 \text{ cm}$$

$$= 14.5 \text{ cm}.$$

Reflex Response to Laryngoscopy and Intubation

- During laryngoscopy, there occurs sympathetic stimulation which can cause tachyarrhythmia and hypertension.
- Intubation can precipitate laryngospasm, particularly if airways are hyper-reactive or patient is in light anesthesia.
- *Methods which can be used to blunt these responses are:*
  Adequate depth of anesthesia, opioids *(Opioid of choice is sufentanil)*, Intravenous/topical lignocaine, β-blockers (esmolol)/calcium-channel blockers.

Other Types of Tubes in Common Use

RAE preformed tubes (RAE after the name of 3 scientists—Ring, Adair and Elwyn) (also popularly called as oxford tubes)
- *South facing:* Used for upper lip, palate and upper dental surgery.
- *North facing:* Used for lower lip, tongue or lower dental surgery.

Spiral embedded (also called as flexometallic tube): *These are non-kinkable, non-collapsible, and therefore are very useful for head and neck surgeries where acute flexion/extension of neck is required.*

Microlaryngeal and laryngotracheal surgery tube (MLT, LTS tubes): Used for microlaryngeal surgeries (these are small size tubes with cuff).

Double Lumen Tubes (Fig. 3.19)

Double lumen tubes (DLT) are used when one lung ventilation/lung separation is required. Most commonly used DLT is Robert Shaw disposable DLT. They have two lumens, tracheal lumen and bronchial lumen. Based on bronchial lumen, they are named right sided (means bronchial lumen in right bronchus) or left-sided (means bronchial lumen in the left bronchus).

Indications for One Lung Ventilation/Lung Separation

Absolute: (1) To prevent spillage of contents of one lung (like pus, blood) to other side; (2) Unilateral lavage to prevent spillage of lavage fluid to healthy lung; (3) Massive bronchopleural fistula or large

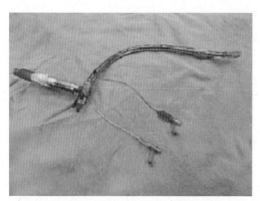

Fig. 3.19: Double lumen tube (Note 2 cuffs, 2 pilot system and 2 ventilation ports) *(For color version, see Plate 4)*

cyst/bulla where positive pressure ventilation can cause pneumothorax.

Relative: Any surgery on the lung (or thoracic aorta or esophagus) is considered as relative.

Complications of Double Lumen Tubes

- *Hypoxia: The most common cause of hypoxia is ventilation perfusion mismatch* (non-ventilated lung behaves like shunt). *Malposition of tube* (bronchial lumen in wrong bronchus) used to be the most common cause of hypoxia however the *confirmation of position of Double lumen tube by bronchoscopy* has significantly reduced the incidence of malposition.
- *Trauma to larynx.*
- *Bronchial rupture:* Due to over inflation of cuff in bronchus.

NASAL INTUBATION

Indications for Nasal Intubation

- Oral surgery
- Oral mass
- Inadequate mouth opening due to any cause like fracture mandible, Temporomandibular joint ankylosis, Ludwig angina, quinsy, tetanus, post-burn contractures.
- For awake intubation, nasal intubation is preferred over oral intubation.
- When tube is to be kept for prolonged periods in intensive care units and patient is going to remain awake most of the time nasal tube is preferred because it is better tolerated by patient.

Advantages of Nasal Intubation Over Oral Intubation

- Better fixation and therefore less chances of accidental Extubation.
- No possibility of tube occlusion by biting.
- Oral hygiene can be better maintained.
- Better tolerated by the patient.

Disadvantages

- Increased chances of bleeding and trauma to nasal structures (to avoid trauma to inferior turbinate bevel of the tube should be towards the septum).
- Increased chances of bacteremia (sinusitis, otitis, meningitis).
- Nasal deformities on long-term use.

Contraindications for Nasal Intubation

- Basal skull fractures and CSF rhinorrhea (there have been case reports of tube slipping into cranium and also CSF leak into nose can cause meningitis).
- Bleeding disorders (nasal and septal mucosa are highly vascular areas).
- Nasal polyp, abscess, foreign body.
- Adenoids
- Previous nasal surgery (relative contraindication).

Contraindications for Both Nasal and Oral Intubation

As such, there is no absolute contraindication to intubation. The very simple rule is "intubate where you can", therefore the relative contraindications are:

- Laryngeal edema—may get aggravated by intubation
- Acute epiglottitis and laryngotracheobronchitis—As airways are hyper-reactive intubation can precipitate laryngospasm.

Checking for Correct Position of Tube

- Auscultation of chest for air entry.
- Characteristic feel of bag.
- Chest inflation on positive pressure.
- *Capnography (measuring end tidal CO_2):* It is the *surest sign.*
- *Fiberoptic bronchoscopy:* It is also confirmatory but practically not feasible in every case.

Complications of Intubation

Perioperative

- *Esophageal intubation:* This is a hazardous complication. If not detected in time can cause severe hypoxia and death.
- Ischemia, edema and necrosis at local site (especially with red rubber tubes).
- Aspiration (if cuff is not properly inflated).
- Bronchial intubation and collapse of other lung.
- Tracheal tube obstruction by secretions, kinking. If not detected in time can cause hypoxia.
- Accidental extubation.
- Trauma to gums, lip, epiglottis, pharynx, larynx and nasal cavity (in nasal intubation).
- Reflex disturbances such as laryngospasm, bronchospasm, tachyarrhythmia and hypertension

Postoperative

- *Sore throat* (pharyngitis, laryngitis): This is the *most common postoperative complication.* It usually subsides in 2–3 days without any treatment.
- Laryngeal edema (usually present after 1 to 2 hours).
- Laryngeal nerve palsies.
- Surgical emphysema, mediastinal emphysema.
- *Infection:* Pneumonia, lung abscess, mediastinitis.
- Lung atelectasis.

Delayed Complications

- Vocal cord granuloma.
- Laryngotracheal web.
- Subglottic or tracheal stenosis.
- Tracheal collapse.
  Delayed complications usually occurs after prolonged intubation in intensive care patients. Therefore, *maximum permissible time for which an endotracheal tube can be kept is 14 days.*

Extubation

Extubation is performed when adequacy of respiration is maintained. *Extubation should be performed during inspiration* (when the laryngeal opening is maximum).

Complications at the Time of Extubation

- Aspiration.
- Laryngospasm and bronchospasm.
- Trauma to airways.
- Hypoxia (If extubation is premature).

Tracheostomy

Indications

- As an elective procedure where prolonged ventilation is required.
- As a switch over procedure from intubation.
- Excessive secretions leading to blockage or frequent change of endotracheal tube.
- As an alternative when intubation is not possible.
- Upper airways obstruction due to laryngeal edema, impacted foreign bodies, laryngeal trauma, Vocal cord paralysis, Ludwig angina, quinsy, laryngitis.
- For laryngeal surgeries.

Tracheostomy Tubes

- *Silver tubes:* Not used now-a-days.
- *Cuffed plastic tubes:* These are most commonly used. Cuffs should be *high volume, low pressure*
- *Montgomery T-tube or Olympic tracheal button:* These devices have no cuff, so they produce less tracheal injury and allow air to pass through mouth for speech.
- Fenestrated tubes for speaking.

Complications

Early Complications

- Malpositioning of the tube during insertion.
- Hemorrhage.
- Surgical emphysema.
- Pneumothorax.
- Injury to trachea, larynx.

Late Complications

- Blockage of tube due to secretions can cause severe hypoxia.
- Infection.
- Tracheal ulceration.

Delayed

- *Tracheal stenosis at the cuff site or at stoma:* To avoid this complication, low cuff pressure (< 15 mm Hg) is advocated.

- Tracheal web.
- Tracheal dilatation.

Care of Tracheostomy Tube

- Careful, aseptic suctioning of secretions at regular intervals should be done. Inner cannula should be changed every 4–6 hours.
- Adjustment of cuff pressure to keep it below 15 mm Hg.
- Humidified oxygen.
- Strict asepsis at the time of change. First change should not be done before 5 days as stoma takes 5 days to establish completely and change before this time can create false tract.
- Conscious patient should be given a bell, pencil and paper.

Minitracheostomy

Useful in emergency situations. Special sets are available. A stab is given in trachea and small size tube is inserted.

Emergency Infraglottic Airway Devices

Cricothyrotomy

Useful in life-threatening situations. Incision is given in cricothyroid membrane. *Disadvantages* are injury to cricoid cartilage and larynx.

Needle Cricothyrotomy

A needle or cannula 12G or 14G is inserted at cricothyroid membrane and oxygen is provided by flushing at high rate or by jet ventilation. Inspiratory and expiratory rate is kept at 1 : 4 instead of normal 1 : 2 allowing for passive expiration through narrow channel.

OTHER EQUIPMENT

OXYGEN DELIVERY SYSTEMS IN NON-INTUBATED PATIENT

Classification

- High flow (fixed performance) delivery systems.
- Low flow (variable performance) delivery systems.

High Flow Delivery System

These devices are *fixed performance* devices because their output is not affected by the changes in patient's tidal volume and respiratory rate and therefore they deliver *accurate oxygen concentration* (error is 1–2%). As they are more accurate in oxygen delivery they are more effective in treating hypoxemia than low flow systems. The major limitation of high flow system is low patient acceptance (due to high flow).

High flow system includes *Venturi mask*, special nebulizers and high airflow blenders. Among these Venturi mask is most commonly used. It works on *Venturi principle* which states that if a gas is passed through a narrow orifice at high pressure it creates shearing forces around the orifice which entrain room air in specific ratio.

Venturi masks are available in different colors. For example, blue color delivers minimum, i.e. 24% oxygen and green color delivers *maximum i.e. 60% oxygen.*

Low Flow Oxygen Delivery Systems

These are *variable performance devices*, i.e. their performance gets changed with the changes in patient respiratory parameters. As their output varies they are *less accurate and less reliable* in terms of oxygen delivery. Therefore, they can be used only used for stable patients.

Low flow systems include nasal cannula, simple oxygen mask (also called as Mary Carterall or Hudson mask), Non-rebreathing mask, rebreathing mask and polymask.

As they are well tolerated by the patients, therefore are frequently used in wards, however, not for very critical patient where accuracy is more important than comfort.

Maximum concentration of oxygen that can be delivered by oxygen mask is 60% (at a flow of 7–8 L) and by nasal cannula is 44% (at a flow of 6 L/min.). Non-breathing mask with oxygen reservoir can deliver as high as 80–100% of oxygen and therefore is now preferred over Venturi mask by majority of clinicians.

Extracorporeal Oxygen Delivery Systems (Oxygenators)

As the name suggests, the gas exchange takes place outside the body. These oxygenators are the part of cardiopulmonary bypass (heart lung machine). Two types of oxygenators in current use are:

1. *Bubble oxygenators* where oxygen is pushed with pressure from below to the blood chamber

in the form of bubbles. These bubbles can cause damage to blood cells, therefore bubble oxygenators are not preferred.

2. *Membrane oxygenators* where blood chamber and oxygen chamber is separated by a membrane; oxygen reaches blood by diffusion through membrane. As there is no damage to blood cells, *membrane oxygenators are preferred over bubble oxygenators.*

HUMIDIFICATION DEVICES

Preservation of humidity is very important. 50% fall in humidity can cause complete cessation of ciliary activity. Moreover, dry gases can cause direct injury to tracheobronchial mucosa.

Various methods used for humidification are:

Humidifiers

Humidifiers can be classified as passive and active humidifiers.

Passive Humidifier

Also called as *artificial nose, condenser humidifier or heat and moisture exchanger (HME) filter* **(Fig. 3.20)**.

These are disposable devices containing hygroscopic layers which preserve heat and water of exhaled gases and deliver it in next breath to the inspired gas. These are placed between endotracheal tube and breathing circuit. Not only they preserve humidity, they also act as filter to prevent contamination. The disadvantage is that they increases the dead space, resistance and can get obstructed due to blood or secretions.

Active Humidifiers

These are further classified as non-heated and heated humidifiers.

Non-heated Humidifiers

These are simple containers (glass/plastic bottles) containing water. The oxygen is passed over it or through it and gets humidified. These are used for delivering humidified oxygen through masks or nasal cannula. The advantage is that they are cheap and simple to use but disadvantage is that they cannot attain 100% humidity (Maximum humidity that can be achieved is 70–75%).

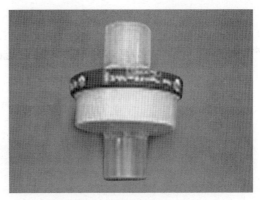

Fig. 3.20: Heat and moisture exchanger
(For color version, see Plate 4)

Heated Humidifiers

These are electrically operated, can deliver fully saturated gases but are expensive and increases the risk of thermal burns.

Nebulizers

Nebulizers are also called *aerosol generators.* They emit water in the form of aerosol (droplets). These are used for producing humidification and delivery of drug directly into respiratory tract. They may be pressure driven or ultrasonic.

The optimal particle size of droplet should be between 0.5 to 5 μm. Particles larger than 5 μm are too big to reach peripheral airways while less than 0.5 μm are too light that they come back with expired gases without being deposited in airways. Drugs delivered by nebulizers are bronchodilators, decongestants, mucolytic agents and steroids.

STATIC CURRENT

Flow of gases in anesthesia machine can generate current, therefore anesthesia masks, circuits, wheels of machines are made *antistatic by adding carbon* to them.

STERILIZATION OF ANESTHESIA EQUIPMENT

- Metallic instruments such as laryngoscope blades, Magill's forceps, and stylet can be autoclaved.
- Non-metallic items such as endotracheal tubes, facemasks, airways are best sterilized

by *ethylene oxide (ETO) gas sterilization.* After ETO, second method of choice for these items is chemical sterilization by 2% glutaraldehyde (Cidex) or orthophthaldehyde (OPA). As silicone resists gas sterilization, silicone containing items such as laryngeal mask airway (LMA) should not be sterilized by ETO. The *only recommended method for sterilizing LMA is autoclaving* at temperature < 134°C.

• For fiberoptic scopes, chemical sterilization by 2% glutaraldehyde or orthophthaldehyde is the preferred method of sterilization.

Before sterilization all equipment should be thoroughly cleaned with soap and water and dried with air.

KEY POINTS

- The most common airway used to prevent the tongue fall is Guedel's airway.
- The major limitation of mask ventilation is that it increases the chances of aspiration.
- Macintosh is the most commonly used laryngoscope.
- Intubation success rates of 94–99% has been reported for video laryngoscopy as a rescue modality after failed direct laryngoscopy.
- Most commonly used video laryngoscopes is C-MAC.
- Fiberoptic laryngoscope/bronchoscope-guided intubation is considered as gold standard technique for the management of difficult/failed intubation.
- Current day anesthetic practice is an era of supraglottic devices.
- Second generation LMA has shown significant decrease in incidence of aspiration as compared to first generation LMA.
- Among the second generation LMA, I-Gel is most frequently used in India.
- Definitive airway management devices includes endotracheal tube and tracheostomy.
- The chief advantage of PVC tube is that their cuff is low pressure and high volume.
- During laryngoscopy, there should be extension at atlanto-occipital joint and flexion at cervical spine.
- Capnography is the surest sign to confirm the correct position of endotracheal tube.
- The traditional approach of not using cuffed tubes in children up to 10 years does not hold true in present day practice.
- The most common cause of hypoxia for double lumen tube is ventilation perfusion mismatch.
- Fixed performance devices deliver accurate oxygen concentration.
- Heat and moisture exchanger (HME) is the most commonly used device to preserve humidity in anesthesia.

Quintessential in Anesthesia

CHAPTER 4

Preoperative Assessment and Premedication

PREOPERATIVE ASSESSMENT

The goals are:

- To reduce the anxiety and educate the patient about anesthesia.
- To obtain information about patient's medical history.
- To perform physical examination.
- To determine which tests are required.
- To plan anesthetic technique.
- To obtain informed consent.
- To give preoperative instructions.

Preoperative evaluation is done with:

History

- Any medical illness in past/present.
- History of allergy to any drug.
- History of medications.
- History of previous anesthesia.
- History of personal habits (smoking, alcoholism or drug abuse).

Physical Examination

- General physical examination (including pulse and blood pressure).
- Systemic examination of cardiovascular system, respiratory system, hepatic system, nervous system, abdomen and spine. In respiratory system examination, other than routine assessment *Breath-holding time* should be assessed in every patient. Patient is asked to hold the breath after full inspiration. Normal is *more than 25 seconds*.

15–25 seconds is borderline.

Less than 15 seconds indicate severely diminished cardiorespiratory reserve.

- *Airway assessment* to rule out difficult airway. It is one of the most important assessments for anesthesiologist. It includes assessment of mouth opening, denture status and neck movements. Out of the many parameters used for airway assessment Mallampati grading, Thyromental distance and neck movements are assessed in every case (*for details of airway assessment and management of difficult intubation see Chapter 5, page no. 53*).

Investigations

Routine investigations: The protocols for routine investigations vary from hospital to hospital, state to state and country to country. *Nowadays, the inclination is towards minimum investigations.* The decision to order preoperative tests should be guided by the patient's clinical history, comorbidities, physical examination findings and the proposed surgery.

Complete blood count: As per western guidelines, complete blood count (CBC) is indicated only for patients with diseases that increases the risk of anemia (like chronic renal failure) or patients in whom significant perioperative blood loss is anticipated. However, due to high prevalence of anemia, CBC is performed in all patients in India.

Renal function test, urine analysis, random blood sugar, liver function test and coagulation profile: Recommended, only if there is positive medical history or examination (contrary to previous guideline of performing RFT in all patients >60 years).

Electrocardiography: Contrary to previous recommendation of ECG in all males > 40 years and all females >50 years, ECG is recommended for patients with positive medical history or undergoing high-risk surgery. Asymptomatic patients undergoing low-risk surgery do not require electrocardiography.

X-ray chest: Advisable only for patients at risk of postoperative pulmonary complications.

Risk Stratification

Based on the preoperative assessment, the patients are classified into *six categories* by *American Society of Anesthesiologist (ASA)*. The morbidity and mortality is highest in grade V patients and minimum in grade I patients.

I   : Normal healthy patient.

II   : Mild-to-moderate systemic disease not limiting functional activity.

III : Severe systemic disease that limits the activity but not incapacitating.

IV : Incapacitating disease that is a constant threat to life.

V   : Moribund patient who has very little chances of survival with or without operation.

VI : Brain dead patients (for organ donation).

The major limitation of ASA classification was that it did not include age, obesity (two major enemies of anesthetist) and risk associated with surgical procedure (morbidity and mortality may be minimum with minimally invasive procedure like cataract but may be very high with highly invasive procedure like thoracic aortic surgery). However, new guidelines by ASA (2014) has at least included obesity in ASA classification (patients with BMI < 40 are considered as grade II risk and >40 as grade III risk).

INSTRUCTIONS

Instructions Related to Modification in Pre-existing Medical Therapy

Oral Hypoglycemics

Oral hypoglycemics should be continued, omitting the morning dose. However, sulfonylurea and metformin have longer half-lives so they need to be stopped 24–48 hours before surgery.

Insulin

Most of the patients are either on intermediate acting or mixed insulin. Adjustments in the doses of insulin are required as per the regime followed. There are different protocols followed by different institutions (*for details see Chapter 23, page no. 206*).

Oral Contraceptives

Estrogen increases the chances of postoperative deep vein thrombosis and thromboembolism, therefore standard dose estrogen containing pills should be stopped 4 weeks before. *Pills containing only progesterone or low dose estrogen need not be stopped.*

Oral Anticoagulants

- *Standard oral anticoagulants, i.e. Warfarin (Coumadin) should be stopped 4 days prior to surgery.* The newer one, i.e. Dabigatran (Pradaxa) should be stopped 3 days prior, Rivaroxaban (Xarelto) and Apixaban (Eliquis) 48 hours prior, and Edoxaban 72 hours prior to surgery. However, before considering for surgery it is mandatory to check whether the effect of oral anticoagulant has been weaned off or not by doing INR before surgery. *INR must be < 1.5 to consider the patient for surgery.*

- If stopping of Warfarin is not possible like in prosthetic heart valves, then switch over to heparin which is stopped 12–24 hours prior to surgery.

- In case of urgency, effect of oral anticoagulants can be reversed with vitamin K but if it is not possible to wait for 6–12 hours (vitamin K takes 6–12 hours to completely reverse the effect of Warfarin), then patient can be taken up for surgery after transfusing fresh-frozen plasma.

Heparin

Low molecular weight heparin (LMWH) {Enoxaparin} should be stopped 12–24 hours prior to surgery (Prophylactic dose 12 hours while therapeutic dose has to be stopped 24 hours prior). *Standard (unfractionated) heparin* has short half-life, therefore stopping *6–12 hours* before surgery is sufficient while long acting such as *Fondaparinux (Arixtra)* should be stopped *48–72 hours* (48 hours for prophylactic dose and 72 hours for therapeutic).

Thrombolytic/Fibrinolytic Therapy (Alteplase, Urokinase, Streptokinase)

Patients can be considered for elective surgery 10 days after the last dose of these drugs.

Antianginal Drugs

All antianginal drugs (including calcium-channel blockers, nitrates) should be continued except antiplatelets.

Antiplatelet Drugs

Aspirin: Although aspirin increases the risk of bleeding but stopping aspirin carries the risk of ischemia, therefore *it is recommended to continue aspirin.*

Clopidogrel (plavis): *Clopidogrel should be stopped 5 days prior to surgery.*

Other less commonly used antiplatelets such as dipyridamole should be stopped 48 hours, ticlopidine 14 days, abciximab 2 days and eptifibatide 8 hours prior to surgery.

In case of emergency surgery, when there is no time to stop antiplatelets, then patient can be taken for surgery after platelet transfusion.

NSAIDs: Usually continued however should be discontinued 48 hours prior to surgery if given with other antiplatelets and continuing other antiplatelet is mandatory. For example, if the patient is on aspirin (for cardiac disease or stroke) and diclofenac then stop diclofenac 48 hours prior and continue aspirin.

Antihypertensives

All antihypertensives on which the patient blood pressure is controlled should be continued except for angiotensin II antagonist and angiotensin-converting enzyme (ACE) inhibitors where morning dose is withheld. Studies have found a higher incidence of significant hypotension in patients who were continued with the morning dose of angiotensin II antagonist and ACE inhibitors.

Antidepressants

Antidepressants (SSRI, tricyclic antidepressants, reversible MAO inhibitors and MAO-B (Selegiline) has to be continued. However, MAO-A inhibitors (which are not used nowadays) can significantly increase the levels of catecholamines, therefore need to be stopped 3 weeks before surgery.

Lithium and Lamotrigine

Although Lithium do enhances the block produced by muscle relaxants but this effect seems to be clinically insignificant therefore in contrary to older guidelines of stopping lithium 48 before surgery current recommendation is to *continue Lithium.* The other drug approved for bipolar disorder, i.e. Lamotrigine has to be continued.

Levodopa

Recent recommendation is to *continue levodopa* otherwise withdrawal can cause muscular rigidity.

Anticholinesterases (Neostigmine, Pyridostigmine)

The continuation of anticholinesterases in perioperative period is debatable. One school of thought advocates discontinuation 4–6 hours prior to surgery but this increases the possibility of myasthenic crisis, therefore the more favorable and acceptable dictum is to continue anticholinesterases with adjustments (reduction) in doses.

Steroids

If patient has taken steroid (prednisone in doses > 5 mg/day or equivalent) for more than 3 weeks (by any route-even topical or inhalational) in last 1 year he/she must receive intraoperative supplementation with hydrocortisone. The reason for supplementation is that if a patient takes prednisone in doses > 5 mg/day or equivalent for more than 3 weeks, there occurs suppression of hypothalamus-pituitary-adrenal axis, the recovery of which takes place in 1 year. Therefore, during this period, the patient may not be able to cope up with the stress of surgery.

Smoking

Smoking inhibits cilia, causes hyperactivity of airways, increases mucous production and decreases immune response. The normal restoration of these effects (particularly recovery of ciliary activity) takes 6–8 weeks, therefore smoking should ideally be stopped *8 weeks* before surgery. However, cessation of smoking any time before surgery is beneficial. The 12 hours of cessation decreases the level of carboxyhemoglobin, shifting the oxygen dissociation curve to right and facilitating oxygen delivery to tissues. Same way, decreases in nicotine levels decreases the chances of arrhythmias.

Antibiotics

Aminoglycosides can potentiate the effect of muscle relaxants but not to an extent that they should be stopped (This is in contrary to the older guidelines of either stopping or switch over to other antibiotic 48 hours prior to surgery).

Herbal Medicines

Herbal medicines (including commercial preparations of ginger, garlic, green tea) can effect drug metabolism, bleeding profile and neuronal functions. Therefore, they should be stopped 1 week prior to surgery.

Viagra (Or Similar Drugs)

To be stopped 24 hours prior to surgery.

Topical Medications (Creams, Ointments)

Discontinue on the day of surgery as the chemicals in these ointments can react with antiseptic solutions used during surgery.

Diuretics

Discontinue on the day of surgery except for thiazides taken for hypertension.

Disulfiram

To be discontinued 10 days before the surgical procedure

Antitubercular Drugs

To be continued but assessment of liver functions is mandatory.

Preoperative Instructions

- *Fasting Instructions: For solid food, 8 hours of fasting is must (fasting period of 6 hours may be considered after a light meal) while clear fluids (water and juices without pulp) can be given up to 2 hours.*
  For neonates and infants, the recommended fasting period for *breast milk is 4 hours* while for formula milk and solids a fasting of 6 hours is required.
- Artificial dentures, limbs, contact lenses should be taken off.

- Jewellery (can cause cautery-related burns), lipstick and nail polish to be removed (can obscure cyanosis).
- Good oral hygiene.
- Informed consent to be taken.
- Premedication.

PREMEDICATION

In the current day practice of anesthesia *patient is premedicated with a purpose not as a routine procedure*. If given, the premedication is given with the following goals:

Goals

- To relieve anxiety.
- To produce hemodynamic stability.
- To induce sedation (good sleep) and reduce metabolic rate.
- To provide analgesia and amnesia.
- To decrease the chances of aspiration.
- To control oral and respiratory secretions.
- To prevent postoperative nausea and vomiting.
- To control infection.

To relieve anxiety: *Relieving anxiety is the most important goal is present day anesthesia.* Nothing can be more helpful in relieving the anxiety of the patient than preoperative visit of the anesthetist clearing the patient's doubts, fears, myths and explaining the anesthetic technique. Benzodiazepines should be used only for the patients where assurance by anesthetist is not sufficient or for pediatric patients. In the current day surgical practice where majority of the patient are getting admitted on the same day of surgery, the *benzodiazepine of choice is Midazolam.*

To produce hemodynamic stability: Clonidine was recommended for hypertensive patient in past but not used now a days.

To provide analgesia: Opioids are given intravenously just before induction to provide analgesia and to attenuate cardiovascular response to laryngoscopy and intubation.

To decrease chances of aspiration: The best way to reduce the chances of aspiration is by keeping the patient fasting. Therefore, the drugs for aspiration prophylaxis, i.e. metoclopramide, antacids and H_2 blockers (ranitidine) *should be employed only for patients who are at high risk of aspiration such as* *hiatus hernia, pregnancy, not routinely for every patient.*

To control secretions

Anticholinergics available to control secretions are atropine, glycopyrrolate and scopolamine. Anticholinergics can cause dry mouth which can be troublesome to patients therefore *they should be used only when required* (like oral surgeries where dry mouth is the requirement of surgery), *not routinely in all patients.*

Glycopyrrolate is a preferred anticholinergic over atropine and scopolamine because it does not crosses the blood-brain barrier therefore is devoid of central side effects.

To prevent nausea and vomiting: Drugs which can be used for antiemetic prophylaxis are:

- Hyoscine.
- 5HT3 antagonist (Ondansetron/granisetron).
- Metoclopramide.

Current day recommendation is to use antiemetic prophylaxis only for the conditions associated with higher incidence of postoperative nausea and vomiting (like middle ear surgeries), *not routinely to all patients. In current day practice 5-HT3 antagonists are the first-line medications for prophylaxis as well as treatment of postoperative nausea and vomiting.*

To control infection: The timing of antibiotic should be adjusted so that the peak blood levels are achieved at the time of skin incision. Therefore, antibiotic prophylaxis must be given *within 60 minutes before skin incision.*

KEY POINTS

- Preoperative assessment is done to obtain history, do physical examination, order investigations, risk stratification (by ASA grading) and give preoperative instructions.
- The decision to order preoperative tests should be guided by the patient's clinical history, comorbidities, physical examination findings and the proposed surgery. Only the investigations which are necessary should be done.
- For solid food 8 hours of fasting is must while clear fluids can be given up to 2 hours.

Medications need to be stopped:
- MAO-A inhibitors (3 weeks before)
- Oral anticoagulants (Warfarin 4 days prior)
- Heparin (Low molecular weight 12 hours before)
- Antiplatelets except aspirin (Clopidogrel 5 days prior)
- Thrombolytic (10 days prior)
- Nonsteroidal anti-inflammatory drugs (NSAIDs) (48 hours prior if used with other antiplatelts)
- High dose estrogen oral contraceptives (4 weeks prior)
- Viagra (24 hours prior)
- Disulfiram (10 days prior)
- All herbal medications (7 days before)
- Smoking (8 weeks before)

Medications for which only morning dose to be omitted:
- ACE inhibitors and angiotensin II antagonist
- Oral hypoglycemics
- Topical creams and ointments
- Vitamins and iron.

Dose adjustment is needed for:
- Cholinesterase inhibitors
- Corticosteroids
- Insulin
- Rest all medications are continued in the same dosages and same regime with morning dose on the day of surgery to be taken with a sip of water.
- In the current day practice of anesthesia patient is premedicated with a purpose not as a routine procedure.

CHAPTER 5

Difficult Airway Management

CAUSES OF DIFFICULT INTUBATION/ DIFFICULT AIRWAY

Inability to Open Mouth

- Submandibular abscess
- Ludwig angina
- Retropharyngeal abscess
- Tetanus (trismus)
- Temporomandibular joint ankylosis
- Maxillary trauma
- Mandibular trauma
- Growth in oral cavity.

Abnormalities of Mandible

- *Micrognathia:* Receding chin
- *Pierre-Robin syndrome:* Hypoplastic mandible
- *Treacher Collins syndrome:* Mandibulofacial dysostosis
- *Goldenhar syndrome:* Hypoplasia.

Abnormalities of Tongue (Macroglossia)

- Pierre-Robin syndrome
- Down syndrome
- Hypothyroidism.

Abnormalities of Soft Palate

- *Pierre-Robin syndrome:* High-arched palate
- *Treacher Collins syndrome:* High-arched palate
- Marfan syndrome
- Achondroplasia.

Neck Abnormalities

- Short neck
  - Neck circumference >43 cm
- *Restricted neck movements:*
  - Rheumatoid arthritis

- Spondylitis (osteoarthritis)
- Disc disease
- Klippel–Feil syndrome (cervical vertebrae fusion)
- Neck trauma
- *Neck contracture:*
  - Post-burn
  - Post-radiotherapy
- *Neck swellings:*
  - Large thyroid gland
  - Cystic hygroma
- *Diabetes mellitus (reduced mobility of atlanto-occipital joint).*

Laryngeal Abnormalities

- Edema
- Tumor
- Stenosis
- Web
- Fixation of larynx to other structures of neck (in malignancies).

Tracheal Abnormalities

- Stenosis
- Tumor.

Thoracoabdominal Abnormalities

- Kyphosis
- Prominent chest or large breast.

Abnormalities of Temporomandibular Joint

- True ankylosis
- *False ankylosis:*
  - Burns
  - Trauma
  - Radiation.

Other Causes

- Protruding teeth (Rabbit teeth)
- Absent denture (slippage of laryngoscope)
- Children (anteriorly placed larynx)
- Basilar skull fracture
- Scleroderma (restricted temporomandibular joint)
- Sarcoidosis (airway obstruction by lymphoid tissue)
- Obesity
- Presence of beard.

ASSESSMENT OF DIFFICULT INTUBATION

Commonly used grades and parameters for assessment of airway include:

- *Mallampati grading:* It is done to assess *mouth opening*. Patient is asked to open the mouth as wide as possible and protrude the tongue. Depending on the structures seen by examiner the classification is as follows **(Fig. 5.1)**:
  Class I: Faucial pillars, soft palate and uvula seen.
  Class II: Base of uvula and soft palate is seen.
  Class III: Only soft palate is seen.

Class IV: Only hard palate is visible (modified Sampson and Young classification).

In Mallampati grade (class) I and II oral intubation can be done comfortably, in grade III with difficulty while oral intubation is not possible in grade IV.

- *Thyromental distance* (distance between thyroid notch to mental prominence with fully extended neck):
  Normal: 6.5 or more (> 3 finger breadth).
  6.0–6.5 cm: Difficult laryngoscopy.
  < 6.0 cm: Laryngoscopy may be impossible.
- *Mentohyoid distance:* Normal > 5 cm (2 finger breadth).
- *Assessment of TM joint function:* Inter incisor gap (mouth opening) should be at least 5 cm (2 finger breadth).
- *Neck movements:* Normal range of flexion and extension varies between 165° and 90°.
  Mallampati grading, thyromental distance and neck movements are assessed in every case.

Grading of Difficult Laryngoscopy (Cotmack and Lehane) (Fig. 5.2)

- *Grade I:* Glottis fully visible.
- *Grade II:* Only posterior glottis visible.

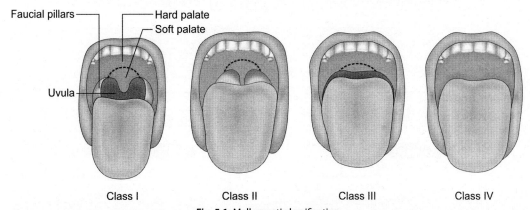

Class I   Class II   Class III   Class IV

Fig. 5.1: Mallampati classification

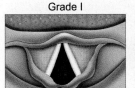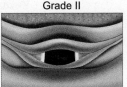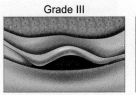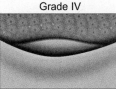

Grade I   Grade II   Grade III   Grade IV

Fig. 5.2: Grading of laryngoscopy

- *Grade III:* Only epiglottis visible.
- *Grade IV:* No recognizable structures.

MANAGEMENT (FLOW CHART 5.1)

Anticipated Difficult Intubation

If difficult airway is anticipated then intubate in *awake state* preferably with fiberoptic broncho-scope under topical anesthesia (xylocaine spray and/or gargles) or nerve blocks (glossopharyngeal and superior laryngeal).

If awake intubation fails then surgery, if possible should be performed under regional anesthesia or alternative methods like mask ventilation, laryngeal mask. If surgery is not possible by above-said methods and deemed necessary, then it should be performed with tracheostomy (if agreeable to patient).

Nonanticipated Difficult Intubation (Patient under Anesthesia)

- *Ventilation with bag and mask possible (cannot intubate but can ventilate situation) {non-emergency}:* While maintaining the ventilation consider reattempt intubation called as *plan A* (maximum 4 times) with manipulations such as changing the position of head and neck, cricoid pressure, using different blades of laryngoscopes, use of stylet or bougies, light

Flow chart 5.1: Difficult airway algorithm

Abbreviations: LMA, laryngeal mask airway; ILMA, intubating laryngeal mask airway

wands or intubation with videolaryngoscopy (Video laryngoscopy have revolutionized the practice of airway management; Intubation success rates can be as high as 94–99% with video laryngoscopy after failed intubation with direct laryngoscopy).

– If plan A fails, then get the surgery done under *plan B* which includes surgery under laryngeal mask airway (LMA) if possible or intubation with the help of intubating laryngeal mask airway (ILMA)

– If plan B fails, then proceed to *plan C* which includes revert back to facemask and get surgery done under facemask if emergency or postpone the case to be done next time as anticipated difficult intubation.

– If any time situation becomes that mask ventilation also fails which can happen due to laryngeal edema, excess secretions), then manage like *plan*

D, i.e. ventilation with bag and mask not possible (cannot intubate, cannot ventilate).

• *Ventilation with bag and mask not possible (cannot intubate, cannot ventilate) {emergency situation}.* It is one of the worst nightmares in the life of an anesthetist. It should be managed in following stepwise manner:

i. Immediate call for help

ii. Retry mask ventilation by holding mask with two hands while assistant maintaining ventilation, put an airway (if not in place). If it fails, then go to step iii

iii. Put LMA and try to get surgery done under LMA if possible or postpone the case to be done next time as anticipated difficult intubation. If LMA also fails, then go to step iv

iv. Cricothyroidotomy which should be replaced by definitive measure, i.e. tracheostomy as soon as possible.

Flow chart 5.2: Cervical spine injury

Airway Management for Cervical Spine Injury (Flow chart 5.2)

Neck manipulation in cervical injury may be life-threatening. *Every head injury should be considered to be having cervical injury until proved otherwise.* During manual management, airway should be managed only by jaw thrust however *if airway is not manageable by jaw thrust alone then head tilt and chin lift can be given* because life takes the priority over cervical spine.

Oral intubation with *'neck stabilization'* with neck in *'neutral position'* should be tried first and is usually successful. Neck stabilization can be done manually and with hard cervical collars. As intubation often requires removal of cervical collar *manual stabilization is always preferred over collar stabilization.* If unsuccessful, then only tracheostomy should be undertaken. LMA, combitube and cricothyroidotomy are reserved as temporary measure for the cases when tracheostomy is not possible due to non-availability of equipment/experienced person or life saving measure where time for tracheostomy is not there.

KEY POINTS

- Airway assessment is one of the most important parts of preoperative assessment, failure to do so can make anesthetist negligent in case of some catastrophe.
- Mallampati grading, thyromental distance and neck movements are the three most important parameters to be assessed in every case.
- Video laryngoscopy have revolutionized the practice of airway management; intubation success rates can be as high as 94–99% with video laryngoscopy after failed intubation with direct laryngoscopy.
- Every head injury should be considered to be having cervical injury until proved otherwise.
- For cervical spine injury intubation should be done after neck stabilization with neck in neutral position.

CHAPTER 6

Monitoring in Anesthesia

Monitoring is the most important part of anesthesia to prevent complications. Although a number of sophisticated monitors are available but *nothing can replace the vigilance of an anesthetist*. The principle to use of monitors is–they should assist you and you should not be fully dependent on them.

CLINICAL MONITORING

- Pulse rate by palpation
- Color and turgor of skin to assess hydration, oxygenation and perfusion
- *Blood pressure:* It is measured either by palpatory method (measures only systolic pressure) or by auscultatory method (Korotkoff sounds). Two common sources of error are:
  - *Inappropriate cuff size:* Oversize cuff underestimates while undersize cuff overestimates BP. The *cuff should cover two-thirds of the length of arm and the width should be 40% greater than patient arm* (Usual width of cuff is 12–15 cm for adults, 6–9 cm for children and 2.5 cm for neonates).
  - *Rapid deflation: Deflation rate should not be more than 3–5 mm Hg/sec.*
- Inflation of chest
- Precordial and esophageal stethoscopy
- Any signs of sympathetic over activity such as lacrimation, perspiration to detect the depth of anesthesia.
- *Urine output:* Urine output is the best clinical indicator for assessing adequacy of perfusion; it should be > 0.5 mL/min.

ADVANCE MONITORING (INSTRUMENTAL MONITORING)

CARDIOVASCULAR MONITORING

Electrocardiography

Electrocardiography (ECG) is the mandatory monitor as it measures heart rate and can detect arrhythmias, ischemia and cardiac arrest. It is not possible to monitor 12 leads in perioperative period therefore, the leads *most preferred are lead II and V_5 because arrhythmias are best detected in lead II and V_5 for ischemia in lead V_5* (Lead V_5 alone can detect more than 80% of ischemic events). It is highly recommended to use monitors which have an option of automatic ST analysis.

Blood Pressure

Blood pressure can be monitored by noninvasive and invasive methods.

Noninvasive Blood Pressure Monitoring

Automated Noninvasive Blood Pressure Monitoring

Automated noninvasive blood pressure (NIBP) monitors are most frequently used in perioperative period to measure blood pressure; these instruments automatically measure blood pressure at set intervals by *oscillometry*. The *maximum interval between two blood pressure recordings should not exceed more than 5 minutes* (This interval of 5 minutes in fact, is not only applicable to blood pressure but to the recording of all vitals). The basic difference in oscillometric principle of BP monitoring is that mean arterial pressure is measured first and then systolic and diastolic pressures are derived by a set algorithm while in all other methods systolic and diastolic pressure are measured first and then mean arterial pressure is derived.

Other noninvasive methods which can be used are arterial Tonometry or using Doppler probes in place of fingers by palpatory methods.

A continuous noninvasive method by using finger cuff was tried but could not become popular due to many reasons.

Invasive Blood Pressure Monitoring

Invasive blood pressure monitoring is done by cannulating one of an artery and connecting the cannula to a transducer which in turn is connected to monitor. Invasive blood pressure (IBP) monitoring is required when surgery or patient condition mandates beat to beat, i.e. continuous monitoring of blood pressure. *IBP is considered as gold standard method to monitor blood pressure.*

IBP can be significantly affected by the dynamics of equipment used for IBP monitoring (tubing, transducer, etc.). Over damping under-estimates while underdamping overestimates systolic blood pressure. Its accuracy should be checked by matching with noninvasive blood pressure (NIBP). The difference in IBP and NIBP should not be more than 5–8 mm Hg (in normal circumstances IBP is higher than NIBP).

Most often transducers are zeroed at the level of heart (usually at mid axillary line). However, it has been found that the *zeroing point 5 cm posterior to sternal border yields more accurate BP recordings.*

As radial artery has collaterals (transpalmar arch) for the blood supply of hand, it is most commonly chosen artery for cannulation. Before doing radial artery cannulation *Allen's test* should be performed to assess the patency of ulnar artery. In Allen's test after exsanguination of patient's hand ulnar and radial arteries are occluded. Release pressure from the ulnar artery while maintaining the pressure on radial artery. Color of hand returning to normal within 5–7 seconds indicates patency of ulnar circulation and it is safe to go ahead with radial artery cannulation. Color returning to normal in > 10 seconds indicates severely compromised ulnar circulation contra-indicating radial artery cannulation. Due to the peripheral location (and hence less chances of ischemic damage), dorsalis pedis is second most preferred artery after radial. Others arteries which can be cannulated are brachial and femoral.

Complications of Arterial Cannulation
- Arterial injury, spasm and distal ischemia
- Thrombosis and embolization
- Sepsis
- Tissue necrosis
- Fistula or aneurysm formation
  To prevent thrombosis, a continuous flush with/without heparin is needed.

Other Uses of Arterial Cannulation
- Taking blood sample for repeated arterial blood gas analysis (ABG)
- Avoid the frequent puncture to take blood sample for investigations.
- Measuring dynamic parameters of cardiac function like stroke volume variation (SVV), Pulse pressure variation (PPV) and cardiac output by using pulse contour devices such as Flotrac. *Measuring dynamic parameters by arterial cannulation may be considered as one of the most recent and useful advancement in the field of monitoring.* As already discussed in the chapter of fluids, dynamic parameters are far more superior to static parameter, i.e. CVP for assessing fluid status and titrating fluid therapy.

Central Venous Pressure Monitoring

Ideal vein for monitoring of central venous pressure (CVP) is *right internal jugular vein* (because it is valve less and in direct communication with right atrium). CVP can also be measured by subclavian, basilic and femoral vein.

Indications
- Major surgeries where large fluctuations in hemodynamics is expected
- Open heart surgeries
- Fluid management in shock
- As a venous access
- Parenteral nutrition
- Aspiration of air embolus
- Cardiac pacing.
  Normal CVP is 3–10 cm of H_2O (or 2–8 mm Hg). In children CVP is 3–6 cm of H_2O. CVP more than 20 cm of H_2O indicates right heart failure.

CVP is increased in:
- Fluid overloading.
- Congestive cardiac failure.
- Pulmonary embolism.
- Cardiac tamponade.
- Intermittent positive pressure ventilation with PEEP.
- Constrictive pericarditis.
- Pleural effusion.
- Hemothorax.
- Coughing and straining.

CVP is decreased in
- Hypovolemia and shock.
- Venodilators.
- Spinal/epidural anesthesia.
- General anesthetics (by causing vasodilatation).

A low CVP with low BP indicates hypovolemia while a high CVP with low BP indicates pump failure.

Technique of CVP Catheterization (through Internal Jugular Vein)

It is introduced through *Seldinger* technique. The patient lies in Trendelenburg position (to decrease the chances of air embolism). The cannula with stylet is inserted at the tip of triangle formed by two heads of sternomastoid and clavicle. The direction of needle should be slightly lateral and towards the ipsilateral nipple. Majority of the clinicians use ultrasound to locate the internal jugular vein. In fact in many countries, it has become mandatory to used ultrasound for CVP insertion.

Once the internal jugular vein is punctured stylet is removed and a J wire is passed through cannula. CVP catheter is railroad over the J wire. *The tip of catheter should be at the junction of superior vena cava with right atrium* (which is usually 15 cm from the point of entry).

An X-ray chest should be performed to check the position of catheter and to exclude pneumothorax.

Complications

Mechanical complications:
- *Arterial puncture: Carotid puncture is the most common acute mechanical complication* (incidence: 2–15%)
- Cardiac arrhythmias.

- *Pneumothorax/hemothorax/chylothorax:* More commonly seen with Subclavian vein cannulation
- *Cardiac perforation/cardiac tamponade:* It is the most important life-threatening complication
- Trauma to brachial plexus, phrenic nerve, and airway.

Thromboembolic complications:
- Arterial or venous thrombosis
- Air embolism
- Catheter or guide wire embolism.

Infectious complications:
- Insertion site infection
- Sepsis
  Infection is the most common late complication.

Pulmonary Artery Catheterization

Because of cost, technical feasibility, complications ranging from *minor arrhythmias* (most common complication, *incidence around 30%*) to life-threatening such as pulmonary artery rupture, severe arrhythmias and death and availability of noninvasive (or less invasive) monitors, pulmonary artery catheterization is hardly done nowadays.

Swan Ganz catheter is used for pulmonary artery catheterization. It is balloon-tipped and flow-directed. The presence of catheter in different parts of heart is confirmed by pressure recordings, pressure tracings and distance from catheter tip. *Entry into right ventricle is confirmed by sudden increase in systolic blood pressure* (pressure in right atrium is 0–8 mm Hg while in right ventricle it is 15–30 mm Hg) while *entry in pulmonary artery is best indicated by sudden increase in diastolic pressure* (diastolic pressure in right ventricle is 0–8 mm Hg while in pulmonary artery it is 5–15 mm Hg).

Uses of Pulmonary Artery Catheterization

- Measuring cardiac chambers pressure (except left ventricle).
- *Calculating cardiac output and stroke volume:* Cardiac output is calculated by using ice cold saline. The most commonly used method to calculate cardiac output is thermodilution method where ice cold saline is injected and change is temperature is noted by a thermistor

in pulmonary artery. The processors then calculate the cardiac output by computerized algorithms. The alternative to thermodilution method are dye dilution (where in place of ice cold saline idocyanine green or lithium is injected and change in their colors is noted to calculate cardiac output) and Fick principle (which uses the oxygen consumed by body to calculate cardiac output).

To decrease the invasiveness of pulmonary artery catheterization, a modified approach transpulmonary thermodilution method is used where ice cold saline is injected in superior vena cava through CVP catheter and thermistor is placed in femoral artery (instead of pulmonary artery) to record the change in temperature.

- Measuring pulmonary artery occlusion pressure (PAOP) (also called pulmonary capillary occlusion pressure). Previously PAOP used to be called as pulmonary capillary wedge pressure (PCWP). PAOP represents left atrial pressure. Normal PAOP is *4–12 mm Hg*. *PAOP is best utilized to differentiate between cardiogenic and non-cardiogenic pulmonary edema (ARDS)*. PAOP < 18 mm Hg indicates non-cardiogenic pulmonary edema while cardiogenic pulmonary edema usually develops at PAOP > 25 mm Hg.
- Taking sample for mixed venous blood (pulmonary artery is considered as best site for mixed venous blood sample). *Oxygen saturation of mixed venous blood is the best guide to assess tissue perfusion (cardiac output)* [Best clinical guide to assess cardiac output is urinary output]. Normal mixed venous O_2 saturation is 75% (only 25% is consumed by tissues); less than 60% indicates significant deficiency in tissue perfusion.

Special pulmonary artery probes are available which can continuously measure the oxygen saturation of mixed venous blood.

- *Titration of fluid therapy:* As PAOP measures preload to left heart, it is definitely better guide for fluid therapy than CVP (which measures preload to right heart). Low PAOP and low stoke volume indicates hypovolemia (less preload to heart so less stroke volume). High PAOP and low stroke volume represents pump failure, i.e. cardiogenic shock (heart to not able to generate stroke volume).

Echocardiography (Transesophageal/Transthoracic)

In present day medicine *transesophageal echocardiography (TEE) and transthoracic echocardiography (TTE) are the best tools to assess cardiac function and detect wall motion abnormality, i.e. ischemia (sensitivity >99%) in perioperative period.*

TTE/TEE can measure all hemodynamic parameters (Cardiac output, stroke volume, stroke volume variation, left ventricular ejection fraction, etc.), can detect structural changes (valvular lesions, shunts), and diagnose cardiac failure (systolic/diastolic dysfunction). TEE is also most sensitive to detect air embolism (can detect as low as 0.2 mL of air).

The advantage of TTE is that it is noninvasive however limited access to thorax limits its use in perioperative period. TEE offers excellent window to visualize heart in perioperative period but is invasive, can be used only for intubated patients in general anesthesia and has potential to cause life-threatening complication such as esophageal rupture (very rarely).

Gastric Tonometry

It measures gastric mucosa pH and CO_2. It is very good indicator of tissue perfusion but is not popular due to complex, time consuming and cumbersomeness of the process.

To summarize

Various methods which can be used in perioperative period to calculate cardiac output and other cardiac functions such as stroke volume, stroke volume variation, etc. are:

Noninvasive

- *Transthoracic echocardiography:* Very simple, cost effective and devoid of any major complication. The major disadvantage is poor window in obese patients and limited access in surgical patients.
- *Thoracic bioimpendance:* Six electrodes are placed over chest which measures changes in lung volume to calculate cardiac functions. Accuracy of this technique is questionable in many patients.

Invasive

- *Transesophageal echocardiography:* Provides best window for measuring and assessing cardiac functions in intraoperative period but can be used only for intubated patients.

- *Pulmonary artery catheterization:* Provides most accurate cardiac output, however, is highly invasive, associated with life-threatening complications such as pulmonary artery rupture and cardiac tamponade.
- *Pulse contour devices:* Any artery (most commonly radial) is cannulated and pulse contour device (Flotrac) is attached which analyses the pulse wave to calculate cardiac functions.
- *Partial CO_2 rebreathing cardiac output* can be done only in intubated patient.

RESPIRATORY MONITORING

Measurement of Oxygenation

Pulse Oximetry

Pulse oximetry is the most basic and mandatory monitor to measure the oxygen saturation of hemoglobin in arterial blood (SpO_2). The probe is applied on fingers nailbed, toe nailbed, ear lobule and tip of nose. *Normal SpO_2 = 95 to 98%.*

Principle of pulse oximetry: Pulse oximeters works on the principle of Beer-Lambert law which states that different solvents absorb infrared (and red light) at different wavelengths. A pulse oximeter probe emits two lights of different wavelength (red at 660 nm and infrared at 940 nm). Oxyhemoglobin absorbs more infrared light while deoxyhemoglobin absorbs more red light. This ratio to red to infrared light is measured and converted in numerical value by a processor in pulse oximeter. Higher ratio of red/infrared suggests more deoxyhemoglobin, and hence low saturation.

Errors:
- *Abnormal hemoglobins:*
  - Carboxyhemoglobinemia: Carbon monoxide has same absorption pattern of red light such as oxygenated hemoglobin therefore will overestimate the real value.
  - Methemoglobinemia: Shows fix saturation of 85%.

  However, pulse oximeters perform accurately in the presence of sickle and fetal hemoglobin.
- *Anemia:* Severe anemia causes underestimation of actual values.

- *Hypovolemia and vasoconstriction (especially in cold):* Difficulty in obtaining actual values and false low SpO_2 reading.
- *Vasodilatation:* Slight decrease.
- *Nail polish (especially blue color):* Impairs the transmission of light therefore shows false reading.
- *Shivering:* Constant movement of finger impairs continuous transmission of light and hence false reading.
- *SpO_2 below 60%:* Below 60% most instruments underestimate the actual value.
- *Skin pigmentation:* Theoretically dark pigmentation can also impair the transmission of light
- Dyes such as methylene blue or indocyanine green. However hyperbilirubinemia has no effect.

Co-oximeters: As discussed that routine pulse oximeters cannot differentiate between normal and abnormal hemoglobin, therefore are unreliable in carboxyhemoglobinemia and Methemoglobinemia. *Co-oximeters are the special types of oximeters which can differentiate between normal and abnormal hemoglobin.*

Photoplethysmography: Pulse oximeter is not only used to measure oxygen saturation, variations in the amplitude of the pulse oximetry waveform can be used to assess fluid status and responsiveness to fluids therapy in mechanically ventilated patients.

Mixed Venous Oxygen Saturation (SvO₂)

The limitation of pulse oximetry is that it measures oxygen saturation of arterial blood; it does not indicate tissue oxygenation. *Mixed venous oxygen saturation is the best indicator of tissue oxygenation.* Normal SvO_2 is 75%. Although the ideal sample site is pulmonary artery but practically sample from superior vena cava or even a peripheral vein may suffice.

Any condition which decrease oxygen delivery to tissues (while the uptake remains normal) like hypoxia, cardiac failure, shock, Anemia, carboxyhemoglobinemia or which increases oxygen uptake like pain, shivering, hyperthermia leads to reduction in SvO_2.

Conversely, conditions that decrease oxygen uptake like sedation, anesthesia, hypothermia, cyanide toxicity or improve oxygen delivery like oxygen therapy, inotropic support, blood transfusion lead to an increase in SvO_2.

Regional Oxygenation (rSo₂)

Mixed venous oxygen saturation indicates the oxygenation of whole body; it does not provide information regarding specific oxygenation of an organ or tissue. At present, the only monitor which is used to measure cerebral oxygenation is *reflectance spectroscopy*. Electrodes are placed over forehead to measure frontal cortical oxygenation (rSo₂). Typical values of rSo₂ range from 55% to 80% (Average of arterial, venous and capillary saturation).

Measurement of Expiratory Gases

Various techniques such as mass spectrometry, Raman gas analysis, piezoelectric oscillation can be employed to analyze and measure the concentration of expired gases, however in current day practice, all monitors use *infrared absorption technique to measure concentration of all expired gases except oxygen and nitrous oxide*. These infrared devices work on the principle of Beer-Lambert law which states that different gases absorb infrared light at different wavelength and absorption in a mixture of gases is proportional to their concentration.

Capnography

It is the continuous measurement of *end tidal (expired) carbon dioxide (ETCO₂)* along with its waveform. Normal is *32 to 42 mm Hg (3 to 4 mm Hg less than arterial pCO₂)*. Capnography uses the same principle of infrared absorption. Capnography is one of the most important and sensitive tool for monitoring in anesthesia.

Methods of monitoring
- *Side stream:* Expiratory gas sample is taken and delivered to sample cell (analyzer). The major disadvantage is that there is delay in response and humidity can block the chamber.
- *Mainstream:* Sample cell is placed in expiratory limb of breathing circuit. The major disadvantage is increased dead space.

Normal waveform **(Fig. 6.1)**: It has four phases:
Phase I: Contains dead space gases with almost no CO₂
Phase II: Transition from phase I (dead space) to phase III (alveolar phase)
Phase III: Alveolar plateau
Phase IV: Down slope at the time of inspiration.

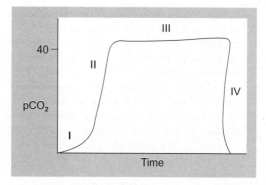

Fig. 6.1: Normal waveform of capnography

Uses of capnography
1. *To confirm intubation: Capnography is the surest technique to confirm intubation*
2. To diagnose the following conditions:

ETCO₂ = 0 and flat line on waveform is seen in
- Esophageal intubation
- Accidental extubation
- Complete obstruction
- Disconnection
- Ventilation failure
- *Cardiac arrest (there is no blood to carry CO₂ from tissues to lungs):* It becomes zero after few waveforms (CO₂ present in lungs keep on exhaling for few breaths).

Decrease in ETCO₂ is seen in:
- Pulmonary embolism by air, fat or thrombus (it may become zero, if embolus is large enough to block total pulmonary circulation).
- Decreased production of CO₂ like in hypothermia
- Decreased perfusion (and hence decrease delivery of CO₂ to lungs) in hypotension
- Hyperventilation

Increase in ETCO₂ is seen in:
- Exhausted sodalime or defective valves of closed circuit which impairs the absorption of CO₂ or causes inhalation of expired CO₂
- Increase production in hypermetabolic states such as fever, malignant hyperthermia (ETCO₂ may even rise to more than 100 mm Hg), Thyrotoxicosis, Neuroleptic malignant syndrome.
- Decreased ventilation (like in neuromuscular diseases, central respiratory depression by

opioids, thoracic surgeries) leads to retention of CO_2 and hence proportionate increase in expired CO_2

- Bicarbonate administration (Bicarbonate on metabolism produces CO_2)
- *Bronchial intubation:* $ETCO_2$ can significantly increase in bronchial intubation due to increase in ventilation perfusion (V/Q) mismatch.

No change in $ETCO_2$

Bronchospasm/COPD: There is increase in up-sloping (phase II) of waveform but due to high diffusibilty of CO_2 net value of $ETCO_2$ remains normal even in severe bronchospasm

3. To control level of hypocapnia during hyperventilation in neurosurgery.
4. *To assess the performance of CPR:* CPR is considered as gross failure, if it is not able to generate $ETCO_2$ of at least 10 mm Hg.

Different waveforms of capnography encountered in clinical practice

- Normal waveform for mechanically ventilated patient [Fig. 6.2(i)]:
- Normal waveform for spontaneously breathing patient [Fig. 6.2(ii)]:

- Prolonged expiration (increased slope of phase III) for COPD, asthma patient [Fig. 6.2(iii)]:
- $ETCO_2$ baseline not coming to zero [Fig. 6.2(iv)] indicates that patient is inhaling CO_2 which can be because of:
  - Defective expiratory valve (stuck open leading to CO_2 getting mixed with inspiratory gases)
  - Exhausted CO_2 absorbent
- Recovery of spontaneous breath [Fig. 6.2(v)]:
- Cardiac oscillations (effect of pumping of heart on lungs) [Fig. 6.2(vi)]:

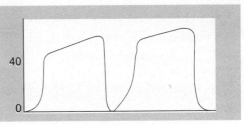

Fig. 6.2(iii): Prolonged expiration for COPD, asthma patient

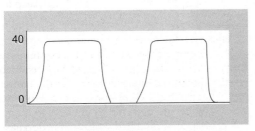

Fig. 6.2(i): Normal waveform for mechanically ventilated patient

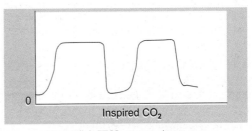

Fig. 6.2(iv): $ETCO_2$ not coming to zero

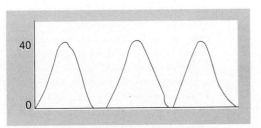

Fig. 6.2(ii): Normal waveform for spontaneously breathing patient

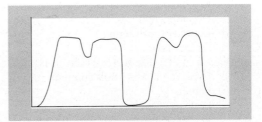

Fig. 6.2(v): Recovery of spontaneous breath

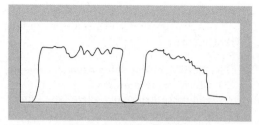

Fig. 6.2(vi): Cardiac oscillations

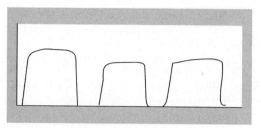

Fig. 6.2(ix): Decreased CO_2

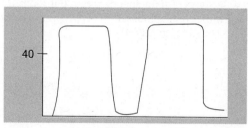

Fig. 6.2(vii): Increase pCO_2

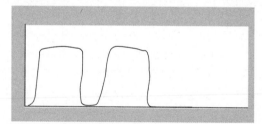

Fig. 6.2(viii): $ETCO_2$ suddenly becoming zero

- Increase $ETCO_2$ **[Fig. 6.2(vii)]** indicating:
  - Hypoventilation
  - Defective valve (in closed position) of closed circuit
  - Malignant hyperthermia
  - Exhausted sodalime
- $ETCO_2$ suddenly becoming zero (flat line) **[Fig. 6.2(viii)]** indicates:
  - Extubation
  - Disconnection
  - Complete obstruction
  - Cardiac arrest
- Decreased CO_2 **[Fig. 6.2(ix)]** indicates:
  - Hyperventilation (most common cause)
  - Embolism
  - Leakage of gas
  - Partial obstruction or partial kinking of tube.

Apnea Monitoring for Nonintubated Patients

Apnea is defined as *cessation of respiration for more than 10 seconds.* It should be detected at the earliest. *For intubated patients, apnea can be detected reliably within seconds by capnography or by airway pressure monitors.* However, detecting apnea in non-intubated patients has always been challenging. Apnea in a non-intubated patient can be detected by either monitoring the airflow at nostrils or by detection of chest movements.

- *Monitoring the airflow at nostrils:* Airflow at nostrils can be detected by placing acoustic probe in nasal cavity, encasing patient head and neck in tight canopy (can be very claustrophobic for conscious patients) or using noninvasive capnography (done by placing a special $ETCO_2$ cannula in nasal cavity).
- *Detection of chest movements:* The methods employed to detect chest movements are:
  - *Impedance plethysmography (Respiratory inductance plethysmography):* The thorax is encircled by elastic bands containing conductor coil and movements are detected by changes in impedence. A modified version of impedance plethysmography called as photoplethymography is more sensitive.
  - *Transthoracic impedance pulmonometry (also known as electrical impendence pulmonometry):* A small current delivered through ECG leads can continuously detect transthoracic electric impedance which is converted to respiratory rate by software present in monitor. All advanced ECG monitors have this parameter incorporated in them. *Electrical impendence pulmonometry is the simplest and most commonly used method to*

detect apnea in a non-intubated patient. However, *measurements of respiratory rate by using nasal ETCO$_2$ cannulas have yield more accurate results than techniques using thoracic impedance technology.*

The major limitation of these monitors is that they cannot detect obstructive apnea; patient with upper airway obstruction may still have paradoxical chest movements and the monitor may continue to detect these paradoxical movements as chest movements.

- Pulse oximeters do not directly detect apnea but are very important indirect indicator of apnea not only in non-intubated patients but in intubated patients too.

Oxygen Analyzers

In present day practice, *oxygen analyzers are the mandatory monitors* because they monitor the final value of oxygen delivered to the patient. That's why they are fitted in inspiratory limb of anesthesia circuit as near as to the patient.

Airway Pressure, Flow and Volume Monitoring

Most of the modern anesthesia machines have sensors for measuring airway pressure, flow and volume. Airway pressure *should be less than 20 to 25 cm of H$_2$O.* High airway pressure indicates either obstruction in tube or circuit or bronchospasm while low pressure indicates disconnection or leaks. Similarly, low tidal volumes indicate leaks or disconnections. *Combination of airway pressure, volume and flow monitoring, oxygen analyzers along with Capnography has bring the revolution in the safety of general anesthesia*; life threatening complications such as accidental extubation, esophageal intubation, ventilator failure, tube disconnection from circuit and complete tube obstruction can be detected within seconds.

Blood Gas Analysis

For sampling, glass syringes are preferred over plastic syringes. Syringe should be heparinized and samples should be stored in ice if the sample is to be sent at far place.

Usually, sample is taken from radial or femoral artery. Blood gas analysis is particularly needed in thoracic surgeries, hypothermia and hypotensive anesthesia. Modern analyzers give results within 1 to 2 minutes and require as low as 0.2 mL of blood.

Normal values on room air
pH = 7.38 to 7.42
Partial pressure of oxygen (pO$_2$) = 96 to 98 mm Hg
Partial pressure = 35 to 45 mm Hg of carbon dioxide (pCO$_2$)
Oxygen saturation (SpO$_2$) = 95 to 98%
Base deficit = –3 to + 3
Blood gas values of mixed venous blood
pO$_2$ = 40 mm Hg
pCO$_2$ = 46 mm Hg
Oxygen saturation = 75%
Mixed venous oxygen better indicates cardiac output, i.e. tissue oxygenation while arterial oxygen is the better indicator of pulmonary function. (For details of ABG see Chapter 40).

Lung Volumes

Lungs volumes are measured by spirometry *(for details refer to Chapter 1).*

TEMPERATURE MONITORING

Hypothermia is the most common thermal perturbation seen during anesthesia.
The reasons are:

- Most anesthetics are vasodilators, causes heat transfer from core to periphery, and consequently heat loss and hypothermia. Moreover, they inhibit centrally mediated thermoregulation and decrease the threshold for response to hypothermia from 37°C (normal) to 33°C to 35°C.
- Cold environment (air-conditioned operation theaters).
- Cold intravenous fluids.
- Heat loss from the body by convection, radiation and evaporation.

During general anesthesia core temperature decreases by 0.5–1.5°C in first hour and heat loss may be as high as *30 kcal/hour*

Hypothermia may be defined as core temperature less than 35°C. It is divided into:

- *Mild:* 28°C to 35°C.
- *Moderate:* 21°C to 27°C.
- *Profound or severe:* < 20°C.

Systemic Effects of Hypothermia

- *Cardiovascular system*: Bradycardia, Hypotension and ventricular arrhythmia's at temperature < 28°C. *Hypothermia triples the incidence of morbid cardiac outcomes*
- *Cerebral*: Decreases cerebral metabolic rate leading to progressive slowing of EEG and complete silence at profound hypothermia.
- *Respiratory system*: Decreased minute volume and respiratory arrest below 23°C. Oxygen dissociation curve is shifted to left.
- *Blood*: Increased blood viscosity, impaired coagulation and platelet function leads to increased blood loss, and consequently increases the chances of blood transfusion by 20%.
- *Acid-base balance*: Increased solubility of blood gases, therefore less values on blood gas analysis. Acidosis occurs because of lactic acid production.
- *Kidney*: Decreased GFR, no urine output at 20°C.
- *Endocrine system*: Decreased adrenaline and nor-adrenaline. Hyperglycemia occurs because of decreased insulin synthesis.
- *Drug metabolism*: Markedly decreased by perioperative hypothermia. Hypothermia also reduces the minimum alveolar concentration (MAC) of inhalational agents.
- *Effect on wound*: Hypothermia not only delays the wound healing but also *increases the chances of wound infection by 3 times.*
- *Thermal discomfort* in conscious patient.

Indications for Temperature Monitoring

As the possibility of developing hypothermia is high in intraoperative period, *temperature should be monitored in patients receiving general anesthesia >30 minutes and in all patients whose surgery lasts > 1 hour (irrespective of type of anesthesia)*, all cardiac surgeries, infants and small children, patients subjected to large evaporative losses such as burns, febrile patients and patients prone to develop malignant hyperthermia.

Temperature can be measured as surface temperature, core temperature and rectal temperature. Core temperature > rectal temperature > surface temperature.

Core Temperature Monitoring Sites

- *Esophagus:* Considering all factors such as economy, accessibility, safety and performance *lower end of esophagus is considered as best site for core body temperature* measurement. The *most accurate measurement of core body temperature is provided by pulmonary artery*, however, is not employed routinely due to cost, technical infeasibility and complications.
- *Pulmonary artery:* This provides most accurate measurement but use is restricted only to patients who have Swan Ganz (pulmonary artery) catheter already in place.
- *Nasopharynx:* It measures not only core temperature but also brain temperature (because of close proximity of carotid artery) but there is associated risk of epistaxis.
- *Tympanic membrane: Most accurately measures brain temperature* but the associated risk of tympanic membrane perforation deters its routine use.

Treatment of Intraoperative Hypothermia

- Warm intravenous fluids.
- *Increase room temperature: The ideal operation theater temperature for adults is 21°C and for children is 26°C.*
- Cover the patient with blankets.
- *Surface warming by warm air provided by special instrument (Bair Hugger airflow device) is the most effective method of treating hypothermia in perioperative period*

Uses of Induced Hypothermia

Hypothermia decreases basic metabolic rate (BMR) and oxygen consumption of the body. *Each degree (°C) fall in temperature reduces the metabolic rate by 6 to 7%.* However, for clinical purposes only mild hypothermia is produced (temperature is kept between 32°–36°C). Hypothermia is induced for:

- Brain protection in cardiac arrest.
- Tissue protection against ischemia during cardiac surgery.
- Neonatal asphyxia

NEUROMUSCULAR MONITORING

Neuromuscular monitoring is usually required for patients suffering from neuromuscular diseases and muscular dystrophies or in patients who had received long-acting muscle relaxants.

A nerve is stimulated by placing electrodes over its course and the response (visual and tactile or electromyographic) is observed in the muscle supplied by it. As the effect in *Corrugator Supercilii* and *Orbicularis oculi (supplied by facial nerve)* parallels with the laryngeal muscles they *are the ideal muscles for monitoring (Corrugator Supercilii considered more ideal than Orbicularis oculi).* However, due to technical infeasibility of applying electrodes over face, they are not used routinely; *most commonly used muscle for neuromuscular monitoring is adductor pollicis supplied by ulnar nerve.* Other nerves which can be used are median, posterior tibial and peroneal.

Stimuli Used for Neuromuscular Monitoring

- *Single twitch:* A single stimulus is given for 0.2 milliseconds. Both depolarizing and non-depolarizing muscle relaxants will cause depression of single twitch in dose-dependent manner.
- *Train of four:* Train of four is the most commonly used modality for neuromuscular monitoring in clinical practice **(Fig. 6.3)**. The monitor delivers 4 stimuli, each of 2 Hz for 2 seconds and recordings are taken. Four responses recorded are labeled as T_1, T_2, T_3 and T_4 **[Fig. 6.3(i)]**. The ratio of T4 to T1 (called as TO4 ratio) is automatically calculated by monitors. In normal condition, the amplitude height of fourth and first response will be same, i.e. T_4/T_1 ratio will be 1.

It is observed that with depolarizing muscle relaxants all four responses decrease simultaneously in amplitude, i.e. T_4/T_1 remains 1 **[Fig. 6.3(ii)]** to finally become 0 when all four responses becomes absent (required for intubation). With non-depolarizing muscle relaxants, first there will be decrease in T_4/T_1 ratio followed by *FADING* which means T_4 response will disappear first, then T3 and so on. This is called as TO4 score. If only one response is seen means TO4 score is 1 and if 2 responses are seen means TO4 score is 2 **[Fig. 6.3(iii)]**. The reason for fading seen with non-depolarizers is not only slow and progressive blockage of acetylcholine receptors at neuromuscular junction but also slow and progressive blockage of acetylcholine mobilization at prejunctional level.

Absence of T4 response **[Fig. 6.3(iii)c]** means *75% blockade of receptors which is sufficient for most of surgeries.* Absence of T3 **[Fig. 6.3(iii)d]** means 80% blockade and absence of T2 **[Fig. 6.3(iii)e]** means 90% block (Diaphragm is completely blocked at this level). *Intubation requires complete absence of all 4 responses (100% block).*

Train of four ratio is best utilized to assess reversal. The ratio of 0.7 (i.e. fourth response has a 70% height of first response) indicates adequate recovery but *recovery is guaranteed only at a ratio of >0.9.*

Train of four is also very useful in diagnosing phase II block (which is seen in over dosage of succinylcholine or abnormal plasma cholinesterase activity). *If the patient on*

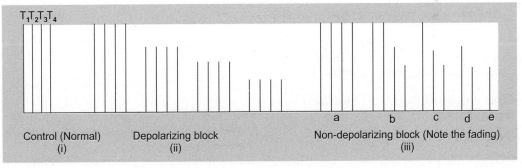

Fig. 6.3: Neuromuscular monitoring (Train of four response)

succinylcholine shows fading, it is pathogno-monic of phase II block.

- *Tetanic stimulation:* A sustained stimulus of 50–100 Hz is given for 5 seconds. Depolarizers will exhibit diminution of all responses while non-depolarizers will show fading followed by post-tetanic facilitation. This facilitation occurs as a result of response generated by increased acetylcholine released from prejunctional area by tetanic stimulus.
- *Post-tetanic count (PTC):* A stimulus is given just after the tetanic stimulation. As discussed, tetanic stimulation will increase acetylcholine levels at neuromuscular junction. This increased acetylcholine will replace some molecules of non-depolarizers from its binding site on receptors producing a response while on the other hand the depolarizers produces relaxation by making the membrane refractory due to continuous stimulation, therefore will not respond to increased acetylcholine. *Absence of PTC with non-depolarizers indicates a very intense block.*
- *Double burst stimulation (DBS 3, 3):* As the name suggests, two sets, each consisting of 3 stimuli of high frequency (50 Hz), are given at a gap of 750 milliseconds. The results are similar to other responses with non-depolarizers exhibiting fading.

  Tetanic, post-tetanic count and double burst stimulus are very high intensity stimuli, therefore are used to assess deep blocks or where neuromuscular monitoring is done by visual observation of movement (like adduction of thumb after stimulating ulnar nerve).

  To conclude: Adductor pollicis (supplied by ulnar nerve) is the most commonly chosen muscle and Train of four is the most commonly used stimulus for neuromuscular monitoring. *Fading, post-tetanic facilitation and post-tetanic count are only exhibited by non-depolarizing muscle relaxants.*

CENTRAL NERVOUS SYSTEM (CNS) MONITORING

CNS Monitors

Electroencephalogram (EEG)
Uses of EEG
- To monitor the depth of anesthesia

- To assess cerebral ischemia during neuro-vascular surgeries (especially carotid endarterectomy)

Effect of anesthetic agents and modalities on EEG:
- All inhalational and intravenous anesthetic agent produces *biphasic* pattern on EEG, i.e. at lower doses, they causes excitation (high frequency and low amplitude waves) followed by depression (high amplitude and low frequency waves) at high doses with the following exceptions:
  - Opioids only produce depression.
  - Nitrous oxide and ketamine only produces excitation.
  - Opioids, benzodiazepines, dexmedeto-midine and halothane cannot produce complete suppression (i.e. isoelectric EEG or electrocortical silence or burst suppression) even at higher doses.
- Similar pattern has been seen with hypoxia and hypercarbia, i.e. early (mild) hypoxia and hypercarbia produces excitation while advanced hypoxia and hypercarbia produces depression of EEG.
- *Hypothermia and cerebral ischemia* produces only progressive depression of EEG.

Evoked Responses
- *Somatosensory evoked response (SSER):* Useful for surgeries which put sensory tracts at risk like spine surgeries, repair of thoracic and abdominal aorta aneurysm, brachial plexus exploration or surgery of brain area which involves thalamus or sensory tract.
- *Brainstem auditory evoked response (BAER):* Useful for procedures involving auditory pathways (like resection of acoustic neuroma) and posterior fossa surgeries.
- *Visual evoked response (VER):* Useful for procedures which put visual tracts at risk such as optic glioma, pituitary tumors etc.
- *Motor evoked response (MER):* Useful for surgeries which put motor tracks (at spinal cord or brain) at risk

Effect of anesthetic agents and modalities on evoked responses:
- All inhalational agents, barbiturates, propofol, benzodiazepines, neurological injury, ische-mia, hypothermia, hypoxia inhibit evoked

responses, i.e. decreases the amplitude and increases the latency (response time).
- Etomidate, ketamine, opioids and dexmedetomidine do not have any clinically significant effect on evoked responses.

Monitoring the Depth of Anesthesia

Clinical Signs

Signs of light anesthesia are:
- Tachycardia, Hypertension.
- Lacrimation, Perspiration.
- Movement response to painful stimuli.
- Tachypnea, breath-holding, coughing, laryngospasm, bronchospasm.
- Eye movements.
- Preserved reflexes (like oculocephalic, corneal)

Monitors

Electoencephalography (EEG)

Light anesthesia (subanesthetic depth) is indicated by waves with high frequency and low amplitude (Beta waves in frontal area). With the increasing anesthetic depth, the waves become larger in amplitude and slower in frequency (appears like alpha waves). Further increase in depth causes further slowing of EEG (theta and delta waves). To conclude, it can be said that *beta waves in prefrontal area indicate light anesthesia while theta and delta waves indicate deep anesthesia.*

Due to technical infeasibility, difficult interpretation, artifacts, interpretation effected by multiple factors, EEG cannot be employed routinely to monitor the depth of anesthesia. However, there are EEG based monitors which can be utilized to monitor the depth of anesthesia.

EEG-based monitors

- *Bispectral index (BIS) monitor:* It was the *first scientifically validated and commercially available monitor to monitor the depth of anesthesia.* It analyzes multiple facets of real-time EEG to generate a score by set algorithm. It exhibits a score of 100 for fully awake state and 0 for completely silent brain. *Bispectral index score (BIS) score of 45–60 indicates adequate depth.*
- *Patient state index:* It is same like BIS index, however, a score of 25–50 indicates adequate depth.

- *Narcotrend:* It analyzes EEG to give 6 stages, from A to F. A represents awake state while F represents silent EEG.
- *Entropy:* Entropy, which measures the degree of disorder and synchrony in EEG to calculate entropy score, is a new monitor.

As ketamine, nitrous oxide and dexmedetomidine do not causes depression of EEG therefore EEG-based monitors cannot be utilized to monitor the depth of anesthesia with these agents.

End-tidal anesthetic concentration

In spite of studies showing that maintaining end-tidal concentration of inhalational agents between 0.7 and 1.3 MAC is as effective as BIS to monitor the depth of anesthesia, it is not considered as highly reliable because it is an indirect measure of level of consciousness. Moreover, it can be used only to monitor depth with inhalational agents (cannot be used for total intravenous anesthesia).

Auditory-evoked response

Although difficult to monitor but is considered as reliable as BIS index to monitor the depth of anesthesia.

Cerebral Blood Flow Monitors

- Xenon^{133} wash out—very cumbersome device
- Transcranial Doppler—*very simple and non-invasive method to monitor cerebral blood flow*
- Jugular vein oxygen saturation
- Cerebral oximetry by special probes applied at forehead
- *Thermodilution:* It is invasive method, 2 thermistors of different temperature are placed in brain and difference in temperature is noted to calculate blood flow.

Monitoring Nociceptin

Till date, we do not have a monitor which can measure the intensity of pain during general anesthesia and we have to rely on clinical signs such as hypertension and tachycardia.

MONITORING BLOOD LOSS

Estimation of blood loss is done by weighing blood-soaked swabs, sponges (Gravimetric method) and estimation of blood loss in suction bottle (Volumetric method). However, the most accurate method is *colorimetric method.*

On an average (a rough guide):
- Fully soaked swab means 20 mL of loss.
- Fully soaked sponge means 100–120 mL of loss.
- A fist of clots means 200–300 mL of loss.

KEY POINTS

- In spite of availability of sophisticated monitors nothing can replace the vigilance of an anesthetist.
- The most preferred leads for ECG monitoring are lead II and V_5. Arrhythmia are best detected in lead II and ischemia's in lead V_5.
- The maximum interval between two blood pressure recordings should not exceed more than 5 minutes.
- Invasive blood pressure monitoring is considered as gold standard monitoring of blood pressure.
- As radial artery has collaterals (transpalmar arch) for the blood supply of hand, it is most commonly chosen artery for cannulation.
- Measuring dynamic parameters like stroke volume variation by arterial cannulation may be considered as one of the most recent and useful advancement in the field of monitoring.
- PAOP is best utilized to differentiate between cardiogenic and noncardiogenic pulmonary edema (ARDS).
- Oxygen saturation of mixed venous blood is best guide to assess tissue perfusion (cardiac output).
- In present day medicine transesophageal echocardiography (TEE) and transthoracic echocardiography (TTE) are the best tools to assess cardiac function and detect wall motion abnormality, i.e. Ischemia in perioperative period.
- Transesophageal echocardiography provides the best window for measuring and assessing cardiac functions in intraoperative period.
- Co-oximeters are the special type of oximeters which can differentiate between normal and abnormal hemoglobin.
- In current day practice all monitors use infrared absorption technique to measure concentration of all expired gases except oxygen and nitrous oxide.
- Capnography is the surest technique to confirm intubation.
- Electrical impendence pulmonometery is the simplest and most commonly used method to detect apnea in a non-intubated patient.
- Hypothermia is the most common thermal perturbation seen during anesthesia.
- Temperature should be monitored in patients receiving general anesthesia >30 minutes and in all patients whose surgery lasts > 1 hour (irrespective of type of anesthesia).
- Lower end of esophagus is considered as best site for core body temperature measurement. However, the most accurate measurement of core body temperature is provided by pulmonary artery.
- Each degree (°C) fall in temperature reduces the metabolic rate by 6 to 7%.
- Most commonly used muscle for neuromuscular monitoring is adductor pollicis supplied by ulnar nerve.
- Train of four is the most commonly used modality for neuromuscular monitoring in clinical practice.
- Fading, post-tetanic facilitation and post-tetanic count are only exhibited by non-depolarizing muscle relaxants.
- Bispectral index (BIS) monitor is the first scientifically validated and commercially available monitor to assess the depth of anesthesia.

Fluids and Blood Transfusion

FLUIDS

Fluids are divided into crystalloids and colloids.

Crystalloids

- Ringer lactate (RL)
- Normal saline (NS)
- Glucose solutions
- Dextrose with normal saline preparations (DNS)
- Hypertonic saline.

Colloids

- Dextrans
- Albumin
- Gelatins
- Hydroxyethyl starch

- Blood.

Table 7.1 shows differences between crystalloids and colloid solutions.

CRYSTALLOIDS

Balanced Salt Solutions

Ringer Lactate Solution (RL; Hartmann Solution)

Composition of ringer lactate is:

Na^+	131 mEq/L
Cl^-	111 mEq/L
K^+	5 mEq/L
Ca^{2+}	2 mEq/L
Lactate	29 mEq/L
pH = 6.5	

■ **Table 7.1:** Differences between crystalloids and colloid solutions

Crystalloids	Colloids
• May be isotonic (NS and 5% dextrose), hypertonic (DNS and hypertonic saline)	• Hypertonic solutions
• Intravascular half-life 30 minutes so expands plasma volume for less time	• Expand plasma volume for 2–4 hours
• Cheap	• Expensive
• Crystalloids should be replaced in a ratio of 1.5:1. For example, blood loss of 100 mL should be replaced with 150 mL of crystalloid	• Replaced in 1:1 ratio (100 mL of blood loss should be replaced with 100 mL of colloid)
• Can precipitate edema by easily diffusing to interstitial compartment	• Decreases cerebral edema and pulmonary edema by increasing intravascular oncotic pressure
• Does not interfere with clotting or causes renal dysfunction	• Colloids in high doses can interfere with clotting (by primarily decreasing factor VIII level) and causes renal dysfunction
• No such effect	• Dextrans can cause rouleaux formation and interfere with blood grouping
• Allergic reactions are rare	• Allergic reactions are common

Ringer lactate is slightly hypotonic (Osmolarity 273 mosm/L). Lactate is metabolized to bicarbonate.

As RL contains calcium blood should not be given through the same drip set.

Plasmalyte

The composition of plasmalyte is:

Na^+	140 mEq/L
Cl^-	98 mEq/L
K^+	3 mEq/L
Mg^{2+}	3 mEq/L
Acetate	27 mEq/L
Gluconate	23 mEq/L

Acetate and gluconate are metabolized to generate bicarbonate.

The concerns that lactate in ringer lactate can cause lactic acidosis lead to evolution of plasmalyte. However, this concern may be only applicable to liver failure patients who cannot metabolize lactate. As plasmalyte has low potassium it may be preferred for renal failure patients otherwise for a normal patient plasmalyte offer no substantial advantage over Ringer lactate and is almost 3 times more expensive making *Ringer lactate to be the preferred crystalloid.*

Normal Saline

It is 0.9% NaCl isotonic solution.

Na^+	154 mEq/L
Cl^-	154 mEq/L

As normal saline contains high sodium and chloride it can cause hypernatremia and hyperchloremic metabolic acidosis (increase chloride decreases bicarbonate). It is only preferred over ringer lactate for treating:

- Hypochloremic metabolic alkalosis.
- Brain injury (Ca^{2+} in ringer lactate can increase the neuronal injury).
- Hyponatremia.

Glucose Solutions (5% Dextrose)

These are isotonic but with the metabolism of glucose inside body they become hypotonic.

Blood cannot be given through the same drip set otherwise rouleaux formation will cause clumping of RBCs.

Dextrose Normal Saline (DNS)

- DNS is hypertonic.

- 1/5 NS + 4.3% dextrose and 5% dextrose + 1/4 NS are isotonic solutions. These are used as maintenance fluids.

Hypertonic Saline

Used for treating:

- Hyponatremia.
- Cerebral and pulmonary edema; 3% hypertonic saline is now even preferred over Mannitol.

COLLOIDS

Dextrans (Lomodex)

Available as Dextran 70 (molecular weight 70,000 Daltons), 150 (molecular weight 1,50,000 Daltons) and 40 (molecular weight 40,000 Daltons).

- Dextrans are polysaccharides.
- These solutions can be stored for 10 years.
- Half life of dextrans is 2–8 hours.

Advantages

- Dextrans are neutral and chemically inert.
- Low molecular weight dextran (Dextran 40) improves microcirculation therefore useful for vascular surgeries.

Drawbacks

- Dextrans interfere with blood grouping and cross matching.
- Interferes with platelet function.
- Can cause severe anaphylaxis.
- Large molecular weight dextrans can block renal tubules.
- ARDS (rarely) because of direct toxic effect on pulmonary capillaries.

Albumins

Available as 5% and 25% solution. Albumins have an intravascular half-life of *10–15 days* but are quite expensive. Albumin is more useful if there is protein loss like in peritonitis, liver failure, burns and protein losing enteropathies/nephropathies.

Gelatins (Haemaccel)

- Molecular weight: 30,000.
- Available as *3.5% solution.*
- Composition of Haemaccel: *Each liter contains:*
- Gelatin: 35 g

- Sodium: 145 mEq
- Chloride: 145 mEq
- Potassium: 5 mEq
- Calcium: 12 mEq

Expand plasma effectively for 2 hours (25% may be present in blood after 12 hours).

At clinically used doses gelatins do not interfere with blood grouping, platelet function and clotting but at high doses they can also interfere with clotting. There is always a possibility of severe anaphylactic reactions.

As haemaccel contains high calcium therefore *citrated blood should not be mixed.*

Hydroxyethyl Starch

Two kind of hydroxyethyl starches available are Hexastarch and Pentastarch. *Hydroxyethyl starch (Haes-Steril) are the most commonly used colloids in current day practice.* They are available as 6% and 10% solution. They have prolonged half-life and *expand plasma effectively for 4 hours.*

Although at clinically used doses they does not interfere with clotting but at *high doses (>20 mL/kg) they also interfere with clotting and can cause renal dysfunction.* Allergic reactions are less common. Allergic reactions and interference with clotting are almost same with Pentastarch and Hexastarch.

Hextend

Hextend is another hydroxyethyl starch which also has glucose and lactate and is considered to effect coagulation less than hydroxyethyl starch.

FLUID MANAGEMENT

Fluids are required in intraoperative period for maintenance and replacement (for losses).

Maintenance Fluids

Hourly maintenance requirement is calculated by formula of *4-2-1.*

Up to 0–10 kg	= 4 mL/kg/hr
10–20 kg	= 2 mL/kg/hr
> 20 kg	= 1 mL/kg/hr

Example: For a patient of 50 kg hourly fluid requirement will be calculated as:

Up to 10 kg @ 4 mL/kg	= 40 mL
10–20 kg @ 2 mL/kg	= 20 mL
20–50 kg @ 1 mL/kg	= 30 ml
Total	= 90 mL

@ = at the rate of

Selection of fluid for maintenance: Anesthesia and surgery are the stressful situations which releases GH, cortisol and catecholamine leading to hyperglycemia. Therefore, balance salt solutions without dextrose should be used, *Ringer lactate, being considered as fluid most near to normal body composition, is the fluid of choice for maintenance.*

As thought previously, children are not so prone for hypoglycemia; therefore dextrose containing solutions along with hyperglycemia of stress can cause hyperglycemia and its consequences in pediatric population too. *Therefore, even for children the fluid of choice for maintenance is Ringer lactate.* As children are prone for fluid overload therefore *they should receive only two-third of the fluid calculated by 4-2-1 formula.*

Replacement Fluids

Hemorrhagic shock with loss > 20% of blood volume should be managed by blood replacement. Non-hemorrhagic shock and hemorrhagic shock with volume loss < 20% is managed by crystalloids/colloids. *Crystalloids are preferred* over colloids due to the following reasons:

- Crystalloids not only replace intravascular volume but they also replace extravascular volume (and cellular hydration depends on extravascular volume).
- Crystalloids do not interfere with clotting while all colloids in high doses can interfere with clotting.
- Colloids can cause renal dysfunction
- Colloids are expensive
- There is risk of anaphylactic reaction with colloids.

  Contrary to the previous belief that 2/3rd of the crystalloid crosses the endothelium to enter the extravascular space (interstitium) and therefore should be replaced in a ratio of 3:1 to intravascular volume loss, it has been now been proven that only 40–50% of crystalloids crosses the endothelium. Therefore, *crystalloids should be replaced in a ratio of 1.5:1.* For example, blood loss of 100 mL should be replaced with 150 mL of crystalloid

  Therefore, it can be well concluded that *colloids are only reserved for severe shock* where maintenance of intravascular volume is vital. Mild to moderate shock should be managed by crystalloid.

Crystalloids of choice for replacement are balanced salt solutions (Ringer lactate preferred) while colloid of choice is albumin. However, due to very high cost and possibility of bacterial contamination albumin is not used and hydroxyethyl starches are continued to be the most popular choice in most of the world including India.

Calculation of intraoperative fluid: It includes maintenance fluids (calculated by 4-2-1 formula) + fasting deficit (maintenance fluid × hours of fasting, 50% given in 1st hour, 25% in 2nd and 25% in 3rd hour) + 3rd space loss (vary from 2–6 mL/kg) + compensatory intravascular expansion (as compensation to effect of anesthesia of decreasing cardiac output) + losses.

As a rough guide during surgery, fluid is given at rate of 10–12 mL/kg in 1st hour and later at a rate of 5–7 mL/kg /hour + losses.

Guiding Parameters for Fluid Therapy

Studies done over last few years have shown that fluids given randomly without guiding parameters (maintenance by 4-2-1 formula and replacement in 1:3 ratio) causes fluid overloading. This lead to the concept of *goal directed therapy (GDT).* GDT means giving fluids by measuring dynamic cardiac functions such as:

- Flow time through aorta (target should be >400 milliseconds)
- Stroke volume and pulse pressure variation (means variation in stroke volume and pulse pressure during inspiration and expiration). *Variation >10–15% confirms hypovolemia*
- Cardiac output.

These dynamic parameters can be measured by esophageal Doppler, transesophageal echocardiography or simply by pulse contour devices like Flotrac (these devices analyses the radial pulse contour to derive these dynamic parameters).

In the absence of above said monitors pulmonary artery occlusion pressure (PAOP) can be used. PAOP < 8 indicates severe hypovolemia and > 18 indicates fluid overload.

Although the static parameter, i.e. CVP is most commonly used (due to technical feasibility and cost) however, the dynamic parameters like stroke volume variation, pulse pressure variation, cardiac output and PAOP are far more superior to CVP for determining the fluid status and titrating the fluid

therapy. Among the dynamic parameters stroke volume variation is considered as most reliable to assess fluid status and titrate fluid therapy.

Practical Guideline for Fluid Therapy

The practical recommendation is that normal Patients undergoing minor to moderate surgeries are given maintenance fluids by 4-2-1 formula and replacement fluids in ratio of 1:1.5 however the patients suffering from major morbidity (especially cardiac and renal) and undergoing major surgeries should receive fluid by GDT.

Fluids for Certain Clinical Situations Commonly Encountered

- *Renal failure:* Fluids should be guided by cardiac monitoring (goal directed therapy). Crystalloid without potassium (Hemosol) is preferred. Normal saline by causing hyperchloremic acidosis can cause hyperkalemia therefore should not be used. *Colloids (particularly hydroxyethyl starch) cause renal dysfunction and therefore must not be used.*
- *Liver failure:* Fluids should be guided by cardiac monitoring. Metabolism of lactate and acetate is reduced so balance salt solutions should be used carefully. Albumin is preferred.
- *Cardiac failure:* Fluids (either crystalloids or colloids) must be guided by cardiac monitoring. Colloids in low volume may be beneficial by decreasing edema in congestive heart failure.
- *Intestinal obstruction:* Except for upper GI losses (where due to hypochloremic alkalosis Normal saline is preferred) Ringer lactate is the fluid of choice for GI losses.
- *Cerebral edema and pulmonary edema (ARDS):* There is no doubt that colloids are excellent in reducing cerebral and pulmonary edema (by increasing intravascular oncotic pressure) if there is no endothelial injury. Previous concern that endothelial damage leads to extravasation of colloids and aggravate edema has not been substantiated therefore, *if needed, colloids can be safely used in head injury or ARDS.* Hyperglycemia can worsen neuronal injury therefore dextrose containing solutions should not be used in case of cerebral edema.

- *Burns:* The conventional method of giving fluid is as per parkland formula, i.e. for first 24 hours give ringer lactate at a rate of 4. mL/kg/% of burns (of this total fluid 50% is to be given in 8 hours and remaining 50% in next 16 hours) has led to fluid overload therefore current recommendation is to start fluid as per parkland (or any other) formula but immediately start tapering once urine output becomes > 0.5–1 mL/kg/hr. Colloids previously were considered contraindicated in acute phase but now can be given even in acute phase, if necessary.
- *Shock (Hypovolemia):* Crystalloids preferred over colloids and among crystalloids ringer lactate is the fluid of choice. (*For detailed management of shock see Chapter 40, page no. 285*).
- *Sepsis:* There is very high possibility of renal impairment (or impending impairment) therefore colloids should be avoided.

Other Routes of Fluid Administration

In case of emergencies where vein is not accessible:
- *Intraosseous route:* A large needle is inserted in medullary cavity of upper tibia. As per new guidelines this route is now recommended for all ages. All medicines and fluids can be given through this route.
- *Subcutaneous* after administration of hyaluronidase into outer side of thigh. Not considered a reliable route.

BLOOD TRANSFUSION

Indications for Transfusion

Considering the complications associated with blood transfusion, the approach in present day practice is towards the minimum use of blood products (called as restrictive approach to transfusion). The general guidelines for transfusion are:

- Blood loss greater than 20% of blood volume
- Hemoglobin level less than 8 gm% in normal patient
- Hemoglobin level less than 9 to 10 gm% in a patient with major disease like ischemic heart disease.
- *1 unit of blood raises the hemoglobin by 0.8 g% in India while in western countries by 1 g% because in India, 1 unit of blood = 350 mL (301 mL of blood + 49 mL of anticoagulant) while in western countries 1 unit contains 450 mL (out of which 63 mL is anticoagulant). One unit of fresh blood (with 100% RBCs while stored blood has only 70% RBCs) increases Hb by 1 g%.*
- Blood products should not be mixed with 5% dextrose (dextrose can cause hemolysis), ringer lactate and hemaccel (as these solutions contain calcium which with citrate can induce clot formation).

Blood Grouping and Compatibility Testing

Although red cell membrane contains more than 300 antigens and 20 blood group antigens are well known but still the *most important is ABO grouping because most serious mismatch transfusions reactions are usually caused by ABO incompatible blood.*

An individual who lacks particular antigen will have antibodies against that antigen in his/her serum. For example in a person with antigen A on RBC (group A) will have antibodies against B antigen and similarly group B individual will have antibodies against A antigen **(Table 7.2)**.

Compatibility Tests

- *ABO-Rh typing (determining blood group):* First step is to determine patient's blood group in which patient's red cells are tested with serum known to contain antibodies against A or B. Red cells are also tested with anti D antibodies to determine Rh +ve or –ve.

■ **Table 7.2:** Compatibility tests

Blood group	Red cells	Plasma	Can donate blood to	Can receive blood from
A	Antigen A	Anti B antibodies	Group A, AB	Group A, O
B	Antigen B	Anti A antibodies	Group B, AB	Group B, O
AB (Universal recipient)	Antigen A and B	Nil	AB	A, B, O, AB
O (Universal donor)	Nil	Anti A and anti B	A, B, O, AB	O

- *Cross matching:* Patient's (recipient) serum is mixed with donor cells. It involves three phases. In first phase ABO incompatibility is determined. It takes 1–5 minutes. Second phase determines antibodies of Rh system. It takes 30 minutes. Third phase (indirect antiglobulin test) determines incomplete antibodies of other system like Kell, Duffy etc.
- *Antibody screening:* It is done in both donor and recipient plasma to detect antibodies known to cause non-ABO hemolytic reactions.

Type and Screen

In this technique ABO Rh typing (blood grouping) and antibody screening is done (i.e., cross match not done). This is based on the fact that incidence of hemolytic reactions with only type and screen is less than 1% (0.01%). So it is advocated that for surgeries in which chances of transfusion are less than 10% only type and screen is done and if transfusion is required then only cross match should be done.

Emergency Transfusion

If there is no time to determine ABO group (or there is some problem in determining recipient blood group) then O –ve (universal donor) red cells should be used. O –ve red cells are preferred over O –ve whole blood because it is seen that some O –ve donors may have anti-A and anti-B antibodies in their plasma.

Storage of Blood

Blood is stored in the cold part of refrigerator at 4°C (never in the freezer).
- It can be stored for *21 days* if acid citrate dextrose is used.
- It can be stored for *35 days* if the preservative anticoagulant solution used is CDPA-1
  C for Citrate as anticoagulant.
  D for Dextrose as energy source for red cells.
  P for Phosphate as buffer.
  A for Adenine to increase the red cell survival.
  CDPA is most commonly used anticoagulant in India.
- It can be stored for 42 days if anticoagulant preservative solution used is ADSOL (Adenine, glucose, mannitol and sodium chloride) or NUTRICE (Adenine, glucose, citrate, phosphate and NaCl) and Optisol.

Changes in Stored Blood

pH	: Decreases (6.98 at 35th day of storage)
Hemoglobin concentration	: Decreases (70% at 35th day)
Hematocrit	: Decreases (40% at 35th day)
Potassium	: Increases
2, 3 DPG level	: Decreases (< 1 μm/mL at 35th day; normal is 13.2 μm/mL)
Platelets	: Decreases (only 5% at 48 hours)
Clotting factors	: Factor V only 15% at 21 days, Factor VIII only 50% at 21 days. Rest all factors are comparatively stable in stored blood.

Massive Blood Transfusion

It is defined as transfusion of blood more than patient's blood volume (5 liters) in less than 24 hours. It also implies transfusion of more than 10% of blood volume in less than 10 minutes.

Blood Component Therapy

Packed Red Blood Cells (PRBC)

In current day practice it is the packed red cell unit which is always preferred over whole blood due to the following advantages:
- Infectious and allergic problems related to plasma can be avoided.
- Cardiac overload due to whole blood can be avoided.
- Whole blood can be utilized to extract other products like fresh frozen plasma, platelets, cryoprecipitate, white cells, etc.
- Hematocrit of packed cell unit is 70% and the volume is 250 mL.
- The half-life of transfused RBCs is less (60 days).

Frozen RBCs

- These are expensive but the chances of reaction and disease transmission are very low.
- The frozen RBCs can be stored up to 10 years. Intercellular 2, 3 DPG can be retained for years in frozen RBCs.

Fresh Frozen Plasma (FFP)

- In FFP, plasma is frozen within 6 hours of collection.
- Volume is 225 mL.

- FFP contains all coagulation factors and plasma proteins.

Indications of FFP
- Treatment of coagulopathies associated with liver diseases, blood transfusion, etc.
- Reversal of warfarin therapy.
- Antithrombin III deficiency.
- Plasma protein deficiency (fresh frozen plasma is poor man's albumin).
- *Each unit of FFP increases the level of each clotting factor by 2–3% (initial volume of infusion is 10–15 mL/kg)*
- *ABO compatibility with FFP may not be necessary* but highly desirable.

Platelet Concentrates
Volume: 50 mL.

Platelets are the only blood products which are stored at room temperature. Survival at room temperature is 4–5 days while at 4°C it is 24–48 hours.
- *1 unit of platelet increases the count by 5,000–10,000.*
- Transfused platelets generally survive for 2–7 days following transfusion.
- *ABO compatibility is desirable but not necessary* (if large number of units are to be given then ABO compatibility becomes necessary). Rh matching is highly desirables for young female patients to avoid Rh immunization in future pregnancies.
- Since platelets are derived from multiple donors, the chances of disease transmission are high. Single donor platelets (SDP), where multiple units of platelets are derived from single donor by apheresis machine, can largely solve this problem. *One unit of SDP is equal to 5-8 units of random donor platelets (RDP) therefore increases platelet count by approximately 30,000-40,000.*
- As the platelets are stored at room temperature (which promotes bacterial growth), the chances of infection is further increased with platelets.

Cryoprecipitate
Volume: 10 mL.

1 unit of cryoprecipitate contains 80–145 units of *factor VIII* and 250 mg of fibrinogen. Cryoprecipitate also contains factor XIII and von Willebrand's factor. Cryoprecipitate is pooled from many donors so there is maximum chance of disease transmission among all blood products.

Granulocyte Precipitate
Indicated for neutropenic patients.

COMPLICATIONS OF BLOOD TRANSFUSION

Transfusion Reactions
These reactions may be allergic or hemolytic.

Hemolytic Reactions
Hemolytic reactions can be:
- Acute
- Delayed

Acute hemolytic reactions: These are *usually due to ABO incompatibility (mismatch reaction). The most common cause of these transfusion reactions is clerical error.* There is *intravascular hemolysis.* Incidence is 1 in 6,000 to 1 in 40,000 (fatal hemolytic reaction incidence is 1 in 100,000). Blood as low as 10 mL can produce hemolytic reaction.

Clinical manifestations: The awake patient presents with pain and burning in vein (earliest), fever with chills and rigors, nausea and vomiting, flushing, chest and flank pain, dyspnea.

In anesthetized individual it is manifested as tachycardia, hypotension (therefore regular blood pressure monitoring during early transfusion is necessary) *and oozing from surgical site* (more specific).

It is confirmed by hemoglobinuria. The hemoglobin crystals block the renal tubules leading to acute renal failure.

Management
- Stop transfusion.
- Recheck the details of blood slip.
- Send the remaining blood back to blood bank.
- Maintain the urine output (1–2 mL/kg/hr) by mannitol and fluid administration.
- Dopamine in renal doses (2–5 µg/kg/min) improves renal blood flow.
- Alkalinize the urine.
- Hemodialysis.
- Assay urine hemoglobin, platelet count, fibrinogen level and PTT (to diagnose DIC) and replace with blood components accordingly.

Delayed hemolytic reactions: These are *extravascular* hemolytic reactions. These are usually due to Rh system or other systems like Kell, Duffy, etc. These reactions are mild and seen after 2–21 days. These reactions are diagnosed by Coomb's test. The treatment is only supportive.

Treatment: Only supportive.

Allergic Reactions

These are usually mild, manifesting as urticaria and *are mainly due to plasma proteins.*

Treatment: Antihistaminics (Avil) + Steroid.

At times (1 in 150,000) these reactions may be anaphylactic. Management includes:
- Immediately stop the transfusion.
- Adrenaline and steroids.

Febrile Reactions

Incidence is 1–3%. These are *due to infusion of white cell microaggregates.* The incidence of these reactions can be minimized by the *use of microfilter blood sets with pore size of 20–40 µm instead of conventional blood sets with pore size of 170 µm* which permits the infusion of WBC microaggregates or by using blood products with leukoreduction. These febrile reactions are mild and generally require no treatment.

Infectious Complications

Chances of infectious complications are more with pooled products (derived from large number of donors) like cryoprecipitate.

Hepatitis

- Incidence is 1 in 2,00000 to 1 in 9,00000.
- 90% of these are due to *non-A non-B (hepatitis C) virus.*

Acquired Immunodeficiency Syndrome (AIDS)

- Incidence is 1 in 900000.
- It is because of HIV-1.

Other Viral Diseases

Cytomegalovirus (can produce severe infection in immunocompromised patients), Epstein Barr virus, human T cell lymphotropic virus (HTLV-1 and 2) and parvovirus.

Bacterial Infections

Bacterial contamination is the second most common cause of transfusion related mortality. The contamination most commonly occurs with *Pseudomonas* (it can grow at 4°C) but can be due to gram-positive like *Staphylococcus*. Although rare but transmission of syphilis, *brucellosis*, *Salmonella*, *Yersinia* and rickettsial diseases has been reported. Therefore it is strongly recommended that *blood products should be transfused within 4 hours.*

Parasitic

Malaria (Malarial parasite may survive for 3 weeks in stored blood) *Toxoplasma*, Filariasis, trypanosomiasis.

Noninfectious Complications

Fluid Overload and Pulmonary Edema

Seen in cardiac compromised individuals.

Metabolic

Metabolic complications are usually seen after massive transfusion.
- *Hyperkalemia:* Stored blood has high potassium levels.
- *Hypocalcemia:* Citrate chelates calcium however hypocalcemia is not seen during routine transfusion.

  The *indications for calcium replacement* during transfusion are:
  - Blood given at a very fast rate (Liver does not get sufficient time to metabolize citrate)
  - Liver diseases.
  - Massive blood transfusion (citrate load is too high)
  - Severe hypothermia (decreases citrate metabolism).
- Hyperammonemia.

Acid-base Abnormalities

Blood gases show variable results. Acidic pH of stored blood causes acidosis while citrate metabolism causes alkalosis. *In massive transfusion alkalosis is more common* due to citrate intoxication (one molecule of citrate generates 3 molecules of bicarbonate).

Coagulation Abnormalities

Massive blood transfusion causes *dilutional coagulopathies especially dilutional thrombocytopenia* (stored blood has no platelets and concentration of other clotting factors is also less). Dilutional coagulopathies leading to disseminated intravascular coagulation (DIC) *is the usual cause of death after massive blood transfusion.*

Management

Treatment should be initiated only if (not prophylactically after 3–4 units as practiced in past)

- There is bleeding from surgical site which is not getting controlled by surgical hemostasis or there is bleeding from intravenous site, mucous membranes or petechial hemorrhages.
- PT, APTT > 1.5 times of normal
- Fibrinogen < 75 mg/dL
- Platelet count < 50,000

Treatment includes

- Fresh blood (collected and used within 6 hours without refrigeration)—Logistically difficult to obtain but is the *best modality of treatment.* (Provides all coagulation factors and platelets)
- Fresh frozen plasma.
- Specific blood component therapy.
- Platelets.

Hypothermia

Significant hypothermia is only seen with massive transfusion. Blood should be warmed to *37°C* before infusion.

Immune Complications

- Immunomodulation (suppression of immune system). Whether this immunomodulation leads to increase incidence of bacterial infections or malignancy is not known.
- Graft versus host reaction (especially in immunocompromised patients)
- Alloimmunization (production of antibodies) against own RBC, platelets and HLA. Alloimmunization against platelets can produce post-transfusion purpura.

Transfusion-related Acute Lung Injury (TRALI)

TRALI manifest as hypoxia within 6 hours of transfusion. Although it can occur with any blood product, however it is most commonly seen with fresh frozen plasma. Exact pathophysiology is not known but most probably it is due to damage to alveolar capillary membrane by anti-HLA or antileukocytic antibodies.

The management is same like ARDS. Despite majority of the patients recovering within 96 hours *TRALI remains the leading cause of death due to blood transfusion.*

Disseminated Intravascular Coagulation (DIC)

Causes may be:

- Mismatched transfusion reaction.
- Dilutional coagulopathies leading to activation of coagulation system.

Tissue Hypoxia

Decrease in 2,3 DPG in stored blood can shift oxygen dissociation curve to left and at least theoretically can produce tissue hypoxia

Synthetic Oxygen Carriers (Artificial Blood)

- Perfluorocarbon emulsion called as Fluosol-DA.
- Perfluorooctyl bromide.
- Recombinant hemoglobin.
- Recombinant erythropoietin.

These synthetic oxygen carriers may be a good replacement of blood in future. These will be particularly useful in Jehovah's witness patients who refuse to receive the blood transfusion because of their religious beliefs.

AUTOLOGOUS BLOOD TRANSFUSION

As the name suggests, patient's own blood is taken and replaced back when necessary. The main advantage of autologous blood transfusion (ABT) is that there is no risk of disease transmission and transfusion related reaction can be avoided. Three techniques are employed for autologous blood transfusion.

Predonation

3 to 4 units of patient's own blood is taken before surgery [subject to condition that hematocrit should not fall below 35% and hemoglobin

below 11 gm% (most of the centers in India accepts up to 10 gm%)] and stored in blood bank.

Last blood donation should not be scheduled less than 72 hours before surgery (time required for plasma volume to return to normal) and should not be later than 4–5 weeks (maximum time for which blood can be stored with CDPA).

The major disadvantage of this technique is that the incidence of mismatch transfusion reactions remains same (because patient's blood is stored in blood bank and the most common cause of mismatch transfusion reactions is clerical errors)

Normovolemic/Isovolemic Hemodilution

Blood is removed just prior to surgery and volume replaced with crystalloid or colloid to produce hemodilution; *the target Hematocrit should be 25–28%.* (Studies have shown that oxygen delivery to the tissues is better at low hematocrit as compared to normal hematocrit). Blood can be transfused back whenever necessary (preferably within 6 hours to preserve platelet function). Since blood is taken in Operation Theater, there is no risk of mismatch transfusion. Negligible cost of technique, technical feasibility, no risk of mismatch transfusion or any other major complication and improved oxygen delivery to tissues makes

Normovolemic/Isovolemic hemodilution as the most widely used technique for autologous blood donation.

Blood Salvage and Reinfusion

Patient's lost blood is saved (salvaged) in a special device, processed (washed, tissue debris, clots, etc. removed), concentrated and transfused back. The major limitation is the cost of the device. Other complications which can occur are air embolism, renal failure due to blockage of renal tubules by free hemoglobin (produced as a result of hemolysis of red cells by excessive suction pressure), infection and disseminated intravascular coagulation (DIC) (shed blood undergoes varying degree of coagulation and fibrinolysis producing DIC).

Contraindications of Autologous Blood Transfusion

Absolute: Blood should not be saved and transfused back if it is infected or contains malignant cells.

Other relative contraindications are sickle cell disease, patient suffering from coronary artery disease or cyanotic heart disease, and if the likelihood of requirement of blood is less than 10%.

KEY POINTS

- Crystalloids should be replaced in a ratio of 1.5:1 to intravascular volume loss while colloids in a ratio of 1:1.
- Colloids in high doses can interfere with clotting and causes renal dysfunction.
- Ringer lactate is the most preferred fluid for maintenance as well as replacement.
- Children are prone for fluid overload therefore should receive 2/3rd of the calculated dose.
- Colloids can be safely given even if there is endothelial injury like in ARDS or head injury.
- The main aim of blood transfusion is to improve the oxygen delivery of tissues, not the volume replacement (which should be done by fluids).
- In spite of varying controversies the most acceptable trigger point for blood transfusion are blood volume loss >20% and hemoglobin < 8 gm%.
- One unit of blood/packed cells increases hemoglobin by 0.8%.
- Most common cause of mismatch transfusion is ABO incompatibility.
- DIC is the most common cause of death after massive transfusion while acute lung injury remains the leading cause of mortality after transfusion.
- Massive transfusion related dilutional coagulopathies should not be treated prophylactically.
- Platelets are the only blood products which are stored at room temperature.
- Normovolemic/isovolemichemodilution is the most widely used technique for autologous blood donation.

Introduction to Anesthesia

CHAPTER 8

History of Anesthesia

History of anesthesia dates back to 1st AD when Dioscorides used the term anesthesia to describe the narcotic effects of plant *Mandragora*.

The word anesthesia which means no senses was coined by Oliver Wendell Homes. The term *'balanced anesthesia' was coined by John Lundy and Ralph Waters.*

NITROUS OXIDE

First anesthetic gas, i.e. *nitrous oxide was synthesized by Priestley in 1774* (Priestley also synthesized oxygen which he called Dephlogisticated air). First clinical use of nitrous oxide was done by Humphry Davy who used it on himself for toothache and called nitrous oxide as *'laughing gas'.* However, *first public clinical demonstration of nitrous oxide was given by 'Horace Wells' for tooth extraction* (1845), but unfortunately the patient cried in pain. Horace Wells became so frustrated that he became chloroform addict and committed suicide by cutting his femoral artery.

ETHER

It was prepared by Valerius Cordus in 1540 when it was known as *'sweet oil of vitriol'. First public demonstration of ether was given by WTG Morton on 16th October 1846 and that is why 16th October is celebrated as World Anesthesia Day* (**Fig. 8.1**).

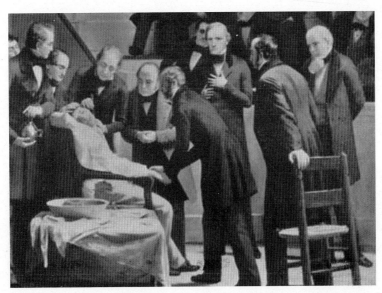

Fig. 8.1: First successful demonstration of ether anesthesia by Morton in Massachusetts General Hospital

CHLOROFORM

It was the John Snow who popularized chloroform using successfully in 4,000 patients. He used chloroform on Queen Victoria for birth of her 8th child.

INTRAVENOUS ANESTHETICS

First intravenous anesthetic used was thiopentone by John Lundy in 1934.

LOCAL ANESTHESIA

- First local anesthetic used was *cocaine* by Carl Koller for anesthetizing cornea (1884).
- First spinal anesthesia in dogs was given by J Leonard Corning while *First spinal anesthesia in human beings was given by August Beir in 1898.*
- First epidural anesthesia was given by Cathelin and Sicard (1901).

MUSCLE RELAXANTS

- Harold Griffith was first to use *'curare'* for muscle relaxation (1942).
- Bovet got Nobel Prize (1949) for using Suxamethonium (Succinylcholine) in practice.

INSTRUMENTS

- First Boyle's machine was invented by Edmund Gaskin Boyle in 1917.
- First endotracheal intubation was done by Ivan Magill.

General Anesthesia

CHAPTER 9

Introduction to General Anesthesia

COMPONENTS OF GENERAL ANESTHESIA

The term anesthesia was given by Oliver Wendell Holmes.

The basic components (TRIAD) of general anesthesia are:

- Narcosis
- Analgesia
- Muscle relaxation.

The anesthesia in present day should be *balanced anesthesia*, a concept laid by John Lundy in 1926. The components of balance anesthesia are:

- Narcosis
- Analgesia
- Muscle relaxation
- Amnesia
- Abolition of reflexes
- Maintenance of normal hemodynamics and physiologic homoeostasis.

The balanced anesthesia can be achieved by combination of different techniques such as general anesthesia with different agents, premedication and regional anesthesia.

GENERAL ANESTHESIA PROTOCOL (FOR A NORMAL HEALTHY PATIENT)

Selected indoor patients may be premedicated with lorazepam or diazepam night before surgery. Benzodiazepines are used to induce good sleep and produce *amnesia*.

On the day of the surgery, patient is directly shifted to Operation Theater. Once the patient lies on operation table, the assistant starts to apply monitors and the anesthesiologist preoxygenates the patient with 100% oxygen for 3 minutes. As 99% of the nitrogen in lungs can be replaced with oxygen *(called as Denitrogenation)* in 3 minutes, preoxygenation increases the oxygen reserve enabling the patient to sustain hypoxia for longer periods.

Once the preoxygenation is complete induction is accomplished with intravenous anesthetics such as Propofol. Intravenous agents are preferred for induction because of their ultrafast action (with 15 seconds). After the patient becomes unconscious, our next aim to secure airway as early as possible. That's why due to its rapid onset, suxamethonium (succinylcholine) is the ideal muscle relaxant for intubation, however, because of the side effects its use is only restricted to rapid sequence or difficult intubation. In normal circumstances, patients are generally intubated with non-depolarizers.

As soon as the effect of muscle relaxants sets in, patient is intubated with cuffed endotracheal tube. Position of the tube is verified by auscultation and capnography. Tube is fixed with adhesive. After confirming the position of tube, positive pressure ventilation (IPPV) is started with bag or ventilator.

Anesthesia is maintained with oxygen (33%) + nitrous oxide (66%) + inhalational agent. As Nitrous oxide depletes ozone, majority of the anesthesiologist in current day practice use air instead of nitrous oxide. Relaxation for surgery is achieved by non-depolarizing muscle relaxant.

At the end of the surgery, the muscle blockade effect of non-depolarizers is reversed with neostigmine + glycopyrrolate, and then the patient is extubated after thorough suctioning of oral cavity.

■ **Table 9.1:** Stages of anesthesia

	Respiration	Tidal volume	Pupils	Eye position and ocular movement	Reflexes abolished
Stage-1 (Stage of analgesia): From analgesia to loss of consciousness	Irregular	Small	Constricted	Divergent (Normal)	Nil
Stage-2 (Stage of excitement): From loss of consciousness to rhythmic respiration	Irregular	Large	Dilated (due to sympathetic stimulation)	Divergent (Roving)	Eyelash
Stage-3 (Stage of surgical anesthesia):	Divided into four planes				
Plane 1 (From rhythmic respiration to cessation of eye movement)	Regular	Large	Constricted	Divergent(Roving initially and fixed till the end)	• Conjunctival • Pharyngeal • Skin
Plane 2 (Cessation of eye movement to respiratory paresis)	Regular	Medium	½ Dilated	Fixed centrally	Corneal
Plane 3 (Respiratory paresis to paralysis)	Regular	Small	¾ Dilated	Fixed centrally	Laryngeal
Plane 4 (Diaphragmatic paralysis)	Jerky	Small	Fully dilated	Fixed centrally	• Carinal • Anal sphincter
Stage-4 (Medullary paralysis)					

STAGES OF ANESTHESIA

Stages were described by *Guedel with ether* (**Table 9.1**). However, in current anesthesia where newer inhalational agent are so fast acting that these stages do not exists therefore there is no need for the students to go in details of the stages and the only salient features to be noted are:

• *Stage of surgical anesthesia is stage III plane 3* because laryngeal reflexes goes in this stage and intubation can be performed. Onset of surgical anesthesia (stage III) is best indicated by *onset of regular respiration.*

• First reflex to go is eyelash, therefore loss of consciousness is tested by absence of eyelash reflex while the last reflex to go is carinal reflex (tested by touching the carina with suction catheter which should initiate cough).

• Initial pupillary dilatation seen in stage II is because of sympathetic stimulation.

• The return of reflexes is in opposite sequence, i.e. first to come is carinal reflex and last is eyelash. Therefore theoretically, it is cough which should come first but swallowing comes earlier because coughing also requires diaphragm and respiratory muscles effort.

CHAPTER 10

Inhalational Agents: General Principles and Individual Agents

Inhalational agents are mainly used in anesthesia for *maintenance of anesthesia*, however, they can also be used for induction, especially in children.

CLASSIFICATION

Agents in Common Use

- Halothane
- Isoflurane
- Nitrous oxide

Newer Agents

- Sevoflurane
- Desflurane

Agents Not in Use

- Enflurane
- Ether
- Trilene
- Methoxyflurane
- Cyclopropane
- Chloroform

MECHANISM OF ACTION OF INHALATIONAL AGENTS

Anesthetic potency of an inhalational agent is directly proportional to its lipid solubility (oil gas partition coefficient). This is called as *Meyer Overton rule*. This rule lead to the *unitary theory of narcosis* which means that all inhalational agents has common lipophilic (lipid soluble) site. However, there were many exceptions to this rule like:

- All lipid soluble agents do not produce anesthesia rather many can even produce convulsions. These agents, which are lipid soluble but do not produce anesthesia are called as *immobilizers*.
- As per Meyer Overton rule all isomers of same agent should have same potency but this is not true. Isoflurane, enflurane and desflurane in spite of being isomers have different potencies. Similarly, homologous series of same compound (with increasing lipid solubility) should be more potent but in fact, it is opposite. This is called as *cut-off effect*.
- It was very well proven that anesthetic agents not only bind to lipophilic (lipid soluble site) site, they also bind to hydrophilic (lipid insoluble) sites.

These exceptions to Meyer Overton rule lead to *shifting of mechanism from lipid sites to protein sites; the most acceptable mechanism is that they directly bind to cellular proteins altering their enzymes.*

Other mechanisms of actions are:

- *Theory of fluidization:* By expanding cellular membrane they cause its fluidization blocking the sodium channels.
- *Critical volume hypothesis:* They expand the cell membrane beyond critical amount altering the membrane function.
- *Enhances GABA (and Glycine) mediated inhibition of central nervous system:* At molecular level, modulation of GABA receptors is considered as principal mechanism of action for all volatile agents except the gases–nitrous oxide and xenon which acts by inhibiting N-methyl-D-aspartate (NMDA) receptors.
- Decrease the concentration of excitatory neurotransmitters in brain.

Site of Action of Inhalational Agents

- These agents mainly act on central nervous system (producing unconsciousness and amnesia) and dorsal horn cells of spinal cord (producing analgesia and immobility).
- Mainly acts on synapses (both pre- and postsynaptic level), however, in high doses can block axonal transmission.

POTENCY OF INHALATIONAL AGENTS

Best estimate for determining the potency of inhalational anesthetic is *minimum alveolar concentration (MAC)* which is defined as minimum concentration of agent required to produce immobility in 50% of the subjects given noxious stimuli, which is skin incision in human beings and tail clamping in rats. More important from clinical point of view is MAC_{95} *(MAC producing effect in 95% individuals)*. MAC_{95} *is 1.3 times of MAC_{50}.*

Another MAC which is sometimes used in clinical practice is MAC_{awake}. It is MAC at which patient is not unconscious but remains amnestic. It is 0.3 times of MAC_{50}.

It is very clear from the definition of MAC that the agent with minimum MAC will be most potent.

MAC for different anesthetic agents in current use is given in **Table 10.1**:

It can be concluded from the **Table 10.1** that *halothane with MAC of 0.74% is the most potent while nitrous oxide with very high MAC of 104% is the least potent among the agents used nowadays.*

Factors Effecting MAC

Factors Decreasing the MAC

- *Age: Maximum MAC in human beings is at the age of 6 months*, thereafter decreasing steadily throughout the life (except a slight increase at puberty).

■ **Table 10.1:** Minimum alveolar concentration (MAC) for different anesthetic agents in current use

Agent	MAC
Halothane	0.74%
Isoflurane	1.15%
Sevoflurane	2.05%
Desflurane	6.0%
Nitrous oxide	104%

- *Temperature:* Decreasing the temperature decreases the MAC. Increasing temperature (up to 42°C) also decreases the MAC.
- *Anemia (Hb < 5 gm%), Hypoxia (pO_2 < 40 mm Hg) and Hypercarbia (pCO_2 > 95 mm Hg)* decreases the MAC, only if they are severe.
- *Alcohol:* Acute alcohol or acute administration of amphetamines decreases the MAC.
- *Pregnancy:* Inhalational anesthetics should be used in lower concentrations in pregnancy.
- Concurrent administration of *Intravenous anesthetics and alpha2 agonists.*
- *Local anesthetics:* All local anesthetics except cocaine decreases the MAC.
- *Electrolytes imbalances* decreasing MAC *are: Hyponatremia, Hypercalcemia and Hypermagnesemia.*

Factors Increasing the MAC

- Hyperthermia > 42°C
- Chronic intoxication of alcohol and amphetamines
- Cocaine, ephedrine
- *Borometric pressure:* Increasing pressure increases the MAC (pressure reversal theory of anesthesia)
- Hypernatremia

Factors Having No Effect on MAC

- Thyroid disorders
- *Sex:* MAC is same for males and females.
- *Obesity:* MAC does not increase in obese patients

UPTAKE AND DISTRIBUTION OF INHALATIONAL AGENTS

Inhalational agents delivered by vaporizer and mixed with carrier gas (oxygen + nitrous oxide or oxygen alone) reach the patient's alveoli; from there they are taken up by blood and reach different tissues. *The concentration in CNS determines the effect of inhalational agent.*

Factors effecting the uptake and distribution are:

Inspired (Delivered) Concentration (FI)

It depends upon the concentration or partial pressure (concentration and partial pressure are used interchangeably) delivered by vaporizer, fresh gas flow, absorption by breathing circuit and ventilation.

Alveolar Concentration (FA)

It depends on inspired concentration and uptake by blood. *Anesthetic tether* is the ratio of delivered concentration to alveolar concentration (FD/FA). It is important that delivered partial pressure (concentration) from the vaporizer must be higher than targeted alveolar pressure. This is called Overpressure. The more overpressure used, the more rapidly anesthetic is delivered.

After equilibrium is achieved between brain and blood, alveolar concentration reflects the concentration in brain. In tissues with high perfusion such as brain, the equilibrium is achieved in 4–8 minutes.

The uptake by blood is directly proportional to blood gas partition coefficient (λ), cardiac output (Q) and alveolar to venous partial pressure ($P_A - P_V$) and inversely proportional to barometric pressure (P)

$$\text{Uptake} = \frac{\lambda \times Q \times (P_A - P_V)}{P}$$

Blood Gas Partition Coefficient (B/G Coefficient)

This is the most important factor determining the uptake of an agent and so the *speed of induction and recovery*. Agents will low blood gas partition coefficient will have high alveolar concentration, e.g. nitrous oxide with blood gas partition coefficient of 0.47 means concentration (or partial pressure) in blood is 47% of alveolar concentration. Since alveolar concentration determines the induction and recovery, *induction and recovery will be fast with agent with less B/G partition coefficient and slower with agents with high B/G partition coefficients.*

Blood/gas (B/G) partition coefficients of different agents are in **Table 10.2**.

It can be concluded from the **Table 10.2** that overall the fastest induction is seen with xenon, but xenon is not yet available for commercial use therefore among the *agents used now a day induction is fastest with desflurane (with B/G coefficient of 0.42) and slowest with halothane (with B/G coefficient of 2.4).*

■ **Table 10.2:** Blood gas partition coefficient of agents in current use

Agent	Blood gas partition coefficient
Xenon	0.14
Desflurane	0.42
Nitrous oxide	0.47
Sevoflurane	0.69
Isoflurane	1.38
Halothane	2.4

Cardiac Output

Increasing cardiac output increases the uptake, decreasing the alveolar concentration delaying the induction. In low cardiac output states such as shock, the agents with high B/G partition coefficient can achieve dangerously high alveolar concentrations, if inspired concentrations are not decreased but the alveolar concentration of agents with low B/G coefficient will not be so high. *That is why in shock, agents with low B/G coefficient such as nitrous oxide, desflurane or sevoflurane are relatively safe.*

Alveolar to Venous Partial Pressure

Once the tissues have taken up the agent, the gradient reverses and the agent enters the venous system and carried back to lungs. If venous partial pressure is high uptake will be less.

Ventilation

Increasing ventilation will increase the alveolar concentration of agents with high B/G coefficient (increased uptake will decrease alveolar concentration so more room for inspired agent). Agent with low B/G coefficient are least affected with increasing ventilation.

AUGMENTED INFLOW EFFECT, CONCENTRATION EFFECT, SECOND GAS EFFECT AND DIFFUSION HYPOXIA

Augmented Inflow Effect and Concentration Effect

If an anesthetic agent is given in high concentration the *alveolar concentration rises more than expected and also the rate of rise is high.* This is called as *concentration effect.* This is seen with nitrous oxide which is given in high concentration. For example, consider a lung containing 70% nitrous oxide, 29% oxygen and 1% halothane. If 50% of nitrous oxide is taken up from alveoli, the remaining concentration of nitrous oxide will be 63% instead of 50% (because decreasing the lung volume to 50% now make 35 parts remaining in total volume of 65 parts yielding a concentration of 63%). This concentration is further increased in the next breath because large uptake of nitrous oxide creates a void (gradient) to indraw more nitrous oxide from machine called as *augmented inflow effect* (nitrous oxide has augmented its inflow from machine).

Second Gas Effect

If another agent such as halothane or Isoflurane is given along with nitrous oxide, by the same mechanism of concentration effect by which nitrous oxide increases its own concentration the concentration of inhalational agent will also increase. This is called as *second gas effect* (one agent effecting the concentration of other).

Diffusion Hypoxia (Fink Effect)

Towards the end of surgery when nitrous oxide delivery is stopped, the gradient reverses and the nitrous oxide from blood gushes in alveoli replacing the oxygen from there causing hypoxia. This is called as *diffusion hypoxia*. To avoid this diffusion hypoxia *100% oxygen should be given for 5–10 minutes after discontinuing nitrous oxide*.

Recovery From Inhalational Agents

Recovery occurs when concentration in brain decreases, therefore it depends on pulmonary exhalation of agent, metabolism and excretion, transcutaneous loss (seen only with nitrous oxide). Recovery is rapid with agents with low B/G coefficient. *Therefore, earliest recovery will be with desflurane (B/G coefficient-0.42) and most delayed with halothane (B/G coefficient-2.4).*

Absorption of Inhaled Anesthetic Agent by Anesthetic Circuitry

Absorption by rubber, plastic and polyvinyl chloride endotracheal tube: In the past, methoxyflurane used to be get maximally dissolved in rubber, plastic and PVC. In current day, practice *maximum absorption in seen with halothane.*

Metabolism

All inhalational agents undergo oxidation (dealkylation or dehalogenation) in liver (halothane also undergoes reduction) by cytochrome P-450 enzymes in phase I reactions and by conjugation in phase II reactions.

All enzyme inducers such as isoniazid, phenytoin, phenobarbitone, ethanol, diazepam increase the metabolism of inhalational agents.

Among the agents available today *maximum metabolism is seen with halothane (20%). Desflurane is negligibly metabolized (< 0.02%) and nitrous oxide does not undergo any metabolism in human body.*

SYSTEMIC EFFECTS OF INHALATIONAL AGENTS (INCLUDING SIDE EFFECTS AND TOXICITY)

Respiratory System

*   *Ventilation:* Initially, all agents decrease the tidal volume and increase the frequency (respiratory rate) but with increasing dose, frequency also decreases finally decreasing the minute volume. Ventilatory responses (to increased CO_2 and hypoxia) are blunted with inhalational agents. Maximum inhibition to ventilatory response is seen with halothane.
*   *Bronchial muscles:* All inhalational agents are *bronchodilators*. Bronchodilatation is not only because of direct effect of agents on bronchial muscles but also by inhibition of central pathways for bronchoconstriction.
*   *Effects on hypoxic pulmonary vasoconstriction (HPV):* All inhalational agents are pulmonary vasodilators (except nitrous oxide which is pulmonary vasoconstrictor) thereby blunt HPV response worsening the ventilation perfusion mismatch.
*   *Effect on ciliary activity: All agents (except ether) inhibit the ciliary activity* thereby reducing capability of patient to cough out secretions in postoperative period.
*   *Airway reflexes:* Airway reflexes are depressed by inhalational agents making the patient vulnerable for aspiration.

Cardiovascular System

*   *Cardiac output:* By causing direct myocardial depression, all new inhalational agents

decrease the cardiac output. The minimum decrease in cardiac output is seen with *Isoflurane.*

- *Systemic vascular resistance (SVR):* By decreasing SVR, all inhalational agents can produce hypotension.
- *Baroreceptor reflex:* All protective cardiovascular responses are blunted by inhalational agents, least with Isoflurane (allowing compensatory reflex tachycardia). Minimum decrease in cardiac output (and that is too get compensated by reflex tachycardia) makes *Isoflurane, an inhalational agent of choice for cardiac patients* (except myocardial ischemia, where theoretically, it can cause coronary steal).
- *Sensitization of heart to adrenaline: Halothane* (and theoretically other agents too *except Isoflurane*) can sensitize myocardium to adrenaline, exogenous to heart.
- *Cardioprotection*: Inhalational agents (particularly Xenon) because of their anti-apoptotic and N-methyl-D-aspartate (NMDA) receptor antagonistic effects have shown cardioprotection in experimental studies, however, more evidence is needed to establish their role as cardioprotective agents in human beings.

Central Nervous System

- All inhalational agents produce dose dependent reduction in cerebral metabolic rate (CMR) and cerebral oxygen consumption (CMO_2). Isoflurane and Sevoflurane can decrease CMR up to 50%.
- *All inhalational agents (including nitrous oxide) increases the cerebral blood flow and hence ICT.* The order of vasodilating potency is—halothane >>Desflurane ≈ Isoflurane > Sevoflurane.

  Due to more favorable effects on cerebral hemodynamics (cerebral blood flow and ICT), better preservation of autoregulation, equivalent reduction in cerebral metabolic rate and smoother recovery *sevoflurane is preferred over isoflurane as a inhalational agent of choice for neurosurgery in current day anesthetic practice.*

- *Neurotoxicity and neuroprotection:* Animal studies showed that babies who received

GA with inhalational agents at very young age developed cognitive impairment later in life. However human studies still remains inconclusive. On the contrary, by the same mechanisms by which inhalational agents produces cardioprotection they can also produce neuroprotection.

Liver

Direct hepatocellular damage is seen with halothane (*and theoretically with Isoflurane and Desflurane) but not with sevoflurane.* Indirectly, all agents can produces some degree of hepatotoxicity by decreasing the blood supply to liver. M*aximal decrease in blood supply to liver is seen with halothane and least with Sevoflurane (followed by isoflurane).*

Renal System

All inhalational agents depress renal function by decreasing the renal blood flow. Direct renal toxicity has been attributed to inorganic fluoride produced by inhalational agents. *Inhalational agents are fluorinated to decrease their flammability.*

The nephrotoxicity produced by fluorinated agents is *vasopressin-resistant polyuric renal failure.* Renal threshold beyond which fluoride levels are toxic is 50 μm and the fluoride level produced by different agents is given in **Table 10.3**.

Hematopoietic System

Nitrous oxide interacts with vitamin B_{12} and inhibits many pathways involved in one carbon

■ **Table 10.3:** Fluoride level produced by different agents

Agent	Fluoride (F⁻) level (produced after 2.5–3.0 MAC hours)
Methoxyflurane	50–80 μm
*Sevoflurane	20–30 μm
Enflurane	20–25 μm
Isoflurane	4–8 μm
Halothane	Produces fluoride only in anaerobic conditions
Desflurane	Does not produce fluoride

*Sevoflurane although produces high fluoride but still does not causes nephrotoxicity even after long exposures because its low blood gas coefficient (0.69) allows its rapid elimination from body.

moiety. It also inhibits the enzyme methionine synthetase and hence the production of thymidate and DNA formation. Due to these effects nitrous oxide can produce *Megaloblastic anemia, aplastic anemia* and *Homocystinuria* on prolonged exposure.

Spinal Cord

Nitrous oxide by inhibiting the production of thymidate can impair myelin formation leading to *subacute degeneration of spinal cord.*

Neuromuscular System

All inhalational agents are centrally acting muscle relaxants (except nitrous oxide). Among the agents used now a day maximum relaxation is seen with Desflurane.

Teratogenicity

Animal studies have shown teratogenicity with inhalational agents (particularly nitrous oxide) however human studies remain inconclusive

Inflammability of Inhalational Agents

Current day inhalational agents are non-inflammable (made non-inflammable by adding fluorine). Inflammable agents used in past were *Ether and Cyclopropane.*

Analgesia

Inhalational agents in current use are not good analgesics except nitrous oxide and xenon which are good analgesics.

Reaction of Inhalational Agents with Sodalime

- *Trielene* can produce dichloroacetylene (which is neurotoxic) and phosgene gas (which can cause ARDS).
- *Sevoflurane* can produce toxic compound called as *compound A* with sodalime and Barylime
- *Desflurane (and other agents too)* can produce *Carbonmonoxide* by reacting with desiccated sodalime and barylime.
- *Sevoflurane* by reacting with desiccated sodalime and Barylime can produce hydrogen fluoride which can cause burns of respiratory mucosa.

Ozone Destruction and Global Warming

Inhalational agents are responsible for ozone depletion and global warming. Its maximum with N_2O followed by desflurane. The best way to reduce this environmental impact is to use closed-circuit anesthesia and avoid N_2O as much as possible.

Uterus

All inhalational agents used nowadays are equally effective uterine relaxants.

Amnesia

All inhalational agents are good amnesic agents except nitrous oxide.

INDIVIDUAL INHALATIONAL AGENTS

Agents in common use:

NITROUS OXIDE

Nitrous oxide is also called as 'laughing gas' (name given by Humpry Davy). It was first prepared by Joseph Pristley in 1774.

Preparation

Prepared by heating ammonium nitrate between 245 and 270°C.

Physical Properties

- It is colorless, non-irritating and sweet smelling.
- Critical temperature is 36.5°C which is above room temperature, therefore can be stored in liquefied state at room temperature.
- It is stored in blue color cylinders at a pressure of 760 psi.
- *1.5 times heavier than air.*
- 35 times more soluble than nitrogen.

Anesthetic Properties

- *It is not a complete anesthetic* (to act as complete anesthetic, the agent must be given in concentration above MAC. MAC of nitrous oxide is 104% and maximum concentration of nitrous oxide which can be given is 66%). Along with the oxygen it acts as a carrier to carry other volatile agents
- Blood gas coefficient of 0.47 makes it an agent with faster induction and recovery.

- Although it is non-inflammable and non explosive, but it can support fire.
- Good analgesic.
- Not a muscle relaxant.
- When given along with other inhalational agents, it increases the alveolar concentration of that agent *(second gas effect)* and its own *(concentration effect)*.
- At the end of surgery sudden stoppage of N_2O delivery can reverse the gradient making it gush to alveoli replacing oxygen from there creating hypoxia called as *diffusion hypoxia,* which can be prevented by giving 100% oxygen for 5 to 10 minutes.

Metabolism

It is not metabolized in human body; excreted unchanged through lungs. A small amount gets excreted through skin (percutaneous excretion).

Systemic Actions

Cardiovascular system: *In vitro* it depresses myocardium but *in vivo* this effect is countered by stimulation of sympathetic system, therefore can be *used safely for cardiac patients and shock.*

Cerebral: Increases cerebral metabolic rate and *raises the intracranial tension.*

Respiratory system: Respiration is minimally depressed

Immunologic system: Effects chemotaxis and motility of leukocytes.

Side Effects

- *Closed gas spaces and nitrous oxide:* Compliant spaces such as gut, pleural and peritoneal cavity and non-compliant spaces such as middle ear cavity and brain can develop very high pressure following nitrous oxide inhalation because 1 mole of nitrogen is replaced with 35 moles of nitrous oxide (35 times more soluble than nitrogen). Therefore nitrous oxide is *contraindicated* in:
  - *Pneumothorax:* Nitrous oxide doubles the pneumothorax volume in 10 minutes and triples in 30 minutes producing severe cardiorespiratory compromise.
  - *Pneumoperitoneum.*
  - *Pneumoencephalus:* Entry of nitrous oxide can significantly increase the intracranial

  tension. Once the patient develops pneumoencephalus nitrous oxide cannot be used for 1 week.
  - *Middle ear surgery and tympanoplasties:* Pressure in middle ear cavity may rise to 20–50 mm Hg which can displace the graft.
  - *Posterior fossa surgeries:* There is increased risk of venous air embolism in posterior fossa surgery and the volume of this air embolus can be significantly increased by ingress of nitrous oxide.
  - *Laparoscopic surgeries:* Chances of air embolism are high in laparoscopies.
  - *Acute intestinal obstruction and volvulus of gut:* Gut has air; ingress of nitrous oxide can increase the gut distension.
  - *Diaphragmatic hernia:* Increased gut distension causes further atelectasis worsening the hypoxia
  - *Eye surgeries:* It can expand sulfur hexa-fluoride bubble increasing intraocular pressure.
  - *Microlaryngeal surgeries (MLS):* By diffusing through the tracheal tube cuff (which is filled with air), it may double or triple the cuff volume aggravating the post-surgical edema, which can cause upper airway obstruction.
- *Hematological system:* It inactivates vitamin B_{12}, impairs methionine and deoxythymidine synthesis which leads to defect in folate metabolism and therefore *bone marrow depression* causing *aplastic* and *megaloblastic anemia*. Vitamin B_{12} inactivation is seen, if nitrous oxide is used for more than 12 hours.

  Another consequence of reduced methionine synthase activity is accumulation of its substrate, homocysteine producing homo-cystinuria. However, whether this increase in homocysteine increases the risk of myocardial ischemia (and atherosclerosis) is not proven.
- *Neurological system:* Vitamin B_{12} deficiency by impairing DNA synthesis can cause *Subacute degeneration of spinal cord* and encephalopathy (sometimes presenting as psychosis).
- *Teratogenic effects:* Teratogenicity and increased risk of abortion has been observed in animals, however, human studies are inconclusive.

- *Environment*: can *deplete ozone layer producing global warming.*
- *Impurities in nitrous oxide cylinder:* Nitric oxide, nitrogen dioxide, nitrogen, carbon monoxide, ammonia. These impurities can cause severe *laryngospasm,* methemoglobinemia and *pulmonary edema.*

ENTONOX

It is mixture of 50% oxygen and 50% nitrous oxide *used commonly for labor analgesia.*
- It is stored in blue colored cylinders with blue and white (or only white) shoulders at a pressure of 2,000 psi.
- It should be stored above 10°C otherwise low temperature can cause separation of oxygen and nitrous oxide and high concentration of nitrous oxide can be delivered. To prevent this, cylinder should be inverted 2–3 times to ensure good mixing.
- Ideally, the cylinder should be stored horizontally.

XENON

Although its anesthetic properties were studied 50 years back but could not be used due to very high cost of manufacturing. Recently, new cheaper methods for its synthesis have again renewed interest in xenon. If the cost of Xenon is reduced it may serve an excellent alternative to nitrous oxide.

Properties

- Noble gas with high density and high viscosity (more than air)
- Chemically inert.
- Blood gas coefficient is lowest (0.14), therefore induction and recovery is fastest (almost 3 times faster than N_2O which has blood gas coefficient of 0.47).
- More potent than nitrous oxide (MAC- 70%)
- Analgesic
- Noninflammable, non-explosive and does not support fire

Systemic Effects

Cardiovascular system: Devoid of any cardiovascular effects.

Respiratory system: Because of high density (almost 6 times of air), it increases airway resistance making it *unsuitable for asthma patients.*

CNS: Depresses sympathetic system, therefore can be utilized to blunt sympathetic response to intubation.

Cardio and neuroprotection: Because of its anti-apoptotic and NMDA-receptor antagonistic property have shown cardio and neuroprotection in experimental studies, however, more human studies are needed.

Metabolism

Xenon does not undergo any metabolism in human body.

Advantages over N_2O

- Rapid induction and recovery.
- More potent
- No teratogenic effect
- No ozone depletion or greenhouse effect (No environmental hazard)
- Analgesia is better than N_2O.
- No expansion of air-filled cavities
- No second gas effect and diffusion hypoxia
- No megaloblastic and aplastic anemia, no subacute degeneration of spinal cord

In conclusion, it can be said that if cost of manufacturing of xenon is reduced, then it will be the most ideal inhalational anesthetic in future

Disadvantages

- Cost (100 times more costly).
- Increased airway resistance
- Priming of breathing circuit with xenon is must, this further increases the cost.

Other noble gases such as krypton and argon also have anesthetic properties but not under normobaric conditions, therefore cannot be used in anesthesia.

HALOTHANE

Halothane is a still widely used inhalational agent in India

Physical Properties

- Colorless
- Pleasant to smell, nonirritant makes *induction to become smooth,* therefore, can be used as an alternative to sevoflurane for induction in children.

- Stored in *amber-colored bottles* and contains thymol 0.01% as preservative (to prevent decomposition by light).
- Non-inflammable, non-explosive.
- Boiling point 50°C.
- Halothane has highest fat/blood coefficient [can get deposited in adipose tissue after prolonged exposure].
- In the presence of moisture halothane can corrode metals of vaporizers (aluminum, brass and tin) and plastic.
- Halothane is significantly absorbed by rubber tubing of circuits.

Anesthetic Properties

- It is potent anesthetic (MAC = 0.74) {in fact, *most potent among the agents used nowadays*}
- *Blood gas coefficient:* 2.4 makes it agent with slow induction and recovery time {*slowest among the agents used nowadays*}
- *Not a good analgesic.*

Metabolism

Halothane undergoes extensive metabolism (20%) by oxidation as well as reduction. Metabolic products are:

- *Trifluoroacetic acid:* It is the major metabolic product
- Chloride (Cl^-).
- Bromide (Br^-).
- Fluoride (F^-) only under anaerobic conditions.

Systemic Effects

Cardiovascular system:
- Halothane causes significant decrease in cardiac output which is because of direct depression of myocardium and bradycardia (beta blocking action).
- Blunts the baroreceptor reflex.
- Blood pressure is decreased by direct action on smooth muscle of blood vessels as well as decreased central sympathetic tone.
- It sensitizes heart to adrenaline (*exogenous to heart*) producing ventricular arrhythmias therefore maximum permissible dose of adrenaline with halothane for local ischemia is 1.5 µg/kg (otherwise 5 µm/kg is the maximum permissible dose) or not more than 30 mL/hr of 1 in 1,00,000 solution. For the same reason, *it is contraindicated in pheochromocytoma.*

So, it can be concluded that *halothane should not be used in cardiac patients.*

Respiratory system:
- Depresses respiration and blunts hypercarbic and hypoxic reflexes
- In spite of being a potent *bronchodilator,* it should be avoided in asthma patients as by sensitizing myocardium to catecholamines, it increases the possibility of arrhythmias in patients on β-agonist and aminophylline. (Inhalational agent of choice for asthmatics in present day practice is Sevoflurane).

Central nervous system: There is marked increase in intracranial tension with halothane.

Renal: Both GFR and urinary flow is decreased because of decrease in cardiac output.

Uterus: Like other inhalational agents in current day practice, it produces similar degree of uterine relaxation.

Thermoregulation: *Postoperative shivering* (halothane shakes) and hypothermia is maximum with halothane as compared to other inhalational agents.

Liver: *Halothane hepatitis,* although rare (1 in 35,000), but is clinically significant as it carries very high mortality (>70%).

The *most important risk factor for halothane hepatitis is multiple and frequent exposures.* Other risk factors are hypoxia, middle age, obesity, female gender and patients suffering from autoimmune diseases.
- Pathologic lesion is *centrilobular necrosis.*

Etiology of halothane hepatitis: There are number of theories:
- Direct hepatocellular injury by metabolites. Reductive metabolites are more dangerous than oxidative.
- Decreased blood supply because of decreased cardiac output.
- *Immunologic mechanism:* This is the *most acceptable theory* because hepatitis is common after repeated exposures, seen more in patients with other coexisting autoimmune diseases and antibodies against liver cells can be detected in serum. Trifluoroacetic acid, which is the major metabolite of halothane,

by it antigenic nature produces antibodies mediating antigen-antibody injury to liver cells.

Based on above observations guidelines for use of halothane are:

- *Avoid repeated use, at least an interval of 3 months is mandatory between two exposures.*
- Avoid in patients with coexisting autoimmune diseases
- As children are more immunocompetent incidence of halothane hepatitis is significantly less therefore halothane can be used safely in children.
- Hypoxia is not permissible with halothane as hypoxia increases severity of hepatic damage.
- *Sevoflurane is the inhalational agent of choice for a known case of halothane hepatitis* because sevoflurane does not produce trifluroacetic acid avoiding the possibility of hepatitis in such a patient where antibodies against trifluroacetic acid are already present.

Contraindications

- History of previous halothane hepatitis.
- Patients with intracranial lesions and head injury.
- Severe cardiac disease
- Pheochromocytoma (as it sensitizes myocardium to adrenaline).

Drug Interactions

- β-blockers and calcium-channel blockers can produce severe depression of cardiac function with halothane.
- Aminophylline can produce serious ventricular arrhythmias with halothane.
- All cytochrome P450 enzyme inducers enhance its metabolism.

ISOFLURANE

It is fluorinated methylethyl ether. It is an isomer of enflurane.

Physical Properties

- *Pungent ethereal odor therefore induction is unpleasant.*
- Vapor pressure is similar to halothane (240 mm Hg).

Anesthetic Properties

It is the agent with moderate potency (MAC 1.15) and moderate induction and recovery time (B/G coefficient 1.38), therefore *inhalational agent of choice for experimental studies*

Systemic Effects

Cardiovascular system: *Hypotension is maximum with isoflurane* (It is the inhalational agent of choice for *controlled hypotension*), however, at the same time, minimally depress myocardium, does not cause bradycardia and baroreceptor reflex is preserved, therefore, *cardiac output is best maintained among all inhalational agents* making *Isoflurane as inhalational agent of choice for cardiac patients* except for myocardial ischemia patients. In MI patients, it can cause *coronary steal* however, coronary steal is just a theoretical phenomenon and Isoflurane can be used in MI patients, if necessary. It does not sensitize myocardium to adrenaline.

Cerebral: Decrease in cerebral metabolic rate, brain's oxygen consumption and not very significant rise in ICT makes Isoflurane as 2nd best choice for neurosurgical procedures.

Liver: Isoflurane on metabolism produces trifluroacetic acid, therefore theoretically can produce hepatitis, however, the amount of trifluoroacetic produced is too minimal to initiate the production of antibodies.

Indications

It is the agent of choice for cardiac patients.

NEWER AGENTS

DESFLURANE

It is the isomer of Isoflurane (chlorine atom replaced by fluorine atom), means it is also an etheral product

Physical Properties

- As it is an ethereal product therefore has pungent odor and unpleasant induction.
- *Vapor pressure is very high* (681 mm Hg) and boiling point is less than 23°C, therefore can boils at room temperature and that is why a

special vaporizer (TEC 6) which is *temperature and pressure compensated* is required for its delivery.

Anesthetic Properties

- Because of the lowest blood gas coefficient (0.42) its *induction and recovery is most rapid* among the agents used nowadays.
- Potency is low (MAC—6%).
- Unpleasant induction may manifests as coughing, breath-holding or laryngospasm.
- Produces *maximum muscle relaxation among the agents used nowadays*.
- Very low fat/gas coefficient therefore excellent for obese patients.

Systemic Effects

Cardiovascular system: As it is an isomer of Isoflurane, therefore at concentrations less than 1 MAC (<6%) its actions are similar to isoflurane with an added advantage that it does not causes coronary steal however, at *concentrations more than 1 MAC (>6%)* (particularly, if this concentration is achieved rapidly) *it stimulate sympathetic system* .

Metabolism

Undergoes *minimal metabolism* (<0.02%), therefore does not produce any fluoride.

Uses

- Because of minimal metabolism *Desflurane is the agent of choice for*:
  - *Prolonged duration surgeries* (no risk of accumulation of any metabolites in spite of prolonged exposure)
  - *Old age* patients who may have impaired hepatic or renal functions
  - *Renal diseases* (does not produce fluoride)
  - *Obese patients*: Least fat/gas coefficient and least metabolism (In obese patients, the metabolism of inhalational agents may be increased by 30–40%)
  - An excellent alternative to Sevoflurane for hepatic patients
- Because of fast recovery, it is inhalational *agent of choice for day care surgery*.
- Because of stimulation of sympathetic system at conc. >6%, it is inhalational *agent of choice for shock patients*.

SEVOFLURANE

Physical Properties

Sweet odor.

Anesthetic Properties

Faster (B/G coefficient 0.69), *pleasant and smooth induction* makes *sevoflurane as an agent of choice for induction in children*.

Systemic Effects

Cardiovascular system: Cardiac output is moderately decreased.

Respiration: Effects similar to other agents, i.e. depresses respiration and blunts ventilatory responses.

Excellent bronchodilatation makes *Sevoflurane as the inhalational agent of choice for asthmatics in present day practice*.

Cerebral:
- Minimum increase in ICT, significant reduction in cerebral metabolic rate and smoother recovery makes *sevoflurane as an inhalational agent of choice for neurosurgery in current day anesthetic practice*.
- Although incidence is very low but *sevoflurane can produce convulsions* (usually at higher concentrations).

Hepatic: It decreases portal blood flow but at the same time, increases hepatic artery blood flow therefore *hepatic blood flow is best maintained*. Does not produce trifluoroacetic acid, therefore, cannot cause immunologic hepatitis. These properties make *Sevoflurane as an inhalational agent of choice for hepatic patients*.

Renal: The clearance of Sevoflurane is so rapid that in spite of producing high fluoride nephrotoxicity has not been reported, however, if the renal functions are compromised, it can cause nephrotoxicity making *sevoflurane* unsuitable for renal patients.

Disadvantages

- *With sodalime and Barylime (Barylime > Sodalime)*, it can produce an olefin called as *compound A*, which can cause nephrotoxicity. The methods to decrease the production of compound A are:

– Use fresh gas flow > 2 liters/min.
– Use Amsorb or lithium containing CO_2 absorbents
- *With desiccated sodalime*, it produces hydrogen fluoride which can cause *burns of respiratory tract.*
- *Sevoflurane with Barylime can produce fire and explosions in breathing circuits*
- Although very rare but can cause *Convulsions.*
- Produces high fluoride.

AGENTS NO MORE IN CLINICAL USE

These agents are no more used in clinical practice therefore details are not required. Only the very important salient features need to be noted.

ENFLURANE

Has been recently obsoleted due to the following reasons:
- *Highly epileptogenic*
- Systemic side effects, i.e. decrease in cardiac output, respiratory depression and increase in intracranial pressure was significant
- Due to slow excretion fluoride may accumulate in renal tubules to cause nephrotoxicity.

ETHER

First public demonstration of ether was given by WTG Morton on 16th October 1846 for the removal of jaw tumor.

Ether is the unique agent with certain advantages and disadvantages.

Advantages of Ether

- It is *very cheap* (almost 800–1000 times cheaper than sevoflurane and desflurane).
- The *only anesthetic till date which can be considered complete*, i.e. has all three basic properties of anesthesia, viz. narcosis, analgesia and muscle relaxation.
- *Safest inhalational anesthetic*: Does not produce any cardiac or respiratory depression, the *only agent which preserves ciliary activity.*
- Can be given by open drop method.
- High safety profile, all anesthetic properties, use without equipment (open drop method) and low cost make ether not only the agent of choice for remote locations (like wars and disasters) and with less experienced hands but also the agent which is *most near to ideal.*

Disadvantages

- *High inflammable and explosive:* There have been death reports following burns by ether.
- Pungent smelling therefore *induction and recovery is very unpleasant.*
- Can be easily decomposed by light and heat, therefore, stored in dark color bottles wrapped in black paper.
- By increasing tracheobronchial secretions it can induce laryngospasm.
- *Very high incidence of nausea and vomiting,* in postoperative period.

■ **Table 10.4:** Summary of anesthetic properties of inhalational agents

Agent	Induction		Analgesia	Muscle relaxation	Amnesia
	Onset	Smoothness			
Halothane	Intermediate	Very smooth	+ / 0	++	+++
Isoflurane	Intermediate	Slightly irritable	+/0	++	+++
Nitrous oxide	Fast	Not used for induction	+++	–	+ / 0
Xenon	Fastest	Not used for induction	+++	–	+/0
Sevoflurane	Fast	Very smooth	+/0	++	+++
Desflurane	Fast	Slightly irritable	+/0	+++	+++
Ether	Slow	Highly irritable	+++	+++	+++

■ **Table 10.5:** Summary of systemic effects of inhalational agents

| | Cardiovascular system | | Central nervous system | | | Respiratory system | | Hepatotoxicity | Nephrotoxicity |
	Heart rate	Mean arterial pressure	CMO_2	CBF	ICT	Ventilation	Bronchial muscles dilatation		
Halothane	↓	↓↓	↓	↑↑	↑↑	↓	+++	+++	-
Isoflurane	↑ (reflex)	↓↓↓	↓↓	↑↑	↑↑	↓	++	-	-
Enflurane	↓	↓↓↓	↓	↑↑↑	↑↑↑	↓	+	-	++
Nitrous oxide	0	0	0/↑	↑	↑	↓	+/0	-	-
Xenon	0	0	0	0	0	0	Bronchoconstriction	-	-
Sevoflurane	↓	↓	↓↓	↑	↑	↓	+++	-	+/-
Desflurane	↑	↓↓ (<6%), (>6%) ↑↑	↓	↑↑	↑↑	↓	+	-	-
Ether	↑	↑	↓↓	↑↑	↑↑↑	↑	++	-	-

- = no effect
0 = negligible effect
↓ = decrease
↑ = increase
+ = minimum
++ = moderate
+++ = maximum

CMO_2 = Oxygen consumption of brain tissue
CBF = Cerebral blood flow
ICT = Intracranial tension

METHOXYFLURANE

- *Overall most potent (MAC 0.16%) and slowest induction and recovery (blood gas coefficient 15)*
- Highly soluble in rubber tubing of closed circuit.
- Undergoes maximum metabolism yielding highest concentration of fluoride (F^-) producing *vasopressin-resistant high output (polyuric) renal failure.*

CYCLOPROPANE

- Highly *inflammable and explosive.*
- Used to be stored in orange color cylinders at a pressure of 75 psi.

TRICHLOROETHYLENE (TRILENE)

- *Most potent analgesic among inhalational agents,* therefore was popular in past for labor analgesia.
- It can react with sodalime producing *dichloroacetylene* which is *neurotoxic* effecting cranial nerves (*most commonly involved are V and VII*) and *phosgene* gas which can cause ARDS.

CHLOROFORM

Number of *cardiac arrest and death has been reported due to ventricular fibrillation.*

For summary of anesthetic properties and systemic effects see **Tables 10.4 and 10.5** respectively.

KEY POINTS

- Inhalational agents are mainly used in anesthesia for maintenance.
- The major changed happened in mechanism of action of inhalational agents is shifting of mechanism from lipid sites to protein sites.
- Best estimate for determining the potency of inhalational agent is minimum alveolar concentration (MAC). Halothane is the most potent while nitrous oxide is the least potent among the agents used nowadays.
- Blood gas partition coefficient indicates induction and recovery. Among the agents used nowadays induction is fastest with desflurane and slowest with Halothane.
- All inhalational in current use decreases cardiac output and depresses respiration.
- Halothane (and theoretically other agents too except Isoflurane) can sensitize myocardium to adrenaline, exogenous to heart.
- Direct hepatocellular damage is seen with halothane (and theoretically with Isoflurane and Desflurane) but not with sevoflurane.
- Inflammable agents used in past were Ether and Cyclopropane.
- Sevoflurane can produce Compound A with sodalime and Barylime.
- Desflurane (and other agents too) can produce Carbonmonoxide by reacting with desiccated sodalime and Barylime.
- Sevoflurane by reacting with desiccated sodalime and barylime can cause burns of respiratory mucosa.
- 35 times more solubility of nitrous oxide than nitrogen makes it absolutely contraindicated in pneumothorax, pneumopericardium, pneumoperitoneum and pneumoencephalus.
- Nitrous oxide can deplete ozone layer and produce global warming.
- Immunologic mechanism of halothane hepatitis warrants to avoid frequent use of halothane; at least an interval of 3 months is mandatory between two exposures.
- Isoflurane is the agent of choice for cardiac patients.
- In the current day practice Sevoflurane is preferred over Isoflurane for neurosurgery.
- Desflurane is agent of choice for prolonged surgeries, old age, renal diseases, obesity, day care surgery and shock.
- Sevoflurane is the agent of choice for induction in children.
- Sevoflurane is the agent of choice for hepatic patients.
- At higher concentrations, sevoflurane can produce convulsions.
- Enflurane was highly epileptogenic.
- Ether is safest, cheapest and only complete anesthetic while on flip side, it is highly inflammable and explosive and induction and recovery are very unpleasant.
- Methoxyflurane can produce vasopressin resistant polyuric renal failure.
- Trielene by reacting with sodalime can produce dichloroacetylene (craniotoxic) and phosgene (ARDS).

CHAPTER 11

Gases Used in Anesthesia

OXYGEN

It was first synthesized by Priestley.

Preparation

Medical oxygen is prepared by fractional distillation of air.

Oxygen concentrators: These are portable devices which can produce oxygen from ambient air by selective absorption of nitrogen on zeolites. Oxygen concentrators are suitable for use in hospitals, home or at remote locations like Warfield.

Storage

- Medical oxygen is stored in cylinders with black body and white shoulders at a pressure of 2,000 psi (pounds per square inch).
- Also stored as liquid oxygen.

Physical Properties

- It is colorless, odorless.
- Specific gravity is 1105 (air: 1000).
- Critical temperature is –119°C therefore liquid oxygen should be stored below –119°C (to keep any gas in liquefied state it has to kept below its critical temperature).
- It supports fire.

Oxygen Delivery Devices

Refer to Chapter 3, page no. 42.

OXYGEN DEFICIENCY (HYPOXIA)

Body Stores of Oxygen

Theoretically it is 1,500 mL, bound to hemoglobin, dissolved fraction and in lungs as functional residual capacity (FRC). Among these only available oxygen is from lungs, i.e. FRC which practically is the only store in body which lasts only for 2–3 minutes.

Classification

- Hypoxic hypoxia: *This is the most common type of hypoxia seen during anesthesia*
- Anemic hypoxia.
- Stagnant hypoxia.
- Histotoxic hypoxia.

Causes of Hypoxia in Anesthesia

For causes of hypoxia see Chapter 14, page no. 136.

Systemic Effects of Hypoxia

- At oxygen saturation (SpO_2) of >80% hypoxia stimulates sympathetic system causing tachycardia, hypertension and increased cardiac output to compensate.
- At SpO_2 60–80% hypoxia causes vasodilatation which causes reflex tachycardia and cardiac output is maintained.
- At SpO_2 <60%, hypoxia is direct cardiac depressant and can produce bradyarrhythmia or even cardiac arrest.

The clinical presentation of hypoxia is *cyanosis* which is produced if *reduced Hb level is more than 5 g/dL* (which roughly corresponds to O_2 saturation <85% or pO_2 < 50 mm Hg), *methemoglobin >1.5 g/dL and Sulfhemoglobin >0.5 g/dL.*

Treatment of Hypoxia

- *Oxygen therapy: Hypoxic hypoxia responds best to oxygen therapy* while there is no benefit to oxygen therapy in histotoxic hypoxia and right to left shunts. In anemic and stagnant hypoxia oxygen therapy does not increase the amount of oxygen carried by the hemoglobin but there occurs rise in dissolved fraction.

If not treated by simple oxygen therapy patient may require mechanical ventilation

- Treat the cause.

EXCESSIVE OXYGEN (OXYGEN TOXICITY)
Systemic Effects of Excessive Oxygen
Pulmonary Toxicity

Prolonged high concentrations can cause pulmonary toxicity. 100% oxygen is usually considered safe up to 8–12 hours in normal adults (in infants and neonates 100% oxygen for more than 2–3 hours can cause pulmonary toxicity). *Pulmonary toxicity depends on alveolar concentration (not on arterial concentration).*

Pathophysiology: Oxygen toxicity occurs because of toxic radicals of oxygen like superoxide and hydroxyl ions, singlet oxygen, hydrogen peroxide. These radicals damage the capillary membrane increasing capillary permeability and *ARDS* like picture. Abnormality in *ciliary transport, absorption atelectasis and tracheobronchitis* are other features of oxygen toxicity. In *neonates* pulmonary toxicity manifests as *bronchopulmonary dysplasia*.

Retrolental Fibroplasia

This is dependent on arterial oxygen concentration. Premature neonates (< 36 weeks) are at greatest risk.

Cerebral Effects

Acute oxygen toxicity may manifest as convulsions.

HYPERBARIC OXYGEN

It means delivering the oxygen above atmospheric pressure {> 760 mm Hg (or > 1 atmosphere (atm.))}. It is delivered by special hyperbaric chambers which are very expensive.

Uses

Theoretically there are many indications for hyperbaric oxygen therapy but practically its use is only restricted to decompression sickness and severe cases of carbon monoxide poisoning.

- *Poisonings:*
  - Carbon monoxide poisoning (half-life of CO at 1 atm. is 214 minutes which can be reduced to 19 minutes at 2.5 atm.). In current day practice its use is reserved only for severe cases, mild-to-moderate cases should be managed by 100% Normobaric oxygen.
  - Cyanide poisoning.
- *Gas bubble diseases:*
  - Decompression sickness.
  - Air embolism.
- *Ischemia:*
  - Crush injuries.
  - Ischemic ulcers.
  - Radiation necrosis.
- *Infections:*
  - Clostridial.
  - Mucormycosis.
  - Refractory osteomyelitis.
- *Others:*
  - Oxygen support during lung lavage.
  - Burns.
  - Cerebral edema.

Hyperbaric Oxygen Toxicity
- *Pulmonary:* ARDS.
- *CNS:* Seizures preceded by facial numbness, twitching, unpleasant olfactory or gustatory sensations. Convulsions occurring after hyperbaric oxygen therapy is called as *Paul Bert effect. Paul Bert effect is usually seen if the pressure used is > 3 atm.*
- *Eye:* Myopia, nuclear cataract and retrolental fibroplasia (in neonates).
- Avascular necrosis of bone.
- Barotrauma.

Safe Levels of Hyperbaric Oxygen and Therapy Schedule

Toxicity depends on three factors:
1. Pressure
2. Time of exposure
3. Oxygen concentration.

Pulmonary effects can be seen at 2 atm. while CNS symptoms manifest above 2 atm.

Hyperbaric chambers may use 100% oxygen or air

- Patients with chronic diseases are usually given 2 hours at 2 atm. once a day.

- Patients with decompression sickness are given 100% oxygen at 2.8 atm. followed by 1.9 atm. interspersed by periods of 5–15 minutes of air breathing.
- Gas embolism patients can be given, air at 6 atm. followed by 100% oxygen at 2.8 and 1.9 atm.

The exact safe levels of hyperbaric oxygen are not defined however *not more than 2.8 atm. should be used with 100% oxygen in chamber and not more than 6 atm. with air (21% O_2) in chamber.* One therapy schedule at a time should be *less than 2 hours.*

NITROUS OXIDE, ENTONOX AND XENON
Already described in Chapter 10.

NITRIC OXIDE
Nitric oxide is the major vasodilatory compound produced in pulmonary and systemic endothelium during the conversion of L-arginine to L-citrulline by nitric oxide synthase. It produces vasodilatation through cGMP.

Because of this pulmonary vasodilatory property inhaled nitric oxide is used for diagnosis and treatment of primary pulmonary hypertension or secondary pulmonary hypertension associated with ARDS (*also see Chapter 40, page no. 292*).

AIR
- Medical air is usually supplied through central supply at a pressure of 60 psi, however it is also available in grey cylinders with black and white shoulders at a pressure of 2,000 psi.
- It can be used as respired gas (as a replacement to nitrous oxide) or as a gas to drive pneumatic devices like ventilators.

CARBON DIOXIDE
In past CO_2 (5%) was used to hasten recovery at the emergence, for glottis opening for blind intubation and for the treatment of postspinal headache however in current day practice it is not used in anesthesia. Currently, it is used only on surgical side for gas insufflation for laparoscopic surgeries and cryosurgeries.

It is stored in grey color cylinders at a pressure of 750 psi.

HELIUM/HELIOX
Helium, mixed with oxygen (79% helium + 21% oxygen) is available as heliox. Heliox is stored in black color cylinders (representing oxygen) with brown and white shoulders (brown representing helium, helium is stored in brown cylinders) at a pressure of 2000 psi.

The most important characteristic of helium is its low density (specific gravity of helium is 341 while that of air is 1,000).

High density of air causes flow to become turbulent in upper airways like trachea and main bronchi producing *maximum resistance to airflow*. If oxygen is mixed with helium (Heliox), the density of gas mixture decreases, decreasing the turbulence and hence resistance to airflow enabling the oxygen to pass even through narrow orifices. Therefore, heliox is used for:

- *Upper airway obstruction* due to any reason like tracheal or bronchial stenosis or foreign body
- Microlaryngeal surgeries to decrease the resistance as small size endotracheal tubes are used.

CHAPTER 12

Intravenous Anesthetics

CLASSIFICATION

Barbiturates
- Thiopentone
- Methohexitone

Nonbarbiturates
- Ketamine
- Propofol
- Etomidate
- Opioids
- Benzodiazepines
- Phenothiazines

Intravenous anesthetics are used in anesthesia for:

1. *Induction: Most commonly used intravenous (IV) anesthetic for induction is propofol.* Indications for induction with thiopentone in present day anesthesia are very limited. Ketamine is used only in specific situations. Since opioids and benzodiazepines are required in very high doses for induction therefore they are seldom used for this purpose.
2. For analgesia (largely opioids).
3. As a sole anesthetic agent for minor procedures, e.g. ketamine or propofol + fentanyl.
4. For amnesia (mainly benzodiazepines).
5. To blunt cardiovascular response to intubation (opioids).
6. For sedation (mainly benzodiazepines).

BARBITURATES

THIOPENTONE

Thiopentone was the first intravenous anesthetic used in clinical practice by Water and Lundy in 1934. It is an ultra short-acting barbiturate. Chemically it is sodium ethyl thiobarbiturate.

Physical and Chemical Properties

- Available as yellow amorphous powder as 0.5 g and 1.0 g vial to which 20 mL of sterile water for injection is added yielding a concentration of 2.5% and 5% respectively (5% solution is further diluted to make it 2.5% solution). The solution is not stable and should be used within 48 hours (but can be used for 1 week if refrigerated or till precipitate appears). It *should not be prepared with ringer lactate* otherwise it will get precipitated due to acidic pH of ringer lactate solution.
- It is sulfur analog of pentobarbitone. *Sulfur is added to increase the lipid solubility.*
- The ultrashort duration of thiopentone is because of methyl group added to it.
- It is available as *sodium salt* to make it water soluble but this increases the alkalinity of solution. pH of sodium thiopentone (2.5%) solution is *10.4 (highly alkaline).*
- 6% anhydrous sodium carbonate is added to powder to prevent the formation of free acid by carbon dioxide from atmosphere.
- It is prepared in the atmosphere of nitrogen.

Anesthetic Properties and Pharmacokinetics

Unconsciousness is produced in one arm brain circulation time, i.e. 15 seconds and induction is largely smooth (however sometimes may be associated with initial excitatory responses).

The *elimination half-life of thiopentone is 10.4 hours* but consciousness is regained after 15–20 minutes because of *redistribution* which means that drug is redistributed from brain to tissues with less vascularity like muscle or fat however repeated doses saturates these tissues and regaining of consciousness after repeated doses depends on metabolism and elimination.

At induction it causes *mild hypokalemia.*

Protein binding: In blood 80–90% of thiopentone is bound to plasma proteins, mainly to albumin.

Metabolism: Thiopentone is metabolized in liver and metabolic products are eliminated through kidneys.

Mechanism of action: It inhibits the function of synapses. Thiopentone (and other barbiturates also) mediates their action through gamma-aminobutyric acid (GABA) receptor (GABA-A subtype) increasing the membrane conductance to chloride ion causing hyperpolarization of membrane. At higher doses it also produces GABA-mimetic action.

The second mechanism of action is the inhibition of the synaptic transmission of excitatory neurotransmitters like acetylcholine and glutamate.

Systemic Effects

Central nervous system
- Unconscious is produced in 15 seconds however the maximum depth is achieved in 60 seconds.
- *Sleep:* It increases stage 2 and decreases stage 3, 4 and rapid eye movement (REM) sleep.
- Cerebral oxygen consumption (CMO_2), cerebral metabolic rate (CMR) and intracranial tension (ICT) are decreased. Therefore, *Thiopentone can be utilized for cerebral protection in case of focal ischemia.* It does not offer any protection in global ischemia seen in cardiac arrest.
- *Anticonvulsant action:* Because of phenyl group, Thiopentone is very potent *anticonvulsant.* In fact, convulsions not responding to other anticonvulsants are controlled with thiopentone.
- *Antanalgesic action:* At subanesthetic doses it acts as *antanalgesic.*
- *Acute tolerance:* Tolerance is seen if initial dose is high.
- In low concentrations it is used for *narcoanalysis*

Cardiovascular system
- It causes *hypotension* which is not only because of central mechanism but also because of direct depression of vasomotor center.
- At high doses it can cause direct myocardial depression.
- Increase in heart rate (10–30%) occurs as compensation to hypotension.

Respiratory system
- If a painful stimulus is given at inadequate depth, severe *laryngospasm* and bronchospasm may occur.
- *Transient apnea* is common after thiopentone. It usually requires no treatment however if gets prolonged (> 25 seconds), gentle intermittent positive pressure ventilation (IPPV) with bag and mask should be given.
- At higher dosage thiopentone depresses respiration after brief recovery from transient apnea, therefore also termed as *double apnea.*

Eye: Thiopentone decreases the intraocular pressure.

Pregnancy: Thiopentone crosses the placenta readily and the *equilibrium with maternal circulation is achieved within 3–5 minutes.*

Thyroid: Thiopentone has got *anti-thyroid* property.

Dose and Recovery

Dose of thiopentone is *5 mg/kg* body weight; Males requiring more than females, obese more than thin and young more than old. Although consciousness is regained after 15 minutes due to redistribution, the drug is eliminated after 10–12 hours (t½ 10.4 hours) therefore patients should not be allowed to carry out important work like driving for next *24 hours.*

Complications

General
- Respiratory depression.
- Cardiovascular depression.
- Laryngospasm and bronchospasm.
- Hiccups and coughing.
- Allergic manifestations which may vary from cutaneous rash, pruritus to severe anaphylaxis.
- Postoperative disorientation, vertigo, euphoria (delirium).

- Some patients complain of onion or garlic taste.

Local

Thiopentone's *high alkalinity* is responsible for local complications.

A. *Perivenous (subcutaneous) and intramuscular injection:* This is commonly seen if thiopentone is injected directly by hypodermic needle or scalp vein set. The high alkalinity leads to *tissue necrosis* and ulceration.
   - Treatment
     - ◆ *Preventive*
       - Always use 2.5% solution.
       - Inject slowly in incremental doses.
       - If patient complains of any pain immediately stop further injection.
     - ◆ *Curative:* 10 mL of 1% lignocaine with 100 units of hyaluronidase to be injected in that area.

B. *Intra-arterial injection:* This is a dreadful complication which can lead to gangrene and loss of limb if not diagnosed and managed timely. *This complication usually occurs if thiopentone is injected in antecubital vein* because in 10% of the cases brachial artery divides above elbow giving a very superficial abnormal ulnar artery which lies just deep to antecubital vein.
   Symptomatology: With injection patient complains of *severe burning pain down the injection site* which is followed by pallor, cyanosis, edema and finally gangrene of limb.
   Pathophysiology: Because of its high alkalinity the thiopentone gets precipitated in acidic pH of blood forming crystals which can cause endothelial damage precipitating *vasospasm* and *thrombus* formation blocking microcirculation. Both these processes can lead to ischemia and gangrene of limb.
   - Management
     - ◆ *Preventive*:
       - Always use 2.5% solution.
       - Inject very slowly and in incremental doses.
       - Avoid thiopentone injection at antecubital fossa (best site to inject thiopentone is dorsum of hand).
     - ◆ *Curative*:
       - *Leave the needle at site*: All therapeutic injections are to be given through this needle.
       - Start dilution with normal saline
       - Inject heparin to prevent the thrombus formation.
       - Inject local vasodilators like papaverine, alpha blockers or 1% lignocaine.
       - *Stellate ganglion block*—will relieve the vasospasm by blocking sympathetic supply of limb.
       - Continue oral anticoagulants for 1–2 weeks.
       - Defer the elective surgery.

C. *Thrombophlebitis*: Due to chemical irritation produced by alkaline solution.

D. *Injury to median nerve*: If the solution is directly injected into nerve.

Contraindications

Absolute:

- *Porphyria*: Thiopentone induces enzyme aminolevulinic acid synthetase which stimulates the formation of porphyrin in susceptible individuals. Therefore, absolutely contraindicated in *acute intermittent* and *variegate porphyria* (can be used safely in porphyria cutanea tarda).
- History of previous anaphylaxis to thiopentone.

Relative:

- As thiopentone decreases the cardiac output therefore should be avoided in shock, hypotension, fixed cardiac output lesions, heart blocks or patient on β blockers.
- *Asthmatics*: Thiopentone can precipitate bronchospasm.
- *Familial hypokalemic periodic paralysis*: It can cause severe hypokalemia in these cases.
- *Hepatic disease*: Only severe hepatic involvement contraindicates its use.
- *Renal disease*: Doses should be reduced.

METHOHEXITONE

- The most striking difference between methohexitone and Thiopentone is that methohexitone is epileptogenic while thiopentone is anticonvulsant making it as an *agent of choice for electroconvulsive therapy (ECT)*.
- Histamine release is less as compared to Thiopentone therefore preferred barbiturate for asthma patients.
- Half-life is short (3–4 hours)

NONBARBITURATES

PROPOFOL

Long half-life and delayed recovery is the main reason for which thiopentone has been almost completely replaced by propofol.

Physical and Chemical Properties

- It consists of a phenol ring with isopropyl group attached deriving it chemical name as 2,6 di-isopropylphenol.
- Propofol is available as 1% and 2% *milky white* solution prepared in soyabean oil making the injection painful. Therefore injection of propofol should be preceded or mixed with lignocaine. *Fospropofol* is a water-based preparation but not widely available.
- Propofol contains egg lecithin and glycerol. As egg is a good media for bacterial growth, chances of contamination of opened vial are very high. In fact, there have been death reports following the use of contaminated solution of propofol. Although the recent formulations of propofol contains antimicrobial agents like disodium edetate or sodium metabisulfite but they also does not guarantee immunity against contamination therefore after opening *it is mandatory to discard the Propofol vial within 6 hours.*

Mechanism of action: It not only act through GABA-A but also inhibit glycine receptors.

Pharmacokinetics:
Induction is achieved in one arm brain circulation time, i.e. 15 seconds. Consciousness is regained after 2–8 minutes due to *rapid redistribution.* Elimination half-life is *2-4 hours*; recovery is rapid and associated with less hangover than thiopentone.

Dose: 2 mg/kg.

Metabolism

Mainly metabolized in liver but significant (30%) *extrahepatic metabolism* also occurs in kidneys. A part of Propofol is also metabolized in lungs. Clearance rate is 10 times more rapid than thiopentone therefore recovery is rapid. All metabolic products of propofol are *inactive.*

Systemic Effects

Cardiovascular system: Hypotension produced is significant and it also impairs baroreceptor response to hypotension.

Respiratory system:
- Incidence of apnea is higher (25–30%) than thiopentone. Respiratory depression is more severe and prolonged than thiopentone.
- Propofol induces bronchodilatation is COPD patients.
- Depression of upper airway reflexes is more than thiopentone and therefore it is preferred for surgeries done under laryngeal mask airway without muscle relaxants.

Cerebral: Like thiopentone it also decreases the metabolic rate of brain and intracranial tension however neuroapoptosis seen in animal models precludes its use for cerebral protection. It is reliable amnestic.

Propofol possess anticonvulsant property and has even been used to treat convulsions. However on the other hand there had been few case reports of grand mal epilepsy being reported with propofol.

Eye: Reduces intraocular pressure significantly (30–40%)

GIT: By decreasing the central serotonin release propofol acts as a potent *antiemetic* agent (even more effective than ondansetron for postoperative nausea and vomiting)

Immunologic: It is *antipruritic* (can be used for the treatment of cholestatic pruritus).
- It has no antanalgesic property.
- It is not a muscle relaxant.

Uses

1. Because of its shorter half life it is the agent of choice for induction.
2. Because of its early and smooth recovery, inactive metabolites and antiemetic effects it is the *IV agent of choice for day care surgery.*
3. Along with opioids (Remifentanil) propofol is the *agent of choice for total intravenous anesthesia (TIVA).*
4. Propofol infusion can be used to produce sedation in ICU.
5. It is the agent of choice for induction in susceptible individuals for *malignant hyperthermia.*

Advantages of Propofol over Thiopentone

- Rapid and smooth recovery.
- Completely eliminated from body in 4 hours therefore patient is ambulatory early.
- *Antiemetic.*
- Antipruritic.
- Bronchodilator.

Disadvantages

- Apnea is more profound and longer.
- Hypotension is more severe.
- Injection is *painful.*
- Solution is less stable (6 hours).
- Chances of sepsis with contaminated solution are high.
- Myoclonic activity may occur.
- Sexual fantasies and hallucinations are additional side effects.
- Expensive than thiopentone.
- Because of maximum inhibition of airway reflexes there are increased chances of aspiration in high risk cases.
- As propofol increases the dopamine concentration in brain its addiction has been reported.
- *Propofol infusion syndrome:* It is rare but is a lethal complication. It is usually seen if propofol infusion is continued for more than 48 hours. It is more common in children. It occurs because of the failure of free fatty acid metabolism caused by propofol. It is associated with severe metabolic acidosis *(lactic acidosis)* acute cardiac failure, cardiomyopathy, skeletal myopathy, hyperkalemia, *lipemia* and hepatomegaly.

Contraindications

- *Obstetrics:* Contrary to the previous recommendations of not using propofol in pregnant patients newer studies have shown that at the doses used for induction *Propofol does not affect the APGAR therefore can be safely used in pregnancy.*
- *Lactation:* The amount secreted in breast milk is too low that Propofol can be safely used during breastfeeding.
- *Children less than 3 years:* Contrary to the previous recommendations of not using propofol in children less than 3 years, in current day practice it can be safely used in children

of any age. However, because of increased possibility of propofol infusion syndrome in children it not recommended for long-term infusion in children less than 16 years.
- *Patient with egg allergy:* Since egg allergy is almost always from egg white (albumin) not from lecithin (which is prepared from yoke), *history of egg allergy is not a contraindication for propofol.* However, it is advisable to not use propofol in patients with history of anaphylaxis to egg.
- *Patients with soy allergy:* Like egg allergy patients with soy allergy can safely receive propofol.

ETOMIDATE

- Chemically it is an imidazole derivative.
- It also acts through GABA.

Advantages

- It is most *cardiovascular stable* among all IV agents.
- Minimal respiratory depression.
- No histamine release.
- It decreases the ICT by almost 50% in patients who have elevated ICT therefore can be used to reduce ICT.

Side Effects (Disadvantages)

- *Adrenocortical suppression* on long-term infusion. Single use only causes temporary adrenocortical suppression which recovers with vitamin C supplementation.
- *Nausea and vomiting: Incidence is 40% which is highest among all intravenous anesthetics.*
- High incidence of *myoclonus* (30–60%).
- Injection is painful.
- High incidence of *thrombophlebitis.*
- It can cause *vitamin C deficiency.*
- Hiccups are common.
- May cause inhibition of platelet function.
- No analgesia.
- It is only porphyrinogenic in rats not in humans therefore *can be safely used in porphyrias in human beings.*

Uses

Etomidate is the intravenous anesthetic of choice for aneurysm surgery and patients with cardiac disease.

BENZODIAZEPINES

Benzodiazepines (BZs) are used in anesthesia for:

1. *Premedication:* To reduce anxiety.
2. *Amnesia:* Amnesia produced by BZs is anterograde.
3. As a sole agent to non-painful procedures like bronchoscopy, gastroscopy under local analgesia (BZs elevates the seizure threshold of local anesthetics).
4. *As induction agent:* Rarely used.
5. To prevent hallucinations by ketamine.
6. To control convulsions.

Pharmacokinetics

See **Table 12.1.**

Mechanism of Action

Benzodiazepines mediates their action through GABA receptor (GABA-A subtype) increasing the membrane conductance to chloride ion causing hyperpolarization of membrane (GABA facilitatory).

Systemic Effects

CNS: *Mainly acts on reticular activating system* (RAS) and amygdala (limbic system) producing *sedation, anxiolysis* and *amnesia.* They also act on medulla producing muscle relaxation and on cerebellum producing ataxia.

- BZ's are *anticonvulsants.*
- They are *not analgesics.*
- Produce *muscle relaxation* by acting at medullary and spinal cord level (central action).
- Reduces cerebral metabolic rate, brain oxygen consumption and intracranial pressure.
- Initial regain of consciousness seen after 10–15 minutes is due to redistribution.

Effects on sleep: Increases stage 2, decreases stage 3, 4 and REM sleep duration but effects on REM are less marked than barbiturates. *Nitrazepam even prolongs REM.* At higher dose BZs can produce loss of consciousness.

Respiratory system: At higher dose BZs cause respiratory depression which can be significant in old age and children. Very high dose can *cause death due to respiratory depression.*

Cardiovascular system: Minimal reduction in blood pressure, heart rate and cardiac output.

Metabolism

The BZs are metabolized in liver. The major active metabolite of diazepam is desmethyl diazepam. Metabolites are excreted in gut and urine. There is significant enterohepatic circulation.

Diazepam and lorazepam: Hardly used in intraoperative period because of the following reasons:

- Preparation is oil based therefore injection is painful.
- Sleep is not smooth (incidence of dysphoria is highest with diazepam).
- Elimination half-lives are prolonged therefore chances of postoperative respiratory depression are there.

Midazolam: It is 3 times more potent than diazepam. In current day practice *Midazolam is the only BZ used in intraoperative period.*

The *advantages* over diazepam and lorazepam are:

- Water based preparation so injection is painless.
- *Elimination half-life is 2–3 hours* avoiding the risk of respiratory depression in postoperative period.
- Because of shorter half-life midazolam can be *safely used for day care procedures.*
- Reversal with flumazenil is complete (no re-sedation).

■ **Table 12.1:** Pharmacokinetics of commonly used benzodiazepines

	Diazepam	Midazolam	Lorazepam
Route of administration	Oral, IM, IV	Oral, IM, IV, rectal, nasal	Oral, IM, IV
Preparation (intravenous)	Oil based, injection is painful	Water base, painless injection	Oil based, injection is painful
Elimination half-life	30–60 hours	2–3 hours	15 hours

- Since midazolam can be given through oral, buccal, rectal and intranasal route (nasal spray) it can be utilized in pediatric population.

Benzodiazepine Antagonist (Flumazenil): It is a *competitive antagonist* at BZ receptors.

It *antagonizes hypnosis, respiratory depression and sedation but amnesia is minimally reversed (particularly at low doses of flumazenil).*

The *disadvantage* of flumazenil is its *short half-life (1–2 hours)* therefore there are chances of re-sedation with long acting agents like diazepam and lorazepam.

KETAMINE

Ketamine produces *dissociative anesthesia.*

It was synthesized by Stevens in 1962 and first used in humans by Domino and Corsen in 1965.

Physical and Chemical Properties

It is *phencyclidine derivative.* Available as solution of 10 mg/mL and 50 mg/mL. Contains preservative benzethonium chloride.

Anesthetic Properties and Pharmacokinetics

- Onset of action in 30–60 seconds.
- Early regain of consciousness after 15–20 minutes is because of redistribution.
- Elimination half-life is *2–3 hours.*
- Metabolized in liver to form norketamine and hydroxynorketamine which are one-third as potent as ketamine. Products are excreted in urine.

Site of Action

Primary site of action is *thalamo-neocortical projection.*

Ketamine *inhibits* cortex (unconsciousness) and thalamus (analgesia) and *stimulates* limbic system (emergence reaction and hallucinations). It also acts on medullary reticular formation and spinal cord.

Mechanism of action: The main mechanism by which ketamine exerts it effect is by inhibiting N methyl D aspartate (NMDA) receptors. Interaction through opioid (μ) receptors has also been postulated.

Systemic Effects

It produces dissociative anesthesia, a state which dissociates the individual from surroundings and himself, i.e. individual is in *cataleptic state.*

Central nervous system

- Increases brain oxygen consumption, metabolic rate and *intracranial tension.* However, on the other hand as a NMDA antagonist it offers neuroprotection. Therefore, it can be used safely in head injury patients who are mechanically ventilated (In mechanically ventilated patients hyperventilation can be instituted to negate the rise in ICT produced by ketamine).
- *Very potent analgesic*
- *Emergence reactions:* These are seen at emergence. The incidence is 10–30%; less incidence in children and old age. Emergence reactions include vivid dreaming, illusions, extracorporeal experiences like floating out of body, excitement, confusion, euphoria, fear.
- *Hallucinations:* It produces both auditory and visual hallucinations (mainly auditory). Incidence is *30–40%. Hallucination is the most common side effect of ketamine.*

  Hallucinations and emergence reactions can be *decreased by giving benzodiazepines* along with ketamine. Opioids, barbiturates, propofol and inhalational agents also decrease the incidence of emergence reactions and hallucinations.

Cardiovascular system

- Ketamine stimulates sympathetic system causing *tachycardia* and *hypertension* therefore is the *intravenous anesthetic of choice for shock.* However in debilitated patients in whom catecholamines have been depleted, ketamine can cause direct myocardial depression. Benzodiazepines attenuate this hemodynamic response (tachycardia, hypertension and increased oxygen demand of myocardium) of ketamine.
- Ketamine not only increases the systemic vascular resistance (SVR) but also increases pulmonary artery pressure.

Respiratory system
- At clinically used doses it maintains respiration however can cause respiratory depression at higher doses especially in children.
- It is such a *potent bronchodilator* that it can be used in the *treatment of refractory status asthmaticus* unresponsive to conventional therapy.
- *Pharyngeal and laryngeal reflexes are preserved* (but silent aspiration can still occur).
- *Tracheobronchial and salivary secretions are increased* producing laryngospasm. Therefore, use of atropine/glycopyrrolate is necessary with ketamine.

Eye: *Increases intraocular tension.* Pupils dilate moderately and there occurs nystagmus.

Gastrointestinal tract (GIT): *Increases intragastric pressure.* Salivary secretions are increased.

Muscular system: *Increases muscle tone.* Patient shows non-purposeful movements but interestingly a contradictory effect of ketamine is potentiation of effects of nondepolarizing muscle relaxants by unknown mechanism.

Dose

It can be given IV, IM, oral, nasal, per rectal and intrathecally. Dose is:
- Intravenous: *2 mg/kg.*
- Intramuscular: 5–10 mg/kg.

Advantages and Uses in Anesthesia

- Induction agent of choice for:
  - *Asthmatics*: Ketamine, in spite of potent bronchodilator is generally avoided due to its side effects (especially vivid reactions) and propensity to increase tracheobronchial secretions. The use of ketamine in present day practice is restricted to *patients in active asthma (wheezing) undergoing life-threatening emergency surgeries*
  - Shock (because it stimulates sympathetic system)
  - Alternative method to inhalational induction in children through intramuscular route.
  - Low cardiac output states like constrictive pericarditis or cardiac tamponade (because it increases cardiac output by stimulating sympathetic system).
  - Right to left shunt like tetralogy of Fallot (ketamine by causing hypertension increases the afterload thereby decreasing the right to left shunt fraction).
  - Can be used as *sole agent* for minor procedures (like incision and drainage), burn dressings.
  - Can be safely used at *remote places* and in inexperienced hands because it does not depress respiration and heart.
  - Preferred agent for patients with *full stomach* (pharyngeal and laryngeal reflexes are preserved).
  - Poor risk patients (ASA IV) (because of safety).
  - *Depressed patients:* They have better recovery after ketamine.

Considering the anesthetic properties *Ketamine can be considered as complete IV anesthetic.*

Disadvantages

- *Vivid reactions* in the form of *hallucinations, vivid dreaming* and *emergence reactions* are the major impedance to the widespread use of ketamine. Patients given ketamine can be found shouting, weeping, singing or even abusing badly in postoperative rooms.
- Increases muscle tone.
- Pharyngeal and respiratory secretions are increased which can cause laryngospasm.
- Increases myocardial oxygen demand.
- All pressures like intraocular, intragastric, intracranial are markedly raised.

Contraindications

- Head injury, as it increases intracranial tension (can be used in mechanically-ventilated patients)
- Ocular surgeries and glaucoma (it increases intraocular pressure).
- Ischemic heart disease (it increases myocardial oxygen demand).
- Vascular aneurysm (it causes hypertension).
- Patients with psychiatric diseases and drug addicts (higher incidence of hallucinations and emergence reactions).

- Hypertensives.
- Hyperthyroidism
- Pheochromocytoma.

S-enantiomer of Ketamine

It is considered superior to conventional ketamine (which is a mixture of S and R isomers) because it has lesser side effects, rapid recovery and better antiapoptotic effect. It is not available in India.

OPIOIDS

Uses in Anesthesia

- Mainly used for *analgesia* in intraoperative and postoperative period.
- Blunting reflex response to intubation.
- Producing sedation in ICU.
- Treatment of pulmonary edema (morphine is agent of choice).
- To abolish shivering (pethidine and tramadol).

Opioid Receptors

Opioids act through specific receptors which have been classified into 4 types: μ (mu), κ (kappa), δ (Delta) and nociceptin (Sigma and Epsilon are no more believed to be in existence in humans). Although opioid receptors are mainly present in brain (where they are called as supraspinal receptors) and spinal cord (substantia gelatinosa of dorsal horn cells) however their presence at extra CNS sites like GIT is well documented.

- *μ (mu) Receptors:* These are the *most important receptors for the action of opioids.* These are further divided into μ_1 and μ_2.
  μ_1: Mediates *analgesia* (*mainly supraspinal* but spinal also), sedation, bradycardia, miosis, urinary retention, prolactin and growth hormone release and muscle rigidity.
  μ_2: Mediates *respiratory depression,* constipation and physical dependence.
- *κ (kappa) Receptors:* Mediates *analgesia* (*mainly spinal* but supraspinal also), sedation, constipation, psychotomimesis (hallucinations), dependence and diuresis (contrary to μ which causes urinary retention)
- *δ (Delta) Receptors:* Mediates *analgesia* (*mainly spinal* but supraspinal also).
- *Nociceptin (also called as orphanin FQ):* Endogenous opioids mediate their action through nociceptin.

Classification

A. On the basis of source of synthesis
   Naturally occurring:
   – Morphine
   – Codeine
   – Thebaine
   Semisynthetic:
   – Heroin
   – Dihydromorphone
   – Oxymorphone
   – Pentamorphone
   Synthetic:
   – Butorphanol
   – Levorphanol
   – Pentazocine
   – Pethidine
   – Fentanyl, Alfentanil, Sufentanil, Remifentanil
   – Tramadol
   – Buprenorphine

B. On the basis of receptor interaction
   Pure agonist:
   – Morphine
   – Fentanyl
   – Alfentanil
   – Sufentanil
   – Remifentanil
   – Pethidine
   Agonist-antagonist (Mixed opioid):
   – Pentazocine
   – Nalbuphine
   – Nalorphine
   – Butorphanol
   – Levallorphan
   – Dezocine
   – Meptazinol
   – Buprenorphine
   Pure antagonist:
   – Naloxone
   – Naltrexone
   – Nalmefene
   – Methylnaltrexone (peripheral antagonist)
   – Alvimopan (peripheral antagonist)

Opioids and Receptor Interaction

- *Pure agonists* are agonist at all receptors with highest propensity for mu receptors.
- Up to a certain dose (like 60 mg for pentazocine and 1.2 mg for buprenorphine)

Agonist-antagonist are agonist at κ, μ (partial or full) and δ and thereafter becomes antagonist at mu (μ) receptors.

As they exhibit agonistic action only up to a certain dose, the analgesia and respiratory depression achieve plateau after this dose, this effect is called as *ceiling effect. Ceiling effect is the most important characteristic of agonist-antagonists.* As the mixed opioids are antagonist at mu receptors in high doses, they can be used to reverse pure antagonist at high doses.

- *Pure antagonist* are antagonist at all receptors with highest propensity for mu receptors.

Mechanism of Action of Opioids

Supraspinal: Opioids bind with receptors in *rostroventral region of medulla* and cause stimulation of *off cells* present there, thereby blocking nociceptive stimuli transmission.

At *spinal level* they act with their receptors present in *substantia gelatinosa* of dorsal horn cells and inhibit the release of excitatory transmitters.

At cellular level opioids bind to receptors to stimulate G protein synthesis and cAMP which causes ↑ K^+ producing hyperpolarization of membrane and ↓ Ca^{2+} decreasing excitability.

At high concentrations they can directly inhibit NMDA receptors.

Systemic Effects (Morphine as Prototype)

Cardiovascular system
- *Hypotension*: Hypotension occurs because of decreased central sympathetic tone and direct vasodilatation.
- *Bradycardia* (except pethidine and pentazocine which causes tachycardia).
- *Shifting of blood from pulmonary to systemic circulation;* it is for this property morphine is used in the treatment of left ventricular failure.
- Meperidine can directly depress myocardial contractility.
- The oculocardiac reflex, which is caused by traction on the extraocular muscles during squint surgery, is augmented by newer opioids, particularly with alfentanil.

Respiratory system
- Opioids inhibit the respiration; both volume and rate are decreased (Rate > volume).

Respiratory depression is the *most common cause of death in morphine poisoning.* Children and old age patients are more prone for respiratory depression.
- Opioids inhibit the ventilatory response to hypoxia and hypercarbia.
- Morphine can inhibit ciliary activity.
- Opioids inhibit airway and tracheal reflex *(maximum with sufentanil)* and therefore used to attenuate the reflex response to intubation and to treat cough (codeine).
- *Bronchi:* Directly acting on bronchial muscles opioids are bronchodilators (particularly fentanyl) however can cause bronchoconstriction by releasing histamine.

Delayed and recurring respiratory depression: Delayed (late) and recurring respiratory depression is exhibited by all pure agonists. The reasons are:
- Sequestration by stomach and reabsorption in blood (particularly seen with fentanyl) produces second phase to respiratory depression and that is why this recurrence of respiratory depression is also termed as *Biphasic respiratory depression.*
- Opioids get deposited in skeletal muscle and later get released into circulation on muscular activity like rewarming, motion and shivering.

Central nervous system
- *Analgesia:* Produced at supraspinal as well as spinal level. Visceral pain is relieved better than somatic pain.
- *Sedation:* Sedation at lower dose can progress to deep coma at high dosage.
- *Cerebral metabolic rate (CMR), cerebral O_2 consumption, intracranial pressure (ICP) and cerebral blood flow (CBF).* Generally opioids decrease CMR, CBF and ICP in a resting brain however they may increase CBF and ICT in head injury and intracranial space occupying lesions (ICSOL).
- *EEG:* Opioids in increased doses produce high voltage slow waves (Delta) on EEG *but cannot cause flattening of EEG as there occur ceiling effect.*
- Stimulation of chemoreceptor trigger zone (CTZ) causes *nausea and vomiting* (at very high dose they inhibit vomiting by inhibiting vomiting center).
- Mood changes, mental clouding.

- Inhibits temperature regulating centers causing hypothermia.
- *Convulsions:* Morphine, pethidine and remifentanil can cause general tonic clonic seizures while with other agents there may occur focal seizures.

Muscular system

Opioids can cause muscle rigidity which sometimes becomes so severe in thoracic muscles that it causes hypoxia. This is called as *Wooden chest syndrome or stiff chest syndrome. Muscle rigidity is most commonly seen with alfentanil.* The treatment of muscle rigidity includes naloxone, benzodiazepines (for mild cases only) and muscle relaxants and elective ventilation (for severe cases).

Endocrine system

Stress hormones like adrenocorticotrophic hormone (ACTH), follicle-stimulating hormone (FSH), LH and cortisol synthesis is decreased by opioids while the synthesis of antidiuretic hormone (ADH), growth hormone (GH) and prolactin is increased.

Stress response: Opioids are not only capable of reducing the stress by modulating nociception but endogenous opioid (β endorphins) themselves can serve as stress reliving hormones.

Gastrointestinal tract (GIT): Opioids inhibit the gut motility and decrease the gastric emptying causing *constipation (Opioid bowel syndrome)*

Biliary tract: Causes constriction of sphincter of Oddi increasing biliary duct pressure, however the *strict guidelines of not using opioids for biliary colic have been questioned* in current day clinical practice.

Eye: Opioids causes *miosis* and decreases intraocular tension.

Renal: Relaxes urinary bladder causing urinary retention.

Immunosuppression: Immunosuppressive effects of morphine have been documented in studies.

Dependence: It is both physical and psychological.

Tolerance: *Tolerance has been seen to all actions of opioids except constipation and miosis* and tolerance is mainly pharmacodynamic. The chronic use of opioids not only produces tolerance to pain but can produce *hyperalgesia.*

Pharmacokinetics of Morphine

Early wakefulness (15–20 minutes) is because of redistribution while elimination half life is 2–4 hours. Metabolism is mainly in liver (elimination half life in neonates is 10 hours).

Metabolites, morphine-3-glucuronide and 6-glucuronide are active and can produce narcosis and respiratory depression for several days in renal failure.

Morphine can be given by IV, IM, subcutaneous, oral, rectal, transcutaneous, intrathecal and epidural routes.

Dose: 0.1–0.2 mg/kg.

Opioid Agonists

Pethidine (also called as Meperidine)

- Chemically it is an atropine congener therefore has additional side effect like atropine, i.e. blurred vision, dry mouth and tachycardia.
- It is one tenth as potent as morphine.
- Action on smooth muscle is less marked than morphine therefore miosis, urinary retention and constipation are less and that is why Pethidine can be used in biliary colic.
- Pethidine is *directly acting myocardial depressant.*
- Pethidine abolishes shivering therefore is the *drug of choice for shivering.*
- Pethidine has also got local analgesic properties.

Contraindications

- Pethidine is absolutely contraindicated in patients on *monoamine oxidase inhibitors (MAO) therapy.* Patient on MAO inhibitors undergo abnormal metabolism of Pethidine to produce *Nor-Pethidine* which can cause restlessness, hypertension, convulsion, coma or even death.
- Pethidine should not be given to patients with myocardial ischemia because it not only depresses myocardium but by causing tachycardia also increases the myocardial oxygen demand.

Piritramide

It is a synthetic opioid structurally similar to Pethidine. It does not causes nausea and vomiting.

Newer Opioids

Fentanyl

- Fentanyl is the most common used opioid in anesthesia.
- Fentanyl along with bupivacaine or ropivacaine is used as continuous infusion for painless labor and postoperative analgesia.
- It is 100 times more potent than morphine.

The advantages of fentanyl are:

- Due to high lipid solubility it has *rapid onset* (2 to 5 min.) and *rapid recovery* (1–2 hours).
- *It can be given by IM, IV, transmucosal, (fentanyl lollipop), transdermal, (fentanyl patch), intrathecal and epidural route.* Fentanyl patch provides analgesia for 72 hours.
- *It is most cardiac stabile opioid.*

Alfentanil

Alfentanil is analog of fentanyl, 1/5th as potent as fentanyl. *Onset (1.4 minutes) and recovery is more rapid* as compared to fentanyl. *Alfentanil is less preferred because of higher incidence of muscle rigidity.*

Sufentanil

- *Sufentanil is the most potent human opioid (500 times of morphine) available in clinical practice.*
- As sufentanil maximally inhibit airway reflexes *it is the agent of choice for inhibiting stress response to laryngoscopy and intubation.*

Remifentanil

It is ultrashort acting opioid metabolized rapidly by *esterases in red cells and tissues.*

   Onset is fastest (1.1 minutes) and recovery is also most rapid among opioids (5–10 minutes) making *Remifentanil as an opioid of choice for day care surgery.*

Disadvantages of remifentanil are:

- Contains glycine which can cause motor weakness making it *unsuitable for postoperative analgesia and painless labor.*
- *Significant hypotension.*

Tramadol

- It is a synthetic derivative of codeine.
- It not only produces analgesia through opioid receptors but also activates spinal inhibition of pain by decreasing the reuptake of norepinephrine and serotonin. The increase in serotonin levels makes tramadol useful for management of chronic pain conditions (chronic pain is often associated with depression) however in acute pain this increase in serotonin produces additional side effects like nausea and vomiting making tramadol a less preferred agent for acute pain management.
- *Seizures* have been reported in patients taking tramadol therefore, it should be used cautiously with the drugs which decreases the seizure threshold like monoamine oxidase (MAO) inhibitors or tricyclic antidepressants.
- Tramadol has also got *local anesthetic and antibacterial* properties.

Other Opioid Agonists

Codeine: Used for suppressing cough.

Heroin: Has got highest addiction potential.

Methadone: Mainly used in prevention of opioid withdrawal symptoms.

Sameridine: Other than opioid actions it has got local anesthetic properties also

Agonist-Antagonist Drugs

Agonist antagonist drugs are less prone for abuse. The best property of these agents is *ceiling* to respiratory depression.

Pentazocine (Fortwin)

- It is agonist at kappa and delta receptors and antagonist at mu receptors.
- Mainly acts on k *receptors* at *spinal level.*
- It is 1/3rd as potent as morphine (30 mg of Pentazocine = 10 mg of morphine).
- Pentazocine stimulates sympathetic system therefore causes *tachycardia and hypertension.*
- Biliary spasm and constipation are less severe.
- Half-life is 3–5 hours.
- Ceiling occurs at a dose of 60 mg.

Buprenorphine

- Buprenorphine is agonist at mu receptors in low doses and antagonist in high doses.
- Buprenorphine has *highest receptor binding potential*
- It is 25 times more potent than morphine.

- It is long acting; the effect of single dose can last for 10 hours
- Ceiling effect is seen beyond 1.2 mg
- *Buprenorphine's local anesthetic properties make it a useful adjuvant to local anesthetics for nerve blocks.*

Butorphanol

Effects are almost similar to pentazocine except *less tachycardia*. Butorphanol patch is commonly used for chronic pain management like cancer patients.

Nalbuphine

It decreases heart rate with no effect on blood pressure therefore cardiac work load is decreased.

Dezocine

Like buprenorphine it is partial agonist at mu (μ) in low doses and antagonist at high doses

Opioid Antagonists

Naloxone

- It is a pure opioid antagonist acting on all opioid receptors with maximum propensity for mu receptors.
- It reverses the actions of all opioids however due to high receptor binding potential reversal with buprenorphine may be partial.
- The duration of action is 30–60 min thereby increasing the chances of *renarcotization* with long acting agents like morphine.
- Naloxone can be given *intra-tracheally*.

Systemic Effects

Cardiovascular system: Naloxone causes sympathetic stimulation and can produce severe hypertension, tachycardia or even pulmonary edema.

Central nervous system: Naloxone has nonspecific *analeptic* effect. Cerebral metabolic rate, oxygen consumption and blood flow is increased therefore increases intracranial tension.

Contraindications (Relative)

- Myocardial ischemia (severe tachycardia and hypertension are detrimental).
- Intracranial lesions.
- *Pheochromocytoma:* Opioid reversal with naloxone can produce ventricular fibrillation and cardiac arrest.

Other Uses of Naloxone

- Diagnosis of opioid dependence.
- Treating neonatal asphyxia if opioids are used during labor.
- The role of naloxone in shock and other conditions like intractable pruritus and thalamic pain syndrome has been doubted in newer studies.

Naltrexone and Nalmefene: These are long acting (8–10 hours) antagonists and can also be given orally.

Peripheral antagonists: *Methylnaltrexone and Alvimopan:* These are quaternary ammonium compounds not crossing the blood brain barrier. Therefore holds very promising role in *reversing the peripheral side effects particularly constipation without reversing the analgesia.*

Endogenous Opioids

- Enkephalins, endorphins dynorphins are the endogenous opioids produced in body. Endomorphin-1 and Endomorphin-2 are the new endogenous opioids however their details are not known.
- Endogenous opioids exert their effect through nociceptin.
- Enkephalins and endorphins mediate supraspinal control of pain while dynorphins mediate pain control at spinal level.
- Enkephalins are responsible for producing acupuncture-mediated analgesia while beta endorphin mediates stress response.

ALPHA 2 ADRENERGIC AGONISTS

Due to the properties like *sedation, anxiolysis, hypnosis, sympatholysis and mild analgesia* α_2 agonist have been very useful in anesthesia. Clonidine had been used for many years as an adjuvant to anesthetics however the side effects like hypotension, bradycardia and withdrawal hypertension restricted the use of clonidine.

Dexmedetomidine

Dexmedetomidine is a new α_2 agonist which is more selective and has lesser side effects as compared to Clonidine. It is very commonly used in anesthetic practice. It can be given nasally and bucally making it useful for children. The uses of Dexmedetomidine in anesthesia are:

- As premedicant (anxiolytic property).
- Adjuvants to reduce the dose of IV (sedative property), inhalational anesthetics (MAC of inhalational agents is decreased) and analgesics (analgesic property). Narcotic requirement has been found to be reduced by 50% in patients who receives Dexmedetomidine infusion.
- To attenuate cardiovascular response to intubation (sympatholytic property).
- For *sedation in ICU*: The mechanically-ventilated patients who were sedated with Dexmedetomidine had smoother and hemodynamically stable weaning.

- For *sedation in operation theater* and diagnostic units. Dry mouth produced by dexmedetomidine serves as an additional advantage in bronchoscopy.
- As a hypnotic agent during surgical procedures like awake craniotomy.
- As an adjuvant to peripheral and central neuraxial (spinal/epidural) nerve blocks.
- For the treatment of addiction of opioids and benzodiazepines.

Side Effects

- Initial hypertension
- Hypotension: *Hypotension is the most common side effect,* seen in almost one-third of the patients.

■ **Table 12.2:** Summary of systemic effects of intravenous anesthetics

	Cardiovascular system		Central nervous system				Respiratory system	
	Heart rate	Mean arterial pressure	CMO$_2$	CBF	ICT	IOP	Ventilation	
Barbiturates								
Thiopentone	↑ (reflex tachycardia)	↓↓	↓↓↓	↓↓↓	↓↓↓	↓	↓↓	Constriction (++)
Methohexital	↑	↓↓	↓↓	↓↓	↓↓	↓	↓↓	Constriction (+)
Nonbarbiturates								
Ketamine	↑↑	↑↑	↑↑	↑↑	↑↑↑	↑↑	↑/↓	Dilatation (+++)
Propofol	0/↑	↓↓↓	↓↓↓	↓↓↓	↓↓↓	↓	↓↓	Dilatation (+)
Etomidate	0	↓	↓↓	↓↓	↓↓	↓	↓	0
Opioids								
Morphine	↓↓	↓↓	↓↓	↓	Variable (↓)	↓	↓↓↓	Constriction (because of histamine release)
Fentanyl, Alfentanil and Sufentanil	↓↓	↓↓	↓↓	↓	Variable (↓)	↓	↓↓	Constriction
Pethidine	↑↑	↓	↓	↓	Variable	↓	↓↓	Constriction/0
Pentazocine	↑↑	↑↑	↑	↑	↑		↓	0
Benzodiazepines								
Diazepam	0/↑ (reflex tachycardia)	↓	↓↓	↓↓	↓	↓	↓↓	0
Midazolam	↑ (reflex tachycardia)	↓↓	↓↓	↓↓	↓	↓	↓↓	0
Lorazepam	0/↓	↓	↓↓	↓↓	↓	↓	↓↓	0

0 = no effect   ↓ = decrease   ↑ = increase

Abbreviations: CMO$_2$, cerebral oxygen consumption; CBF, cerebral blood flow; ICT, intracranial tension; IOP, intraocular pressure

- Bradycardia or even sinus arrest at very high doses.

The effect of dexmedetomidine can be reversed with *atipamezole*.

Although studies have shown the safety of dexmedetomidine being used for many days as continuous infusion however FDA approves its use only for <24 hours.

OTHER INTRAVENOUS ANESTHETICS

Droperidol, Neuroleptanalgesia and Neuroleptanesthesia

The neuroleptanalgesia is produced by a combination of *droperidol and fentanyl* (available in brand name Innovar) in a ratio of 50:1. Addition of nitrous oxide to this combination constitutes neuroleptanesthesia.

The use of neuroleptanalgesia or Neuroleptanesthesia has been disappeared from modern anesthesia practice because of the possibility of *QT prolongation and fatal arrhythmias (torsades de pointes) seen with droperidol* (In fact, FDA issued a black box warning against Droperidol). It can also produce malignant neuroleptic syndrome, hypotension (α blockade) and extrapyramidal side effects.

In past droperidol was used mainly as antiemetic and neuroleptanalgesia/neuroleptanesthesia mainly for neurosurgical procedures requiring arousal patient like stereotactic brain surgery, removal of seizure foci etc.

For summary of systemic effects and anesthetic properties of intravenous anesthetics see **Tables 12.2 and 12.3** respectively.

■ **Table 12.3:** Summary of anesthetic properties

Agent	Analgesia	Induction	Muscle relaxation
Thiopentone	Antanalgesic	Smooth	0
Methohexital	0	Smooth	0
Propofol	0	Smooth	0
Etomidate	0	Smooth	0
Neuroleptanalgesia (Droperidol + Fentanyl)	++	Only somnolence	0 (hyper rigidity may be because of fentanyl)
Opioids	++	Slow (usually not used for induction)	0 (hyper rigidity)
Benzodiazepines	0	Slow (usually not used for induction)	+ (centrally acting muscle relaxant)
Ketamine	+++	Not smooth	0 (hyper rigidity)

0 = no effect   ++ = moderate effect   + = mild effect   +++ = severe effect

KEY POINTS

- Most commonly used IV anesthetic for induction in current day practice is propofol.
- Although elimination half-life of Thiopentone is 10.4 hours but consciousness is regained after 15–20 minutes due to redistribution.
- Thiopentone can be utilized for cerebral protection in case of focal ischemia.
- Thiopentone high alkalinity is responsible for local complications like intra-arterial injection.
- Vasospasm and thrombus formation are the major events responsible for causing gangrene after intra-arterial injection of Thiopentone.
- Thiopentone is absolutely contraindicated in acute intermittent and variegate porphyria but can be used safely in porphyria cutaneatarda.
- Injection of propofol is painful.
- As propofol contains egg lecithin there are high chances of contamination of Propofol.

Contd…

Contd...

- Propofol is the IV agent of choice for day care surgery.
- Propofol is a potent antiemetic agent.
- Etomidate is the most cardiovascular stable among all IV agents.
- The major side effect of etomidate is adrenocortical suppression.
- Midazolam is the only BZ used in intraoperative period.
- Ketamine is the most potent analgesic among IV agents.
- Emergence reactions, mainly hallucinations, are the major limiting factor for restricting the use of ketamine.
- All pressures like intraocular, intragastric, intracranial are raised by ketamine.
- Ketamine is the induction agent of choice for shock, full stomach, low cardiac output states and right to left shunts.
- The most important receptors for the action of opioids are mu receptors.
- The most important characteristic of agonist- antagonists is ceiling to respiratory depression.
- Recurring respiratory depression is exhibited by all pure agonists.
- Muscle rigidity (Wooden chest syndrome) is most commonly seen with alfentanil.
- Tolerance is seen to all actions of opioids except constipation and miosis.
- The chronic use of opioids can produce hyperalgesia.
- Sufentanil is the agent of choice for inhibiting stress response to laryngoscopy and intubation.
- Remifentanil is the opioid of choice for day care surgery.
- Methylnaltrexone and Alvimopan are the peripheral opioid antagonist which can reverse the peripheral side effects without reversing the analgesia.
- Dexmedetomidine is a new $\alpha2$ agonist which is frequently used in anesthetic practice.

Muscle Relaxants

To understand the action of muscle relaxants the basic knowledge of physiology of neuromuscular junction is necessary.

PHYSIOLOGY OF NEUROMUSCULAR JUNCTION (FIG. 13.1)

Neuromuscular junction consists of nerve end, synaptic cleft and muscle end plate.

The neurotransmitter responsible for neurotransmission at neuromuscular junction is *acetylcholine* (ACh). It is synthesized in the nerve cytoplasm by combination of choline which is taken from outside (and this entry of choline is regulated by $Na^+ K^+$ pump) and acetyl coenzyme A, which is synthesized by mitochondria. This reaction is mediated by enzyme *choline acetyltransferase*. The synthesized ACh is stored in *vesicles*. Whenever there is stimulation of nerve these vesicles migrate to surface, rupture and release ACh in synaptic cleft.

Synaptic cleft is 20 nm wide. The ACh molecules bind to ACh receptors at muscle end plate which leads to opening of ion channels, so that ions can move across the membrane and depolarize it producing end plate potential and triggering contraction.

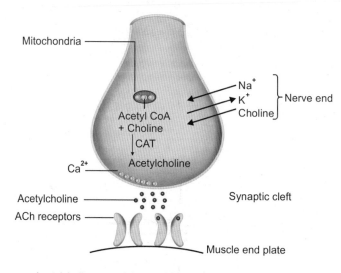

○ Acetylcholine containing vesicles
● Acetylcholine molecules

Fig. 13.1: Neuromuscular junction
Abbreviations: ACh, acetylcholine; CAT, choline acetyltransferase

The acetylcholine is destroyed in less than 1 ms by *acetylcholinesterase (true cholinesterase) which is synthesized by underlying muscle.*

Acetylcholine Receptor (Fig. 13.2)

It is a protein made up of 1,000 amino acids. These receptors exist in pairs. Each pair has 5 subunits. *Alpha (α) subunit is important because ACh, succinylcholine and competitive antagonists (nondepolarizing relaxants) bind to this site.* The receptor has two gates, **(Fig. 13.3)** upper one voltage dependent and the lower one time dependent. For producing muscle end plate action potential both gates should be open. If any one of gate is closed ions cannot pass even through an open channel.

Extrajunctional receptors: These are seen in neonates, infants and denervated (and regenerating) nerves. *These receptors are very sensitive to depolarizing agents and resistant to nondepolarizing agents.*

NEUROMUSCULAR MONITORING

Most commonly chosen muscle is *adductor pollicis,* supplied by ulnar nerve. *The details of neuromuscular monitoring have already been described in Chapter 6, page no. 67.*

Sequence of Muscle Blockade

Due to number of factors different muscles exhibits different sensitivities to muscle relaxants. For example, laryngeal muscles and diaphragm may require more than double doses required to block adductor pollicis. In fact, the *diaphragm is considered as most resistant muscle.* However, in clinical practice it has been seen that central muscle, i.e. muscles of face *(muscle fasciculations after succinylcholine are first seen in eyelids),* jaw, pharynx, larynx, muscles of respiration, abdominal and trunk muscles are blocked earlier than peripheral muscles (limb muscles). This is simply because of early and more blood supply to central muscles delivering more quantity of muscle relaxants to central muscles as compared to peripheral muscles

The sequence of recovery is also same, i.e. first to recover are central muscles (laryngeal, pharyngeal, respiratory and trunk) and last to recover are limb muscles.

This sequence of blockade and reversal has got the clinical significance:

• Adductor pollicis is most commonly monitored for neuromuscular blockade. Relaxation in adductor pollicis means laryngeal muscles have already been blocked and intubation can

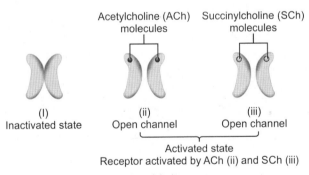

Acetylcholine (ACh) molecules   Succinylcholine (SCh) molecules

(I)
Inactivated state

(ii)
Open channel

(iii)
Open channel

Activated state
Receptor activated by ACh (ii) and SCh (iii)

Fig. 13.2: Acetylcholine receptor

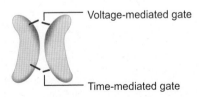

Voltage-mediated gate

Time-mediated gate

Fig. 13.3: Acetylcholine receptor showing two gates

be performed. Similarly at reversal, activity in adductor pollicis indicates recovery of laryngeal, pharyngeal and respiratory muscles and patient can be safely extubated.

- Orbicularis oculi/corrugator Supercilii (*corrugator Supercilii preferred*) are the ideal muscles for monitoring as activity in these muscles corresponds with laryngeal muscles however due to technical infeasibility these muscles are not used routinely.

CLASSIFICATION OF MUSCLE RELAXANTS

Skeletal muscle relaxants are classified into *centrally acting* (acting at cerebrospinal axis) and *peripherally acting* (acting at neuromuscular junction or directly at muscle). The peripherally acting muscle relaxants are further classified into:

A. Depolarizing blockers:
- Succinylcholine (Suxamethonium).
- Decamethonium.

B. Nondepolarizing (competitive) blockers **(Table 13.1)**.

DEPOLARIZING AGENTS

- *Decamethonium:* Not used.
- Suxamethonium [Succinylcholine, (SCh)].

Suxamethonium (Succinylcholine)

It was introduced by Thesleff and Fold in 1952 and was first used clinically by Bovet (for which he got Nobel prize). Chemically, it is dicholine ester of succinic acid.

Pharmacokinetics

It is available in 10 mL vial (50 mg/mL). It undergoes hydrolysis at room temperature therefore should be *stored at 4°C*. Onset of action is within *30–60 seconds* and duration of action is usually *< 10 minutes*. Because of this early onset and short duration *Succinylcholine is the ideal muscle relaxant for intubation* however due to the side effects its use is only restricted to rapid sequence or difficult airway management situations.

Dose: 1–2 mg/kg.

Metabolism

It is immediately metabolized in *plasma by pseudocholinesterase* (Butyrylcholinesterase), which is synthesized in liver and present in plasma in abundant quantities, therefore to prevent its metabolism it *should be given at faster rate.*

Mechanism of Action

At neuromuscular junction succinylcholine acts like acetylcholine binding to the same receptor site, producing the action potential and muscle contraction. Acetylcholine is immediately metabolized by acetylcholinesterase present at neuromuscular junction but succinylcholine metabolism depends on the concentration gradient between plasma and neuromuscular junction making excessive availability of succinylcholine at neuromuscular junction. This excessive succinylcholine produces repeated depolarization and contractions in all muscles which can be directly visualized as *fasciculations.* As a rule of physiology persistent depolarization will make the membrane to become refractory

■ **Table 13.1:** Differences between depolarizing and nondepolarizing block

Depolarizing	Nondepolarizing
1. Also called as phase I block	1. —
2. Block preceded by muscle fasciculations	2. No fasciculations
3. Depolarizing blocking drugs are called as leptocurare	3. Called as pachycurare
4. No fading is seen (fading can be seen at higher doses, i.e. phase II block)	4. Shows fading on neuromuscular monitoring
5. No post-tetanic facilitation	5. Exhibit post-tetanic facilitation
6. Does not require reversal rather cholinesterase inhibitors (neostigmine) can prolong the depolarizing block by inhibiting pseudocholinesterase	5. Reversed by cholinesterase inhibitors like neostigmine

to succinylcholine as well as acetylcholine for a transient period. This transient period is the period of relaxation. This kind of block produced by succinylcholine is termed as *phase I block*.

Systemic Effects

Cardiovascular system: Suxamethonium not only acts on nicotinic receptors but also on muscarinic receptors producing *bradycardia* (however at very high doses it may cause tachycardia due to the stimulation of nicotinic receptors at sympathetic ganglion). Excessive bradycardia can sometimes cause nodal rhythms.

Hyperkalemia: *Hyperkalemia is the most prominent effect of Suxamethonium* which occurs due to excessive muscle fasciculations. In normal circumstances serum potassium increases by 0.5 mEq/L. Hyperkalemia increases the risk of ventricular arrhythmias.

Central nervous system (CNS): By causing contraction of neck muscles thereby blocking jugular venous outflow Succinylcholine *increases intracranial tension.*

Eye: Ocular muscles are multiple innervated muscles which undergo tonic contraction after succinylcholine *increasing the intraocular tension* (IOT).

GIT: *Intragastric pressure is increased* due to contraction of abdominal muscles. By activating GI muscarinic receptors it increases GI secretions and peristalsis.

Muscle pains (myalgia, muscle soreness): This is a common complication seen in postoperative period; incidence is 40–50%. Muscle pains are due to excessive muscle contractions. The incidence of postoperative myalgia can be reduced by:
- *Precurarization*: Precurarization is the technique in which one-tenth dose of nondepolarizing muscle relaxant is given 3 minutes prior to succinylcholine. This small dose of nondepolarizer by blocking some of the receptors will decrease fasciculations and hence myalgia. This technique can also prevent the rise in intracranial and intragastric pressure but does not reliably prevent rise in intraocular pressure (due to multi-innervation of ocular muscles).

- NSAIDs and prostaglandin inhibitor like lysine acetylsalicylate also decrease incidence of myalgia (but not used routinely for this purpose).

Malignant hyperthermia: *Succinylcholine is the most commonly implicated drug.*

Anaphylaxis: Severe hypersensitivity reaction can occur with succinylcholine.

Masseter spasm: Succinylcholine can cause masseter spasm especially in children which may be a precursor sign for malignant hyperthermia.

Contraindications

1. *Hyperkalemia:* Serum K^+ > 5.5 mEq/L is an absolute contraindication for using suxamethonium.
2. Succinylcholine increases the ICT however, the increase is transient and can be revered with hyperventilation therefore *Suxamethonium is not absolutely contraindicated for neurosurgery* and can be safely used if there is clear indication like rapid sequence induction or possibility of difficult airway.
3. Glaucoma and eye injuries (increases intraocular pressure).
   However, if absolutely necessary Succinylcholine can be considered for raised intraocular pressure after pretreatment with nondepolarizers (precurarization).
4. *Newborns and infants*: Newborns and infants have regenerating nerves therefore have extrajunctional receptors making suxamethonium to act on more receptors producing more hyperkalemia.
5. Up to 2–3 months after trauma, up to 6 months after hemiplegia/paraplegia (stroke) and up to 1 year after burns (the greatest risk period is 1 week to 2 months). In these conditions denervated/regenerating nerve develops extrajunctional receptors producing significant hyperkalemia.
6. *Renal failure*: Renal per se is not a contraindication but renal failure is often associated with hyperkalemia.
7. Prolonged intra-abdominal infection-prolonged infection is usually associated with acidosis which is inevitably associated with hyperkalemia.

8. Shock (shock is associated with metabolic acidosis and hence hyperkalemia).
9. Diagnosed case of atypical pseudocholinesterase and low Pseudocholinesterase.
10. *Muscular dystrophies like Duchenne muscle dystrophy or dystrophia myotonia:* Muscles in these patients are so sensitive to suxamethonium that severe life-threatening hyperkalemia can occur. Moreover, these patients may develop permanent contractures if succinylcholine is given and they are one of the highest risk patients to develop malignant hyperthermia.

    In fact, existence of undiagnosed muscular dystrophy is the reason for avoiding suxamethonium in young children.
11. *Tetanus, Guillain Barré syndrome, poliomyelitis or spinal cord injury:* These conditions are associated with hyperkalemia.

Prolonged Apnea after Succinylcholine

It can be because of:
- Low pseudocholinesterase.
- Atypical pseudocholinesterase.
- Phase II block.

Low Pseudocholinesterase

Pseudocholinesterase is a protein synthesized by liver and is present in plasma. Normal serum level is *80 units/mL* and half-life is 12 hours. Pseudocholinesterase level should fall below 75% of normal to produce clinically significant prolongation of suxamethonium effect.

Its levels are *reduced* in:
- Liver diseases because it synthesized in liver.
- As it is a protein therefore, any protein losing enteropathy, uropathy, chronic cachexic diseases like malignancy, newborns, old age, alcoholics, dietary hypoproteinemia or pregnancy (dilutional hypoproteinemia) will decrease its levels.
- *Direct inhibition of pseudocholinesterase:* The following drugs may cause direct inhibition of pseudocholinesterase:
    - Cytotoxic drugs (particularly alkylating agents).
    - *Cholinesterase inhibitors:* Neostigmine, pyridostigmine and echothiophate

inhibits pseudocholinesterase and can prolong apnea up to 60 minutes. (*Cholinesterase inhibitors can reverse the action of non-depolarizers and prolong the block of depolarizers*).
- Metoclopramide.
- Pancuronium.
- Oral contraceptives.
- Bambuterol (a prodrug of terbutaline)
- β-blocker, esmolol.

Treatment
- Continue intermittent positive pressure ventilation (IPPV) and wait for spontaneous recovery as spontaneous recovery occurs in almost all cases after a delayed period.
- *Fresh frozen plasma:* It should be given only if patient is not recovering spontaneously
- Heat treated preparation of cholinesterase is preferred over fresh frozen plasma but available only in few countries.

Atypical (Abnormal) Pseudocholinesterase

It is a genetic disease in which patient has abnormal enzyme which is not able to metabolize Suxamethonium.

Incidence: 1 in 3,000. This is diagnosed by *Dibucaine number.*

Dibucaine is a local anesthetic which can inhibit 80% of normal enzyme and 20% of abnormal enzyme therefore dibucaine number for homozygous typical (normal person) is 80% and homozygous atypical is 20%. *Dibucaine number only indicates the genetic makeup of an individual.* It cannot measure the concentration or efficiency of pseudocholinesterase.

Sodium fluoride can be used in place of Dibucaine (*Fluoride number*).

Treatment

As majority of the patients are heterozygous atypical (i.e. have normal as well as abnormal enzyme) therefore recover spontaneously after 1–2 hours. So continue IPPV and wait for spontaneous recovery. Those who do not recover spontaneously (homozygous atypical) may be given fresh frozen plasma or synthetic preparation of cholinesterase.

Phase II Block

Also called as *dual block*. This is prolonged block seen after *excessive dose of suxamethonium (> 5 mg/kg or > 500 mg)*.

Exact pathophysiology of phase II block is not understood but some of the mechanism may be:

- *Desensitization:* Repeated doses produces structural changes in receptor which undergoes desensitization.
- *Channel blockade:* Succinylcholine molecules enter the open channel and produce prolonged block.
- Calcium mediated injury to end plate.

Diagnosis: *Succinylcholine showing fading on neuromuscular monitoring is pathognomonic of phase II block.*

Treatment
- Maintain IPPV.
- In 50% individuals block may reverse by itself in 10–15 minutes.
- In the remaining cases a trial of neostigmine can be given if there is no response even after 30 minutes. If neostigmine is given early it can worsen the block. Sufficient evidence stating the role of neostigmine in phase II block is still lacking.

NONDEPOLARIZING MUSCLE RELAXANTS

First muscle relaxant, d-tubocurare was used by Harold Griffith.

Nondepolarizing muscle relaxants (NDMR) are used in anesthesia for:

- Maintenance of relaxation (1st dose for maintenance should be full dose but all subsequent doses should be ¼th of the 1st dose).
- *For intubation:* Due to side effects of suxamethonium, in current day practice nondepolarizers are used routinely for intubation (except for certain situations like rapid sequence intubation or difficult airway where suxamethonium is still the drug of choice). The major limitation of nondepolarizers for not using for intubation was their slow onset of action (3–4 minutes). Therefore, numerous methods like priming (giving 1/10th of dose 2–3 minutes prior to main dose) or using

very high doses were devised to enhance the onset of action of action of non-depolarizers however the availability of rocuronium (onset of action in 60–90 seconds) has led to almost complete disappearance of these techniques from modern day anesthesia.

- For precurarization, to prevent postoperative myalgia by succinylcholine.

Mechanism of action: The NDMR are the competitive antagonists at acetylcholine receptor. They bind at the same site (α subunit) at which acetylcholine binds preventing acetylcholine to bind thereby preventing depolarization, action potential and muscle contraction.

All NDMR are quaternary ammonium compounds and highly water soluble, i.e. hydrophilic (not lipophilic) *therefore do not cross blood brain barrier and placenta except gallamine.*

Classification

A. *On the basis of chemical structure*: On the basis of chemical structure they are broadly classified as:

   Steroidal compounds
   - Pancuronium
   - Vecuronium
   - Pipecuronium
   - Rocuronium
   - Rapacuronium

   Benzylisoquinoline compounds
   - d-Tubocurare
   - Metocurine
   - Doxacurium
   - Atracurium
   - Mivacurium
   - Cisatracurium
   - Mivacurium

   Others
   - Gallamine
   - Alcuronium
   - Onium chlorfumrates

   The basic *difference between steroidal and benzylisoquinoline (BZIQ) compounds is that histamine release is seen with BZIQ compounds and vagolytic property with steroidal compounds.*

B. *On the basis of duration of action*: Onset of a nondepolarizer is inversely proportional to potency. More the potency, lesser the dose required, means less molecules delivered at neuromuscular (NM) junction to compete with acetylcholine delaying the onset of action.

Long acting	Intermediate acting	Short acting
D tubocurae	Vecuronium	Mivacurium
Gallamine	Rocuronium	Rapacuronium
Pancuronium	Atracurium	Gantacurium (shortest acting)
Pipecuronium	Metocurine	
Doxacurium (longest acting)	Cisatracurium	

Steroidal Compounds

Pancuronium

The main reason for not preferring pancuronium in current day practice is *cardiac instability*. It releases nor-adrenaline and cause vagal blockade which can cause *tachycardia* and hypertension. By releasing nor-adrenaline it increases the chances of arrhythmias with halothane.

Duration of effect: 30–40 minutes.

Metabolism: Only 10–20% is metabolized in liver. 80–90% is excreted by kidneys therefore *should not be used in renal diseases.*

Vecuronium

It has 2 rings A and D. D ring is similar to pancuronium and A is modified to make its action of shorter duration. It's commonly used muscle relaxant in India.

Pharmacokinetics
Dose: 0.08–0.1 mg/kg,

Onset of action: 2–3 minutes.

Duration of effect: 15–20 minutes.

Metabolism: 30–40% is metabolized in liver. Only 25% is excreted through kidneys. *A significant amount (40%) is excreted in bile therefore it should not be used in biliary obstruction.*

Systemic effects
- As vecuronium is *most cardiovascular stable it is the muscle relaxant of choice for cardiac patients.*
- Long-term use in ICU has resulted in *polyneuropathy* due to accumulation of its metabolite, 3-hydroxy metabolite.

Rocuronium
- It is a derivative of vecuronium with 1/8th potency.
- *The advantage of rocuronium over other nondepolarizing muscle relaxants is its early onset within 60–90 seconds as compared to other relaxants (3–4 minutes).* As rocuronium onset is comparable to succinylcholine *it is nondepolarizer of choice for intubation and precurarization.*
- Rocuronium is preferred over vecuronium for *prolonged use in ICU because it does not produce any active metabolite.*
- *It is the only nondepolarizing muscle relaxant which can be given by intramuscular route.*
Rest of pharmacology is similar to vecuronium except that it has *mild vagolytic* property.

Rapacuronium

Rapacuronium is the analog of vecuronium with less potency. Onset of action is similar to rocuronium (1 minute) but duration of action is short (almost half of vecuronium and rocuronium). Rapacuronium has been withdrawn from market because it produced *intense bronchospasm* in significant number of patients (> 9%).

Pipecuronium

It is a pancuronium derivative with better cardiac stability, however not as cardiac stable as vecuronium. As it does not offer any additional advantage over vecuronium it is hardly used.

Benzylisoquinoline Compounds
A. Agents not used nowaday.

D-Tubocurare

It is named so because it was carried in bamboo tubes and used as arrow poison for hunting by Amazon people.

It is not used in present day practice because of its *highest propensity for histamine and ganglion blockade (and hence severe hypotension).*

Duration of effect: 50–60 minutes.

Metocurine

Possibility of severe anaphylaxis led to its obsoletion. It is an iodine containing compound, therefore persons with allergy to iodine should not be given metocurine.

B. Agents used nowaday.

Atracurium

- Available as atracurium besylate.
- To be stored at 4°C.

Pharmacokinetics

It is an acidic compound therefore can precipitate if given in IV line containing alkaline solution like thiopentone.

Dose: 0.5 mg/kg.

Onset of action: 2–3 minutes.

Duration of action: 10–15 minutes.

Metabolism: It has unique method of degradation. The majority of the drug undergoes spontaneous degradation in plasma called as *Hoffman degradation* (a small amount is metabolized by plasma esterase). Hoffman degradation is a pH and temperature-dependent reaction; higher pH and temperature favor more degradation.

Systemic effects

At higher doses its *metabolic product laudonosine can cross blood brain barrier and can produce convulsions.*

As it is benzylisoquinoline compound it can release histamine which can produce allergic reactions ranging from pruritic rash to angio-neurotic edema, bronchospasm or hypotension.

Uses

As atracurium metabolism is not dependent on hepatic or renal functions it is *relaxant of choice* for

- Hepatic failure.
- Renal failure.
- Newborn (immature hepatic/renal function)
- Old age (impaired hepatic/renal functions)
- If reversal agent is contraindicated (as metabolism of Atracurium is guaranteed there is no risk of accumulation of any active form)
- Neuromuscular diseases like myasthenia gravis.

Cis-Atracurium

- It is an isomer of atracurium with 4 times more potency than atracurium.

- The chief advantage of cisatracurium over atracurium is that *it does not release histamine and laudonosine production is 5 times less than atracurium* therefore *always preferred over atracurium.*
- It is only metabolized by Hoffman degradation; does not undergo any metabolism by ester hydrolysis.

Rest of pharmacology is similar to atracurium.

Mivacurium

Like succinylcholine it is metabolized in plasma by *pseudocholinesterase* therefore prolonged block is expected in conditions causing low Pseudocholinesterase level.

As it is metabolized by pseudocholinesterase it *duration of action is short (5–10 minutes)* making it a muscle relaxant of choice for *day care surgery.*

The major side effect is histamine release.

Doxacurium

Doxacurium long duration of action (60 minutes, *longest acting non depolarizer*), high potency (*most potent nondepolarizing muscle relaxant*) and *almost complete elimination as unchanged drug by kidneys* makes it a least preferred drug by clinicians.

OTHERS

Not used nowaday.

Gallamine

Gallamine is obsolete for more than 2 decades due to following reasons:

- It has got maximum propensity for *vagal blockade (vagolytic)* therefore can cause severe tachycardia.
- *It is the only nondepolarizer which can cross the placenta and cause fetal death therefore absolutely contraindicated in pregnancy.*
- More than 80% is excreted by kidneys therefore *contraindicated in renal diseases.*

Alcuronium

It gets deteriorated on sunlight exposure therefore was available in dark colored ampoules.

Because of the higher risk of anaphylactic reactions it is no more used.

COMPOUNDS UNDER RESEARCH
Mixed Onium Chlorofumarates
Gantacurium

Gantacurium, previously known as AV430A, is a mixed onium chlorofumarates which is still under clinical trials. Preclinical trials has proved it to be having fast onset (< 90 seconds) and *ultra short duration (shortest among nondepolarizers)*; after reversal complete recovery has been reported in 3–4 minutes.

It is rapidly metabolized by forming cysteine adduct followed by ester hydrolysis.

The main side effect, i.e. histamine release is only seen at very high doses (3 times of normal dose). *The properties proven in pre-clinical trials, if maintained after clinical trials also, gantacurium will not be the only nondepolarizer of choice for intubation rather it may emerge as an alternative to suxamethonium for intubation.*

CW 002 is analogue of gantacurium with intermediate duration of action

Changeover of muscle relaxants in the same sitting: It is almost never practiced but if an intermediate acting drug is administered after long acting then duration of intermediate acting drug is prolonged for first two doses.

Addition of muscle relaxants: Two muscle relaxants of same group (steroid + steroid or BZIQ+BZIQ) produces additive effect while addition of different group (steroid+ BZIQ) produces synergistic effect.

Factors Prolonging the Neuromuscular Blockade

- Neonates.
- Old age.
- Obesity.
- Hepatic disease (both depolarizer and NDMR).
- Renal disease (only NDMR).
- *Inhalational agents:* Prolong the block by both depolarizers and NDMR. Inhalational agents decrease the requirement of relaxant by 20–30%. M*aximum relaxation among inhalational agents use now a days is produced by Desflurane.* (Desflurane > Sevoflurane > Isoflurane > Halothane).

- *Antibiotics: Prolong the effect of both depolarizers and NDMR.*
  - Aminoglycosides (Neomycin, streptomycin, gentamicin, kanamycin, polymyxin, and tobramycin), lincosamines (lincomycin and Clindamycin). To reverse the effect of block by aminoglycosides drug used is 4, aminopyridine.
  - Tetracycline.
- *Local anesthetics:* Except procaine local anesthetics prolong the action by stabilizing post synaptic membrane (both depolarizers and NDMR are prolonged).
- *Hypothermia:* Decreases metabolism of muscle relaxants (both depolarizers and NDMR).
- *Hypocalcemia:* Calcium is required for producing action potential. Action of NDMR is enhanced.
- *Hypokalemia:* NDMR block is enhanced.
- Acid base imbalances especially acidosis (Action of NDMR is enhanced).
- Calcium channel blockers (Action of only NDMR is enhanced).
- Dantrolene (Action of only NDMR is enhanced).
- Neuromuscular diseases **(Table 13.2)**.
- *Hypermagnesemia*: Prolongs block by both depolarizers and NDMR.
- Lithium prolongs duration of both depolarizers and non- depolarizers.
- *Cholinesterase inhibitors (neostigmine):* Prolong the action of depolarizers by inhibiting pseudocholinesterase.
- Antihypertensives (Trimethaphan and nitroglycerine)
- Antiarrhythmics (Quinidine, procainamide): Prolongs depolarizers and nondepolarizers.

Drugs which Antagonize Neuromuscular Blockade

- Phenytoin
- Carbamazepine
- Calcium
- Cholinesterase inhibitors
- Azathioprine
- Steroids

These agents only antagonize the effect of NDMR.

■ **Table 13.2:** Altered muscle relaxant responses in muscular diseases

Disease	Response to depolarizers	Response to non-depolarizers	Comments
Conditions with extrajunctional receptors like: • Burns • Hemiplegia • Paraplegia • Denervation muscle injuries • Tetanus • Cerebral palsy.	Increased sensitivity and hyperkalemia	Resistance	Extrajunctional receptors in these conditions are sensitive to depolarizing agents and resistant to nondepolarizers
Myasthenia gravis	Resistance	Increased sensitivity	An autoimmune disease destroying acetylcholine receptors, less competition for nondepolarizers, increasing their sensitivity and less receptors for succinylcholine to act increasing its resistance.
Myasthenic syndrome	Increased sensitivity	Increased sensitivity	Autoantibodies against prejunctional calcium channels, eventually decreasing the production of acetylcholine
Muscle dystrophies like Duchenne myotonias like dsytrophia, congenita	Increased sensitivity and hyperkalemia	Normal or increased sensitivity	Due to multiple reasons sensitivity to depolarizers is significantly increased
Autoimmune diseases like SLE	Increased sensitivity	Increased sensitivity	

REVERSAL OF BLOCK

There are *two rules of reversal*:

1. All patients who have received nondepolarizer must be given reversal agent until unless there is absolute contraindication for using reversal agent.
2. Reversal should be given only after some evidence of spontaneous recovery has appeared like patient has started spontaneous respiration and TO$_4$ shows at least 1 twitch response otherwise reversal agents may enter the open channels and can themselves produce block.

Drugs used for reversal of block by non-depolarizers are cholinesterase inhibitors (anticholinesterases) and gamma cyclodextrins.

A. Anticholinesterases

Anticholinesterases which can be used for reversal of the block of nondepolarizers are:

- Neostigmine
- Pyridostigmine
- Edrophonium
- Physostigmine

These agents except physostigmine are quaternary ammonium compounds therefore do not cross the blood brain barrier.

Mechanism of Action

Cholinesterase inhibitors inactivate the enzyme Acetylcholinesterase which is responsible for break-down of acetylcholine, thus increasing the amount of acetylcholine available for competition with nondepolarizing agent thereby re-establishing neuromuscular transmission. Cholinesterase inhibitors have additional effects others than inhibiting cholinesterase like (i) increase release of acetylcholine from pre-synaptic nerve terminals, (ii) direct agonist (weak) action on nicotinic receptors, (iii) block potassium channels.

The increased acetylcholine will not only act at nicotinic receptors but also on muscarinic receptors producing muscarinic side effects like bradycardia, bronchospasm and increased secretions. Therefore *to prevent these muscarinic side effects some anticholinergic like atropine or glycopyrrolate has to be given with cholinesterase inhibitors.* Glycopyrrolate being devoid of central side effects is always preferred over atropine.

Neostigmine

Neostigmine is the most commonly used reversal agent.

Dose: 0.04—0.08 mg/kg.

The effect begins in 5–10 minutes and peaks in half hour and lasts for one hour. Anticholinergic preferred with neostigmine is glycopyrrolate because both have same onset of action (both are slow acting).

Edrophonium: It has rapid onset (1–2 min) and shorter duration of action. As it has short duration there are increased chances of recurarization with long acting nondepolarizers. The anticholinergic preferred with edrophonium is atropine (both fast acting).

As neostigmine and pyridostigmine inhibit pseudocholinesterase they cannot be used to reverse mivacurium which is metabolized by pseudocholinesterase. Edrophonium does not inhibit pseudocholinesterase therefore is the *reversal agent of choice for mivacurium.*

Pyridostigmine: The onset is slower (10–15 minutes) and duration is longer (> 2 hours). It is *preferred drug for renal failure patients* in whom a prolonged stay of muscle relaxant is expected. This situation is rare in present day anesthesia as for renal failure patients invariably Atracurium or cisAtracurium is used.

B. Gamma Cyclodextrins (Sugammadex)

Cyclodextrins are the reversal agents which directly binds to *steroidal type of nondepolarizing muscle relaxants* to form a complex which gets eliminated unchanged through kidney.

Advantages

- Anticholinesterase are unable to reverse deeper blocks while *sugammadex is effective in reversing profound blockade.*
- The reversal of block with cholinesterase inhibitors is slow (10–15 min.) while reversal

with sugammadex is very fast (2–3 minutes). Moreover there occurs ceiling to the effect of anticholinesterases (there is limit to which acetylcholinesterase can be inhibited)

- As there are no muscarinic side effects, there is no need to use glycopyrrolate or Atropine
- Sugammadex can be given even if there are no signs of spontaneous activity.

Disadvantages

- *Cannot reverse benzylisoquinoline* type of nondepolarizers
- As the Sugammadex—nondepolarizer complex is eliminated unchanged through kidneys it cannot be used in patient with severe renal insufficiency
- Can encapsulate other drugs like oral contraceptives
- *Risk of hypersensitivity reactions* may be one of the major limiting factor preventing wide spread use of sugammadex.

C. L-cysteine

As the fumarates (gantacurium) is inactivated by adduction of cysteine, the administration of exogenous L-cysteine results in complete reversal within 2–3 minutes.

SIGNS OF ADEQUATE REVERSAL

- Regular respiration with adequate tidal volume, i.e. patient is able to maintain oxygen saturation on room air.
- Spontaneous eye opening.
- Spontaneous limb movements.
- Able to protrude tongue.
- Recovery of upper airway reflexes like cough and swallowing.
- *Able to lift head for more than 5 seconds* used to be considered as most reliable clinical test.
- *Sustained jaw clench over a tongue blade is considered as best clinical sign* however it is difficult to perform by patient therefore still most widely used clinical test is head lift.
- Train of four (TO_4) ratio > 0.7 (70%), indicates adequate recovery but *ratio > 0.9 guarantees recovery.* However, most of the clinicians believe that in addition to TO_4 ratio > 0.9, patients must not exhibit any clinical

symptom/sign of impaired neuromuscular recovery like difficulty in swallowing, diplopia, inability to speak, inability to perform head lift or complain of general weakness, to declare guaranteed recovery. *General weakness is considered as most sensitive symptom of inadequate reversal.*

COMMON CAUSES OF INADEQUATE REVERSAL

- Inadequate dose of neostigmine. As there occur ceiling to the effect of neostigmine there is hardly a role of second dose
- Over dosage of inhalational agents (inhalational agents have neuromuscular blocking properties)
- Renal failure, hepatic failure (except atracurium and cisatracurium)
- Hypothermia (decreases metabolism)
- Hypothyroidism (decreases metabolism)
- Electrolyte abnormalities especially hypokalemia and hypocalcemia
- Associated neuromuscular diseases
- Shock (because of acidosis)
- *Acid base abnormalities*: Respiratory acidosis and metabolic alkalosis doubles the dose of neostigmine. It becomes almost impossible to reverse a patient with pCO_2 more than 50 mm Hg.

CENTRALLY ACTING MUSCLE RELAXANTS

These are the drugs which produce muscle relaxation through central mechanism both at supraspinal and spinal level. Polysynaptic reflexes involved in maintenance of muscle tone are inhibited at both spinal and supraspinal level. These drugs also produce sedation. They have no action on neuromuscular junction.

The commonly used centrally acting muscle relaxants are:
- Chlorzoxazone, chlormezanone.
- Diazepam.
- Baclofen.
- Tizanidine, metaxalone.
  Others like mephenesin, meprobamate are no more used intravenously (mephenesin is still used in ointments).

Uses

- Muscle spasms.
- *Tetanus:* Intravenous diazepam is most effective.
- Spastic neurological diseases like cerebral palsy, spinal injuries.
- Close reductions and dislocations in orthopedics.
  For summary of pharmacology of muscle relaxants see **Table 13.3**.

■ **Table 13.3:** Summary of pharmacology of muscle relaxants

	Onset	Duration of action	Metabolism (in liver)	Primary excretion	Histamine release	Vagal blockade	Comments
Depolarizers (Suxamethonium)	Rapid (30–60 sec)	Short (<10 min)	—	Plasma	+	—	Fastest onset, shortest acting muscle relaxant
Steroidal compounds							
Pancuronium	Moderate (3–4 min)	Long (30–40 min)	Only small amount (10%) is metabolized	Renal (90%)	0	++	Tachycardia
Vecuronium	Moderate	Intermediate (20–30 min)	30–40%	Biliary (40%)	0	0	Cardiovascular stable, Contraindicated in biliary obstruction

Contd...

Contd...

	Onset	Duration of action	Metabolism (in liver)	Primary excretion	Histamine release	Vagal blockade	Comments
Rocuronium	Early (60 sec)	Intermediate (20–30 min)	Nil	Hepatic (> 70%)	0	+	NDMR of choice for intubation
Pipecuronium	Moderate	Long	Small amount	Renal	0	+	
Rapacuronium	Early (60 sec)	Small (10–15 min)	Very high (50%)	< 25%	0	+	Intense bronchospasm
Benzylisoquinoline compounds							
d-Tubocurare	Delayed	Prolonged	Insignificant	Renal	+++	0	Maximum histamine release. Maximum ganglion blockade
Metocurine	Moderate	Intermediate	Insignificant	Renal	++	0	
Atracurium	Moderate (2–3 min)	Intermediate (10–15 min)	Nil	Plasma	++	0	Undergoes Hoffman degradation
Cisatracurium	Moderate	Intermediate	Nil	Plasma	0	0	No histamine release, less laudanosine
Mivacurium	Moderate	Small (5–10 min)	Nil	Plasma	+	0	Metabolized by pseudocholines-terase
Doxacurium	Moderate	Prolonged (60 min)	Insignificant	Renal	0	0	
Others							
Gallamine	Delayed	Prolonged	Insignificant	Renal	0	+++	Can cross placental barrier
Gantacurium	Fast	Short	Insignificant	Plasma	0	0	Shortest acting NDMR

The following can be concluded from **Table 13.3**:

- Long acting muscle relaxant are largely eliminated by kidneys. Metabolism by liver is very small. Intermediate acting have rapid clearance because of multiple pathways like metabolism, elimination and degradation.
- *NDMR absolutely contraindicated in renal failure*
  - Gallamine
  - Metocurine
  - doxacurium
  - Pancuronium
  - Tubocurare
- *NDMR relatively contraindicated in renal failure*
  - Vecuronium (only at higher doses)
- *NDMR safe in renal failure*
  - Atracurium
  - Cisatracurium
  - Rocuronium
  - Mivacurium
- *NDMR contraindicated in hepatic failure*
  - Vecuronium
  - Rocuronium
  - Mivacurium

- *NDMR safe in hepatic failure*
  - Atracurium
  - Cisatracurium
- *NDMR contraindicated in biliary obstruction*
  - Vecuronium
  - Rocuronium
- *NDMR contraindicated in pregnancy*
  - Gallamine
- *NDMR of choice for rapid sequence intubation* (muscle relaxant of choice is succinylcholine)
  - Rocuronium

- *NDMR causing ganglion blockade*
  - d-Tubocurare
  - Metocurine
  - Alcuronium
- *NDMR causing vagal blockade*
  - Gallamine
  - Pancuronium
  - Rocuronium
- *NDMR of choice for cardiac patients*
  - Vecuronium.

KEY POINTS

- In clinical practice central muscle are blocked and recover earlier than peripheral muscles (limb muscles).
- Because of early onset and short duration Succinylcholine is the ideal muscle relaxant for intubation.
- Hyperkalemia is the most prominent effect of suxamethonium.
- Succinylcholine is the most commonly implicated drug for malignant hyperthermia.
- Intraocular, intragastric and intracranial pressures are increased by suxamethonium.
- Fading after suxamethonium is pathognomonic of phase II block.
- Continue intermittent positive pressure ventilation and wait for spontaneous recovery is the treatment of choice for low and atypical pseudocholinesterase.
- Benzylisoquinoline releases histamine while steroidal compounds are vagolytic.
- Onset of a nondepolarizer is inversely proportional to potency.
- Vecuronium is most cardiovascular stable muscle relaxant.
- Rocuronium is nondepolarizer of choice for intubation.
- Intense bronchospasm led to withdrawal of rapacuronium from market.
- Atracurium and cisatracurium are metabolized by Hoffman degradation making them relaxant of choice for hepatic and renal failure.
- Cisatracurium does not release histamine and Laudonosine production is 5 times less than atracurium.
- Mivacurium is the muscle relaxant of choice for day care surgery.
- Gallamine is the only nondepolarizer which can cross the placenta therefore absolutely contraindicated in pregnancy.
- Gantacurium onset and duration is almost comparable to suxamethonium.
- To prevent muscarinic side effects, anticholinergic like atropine or glycopyrrolate has to be given with cholinesterase inhibitors.
- Sugammadex is the newer reversal agent which rapidly and completely reverses the block by steroidal type of nondepolarizers but cannot reverse benzylisoquinoline compounds.
- Sustained jaw clench over a tongue blade is considered as best clinical sign however train of four ratio > 0.9 guarantees recovery.

CHAPTER 14

Perioperative Complications of General Anesthesia

Almost all complications which can occur in intraoperative period can also occur in postoperative period. Therefore, complications are classified as perioperative (intraoperative + postoperative). In spite of the debate over the period most of the clinicians consider perioperative period up to 48 hours after surgery.

Most anesthetic complications occur *because of human errors* (may not necessarily amount to negligence).

Although the more turbulent periods in anesthesia are induction and emergence however *maximum complications are reported in maintenance period* necessitating the same vigilance standards in maintenance period as in induction and recovery phase.

Postoperative respiratory depression has been cited as the most common cause of anesthesia related death in perioperative period and the usual cause is transferring the patient to postoperative anesthesia care unit (PACU, newer term for recovery room) without oxygen and reluctance to give oxygen in postoperative period. Therefore *all patients in PACU must receive supplemental oxygen and continuous monitoring of oxygen saturation.*

To prevent complications in PACU vitals should be monitored every 5 minutes for first 15 minutes and thereafter every 15 minutes in stable patients.

MORTALITY

Although majority of studies reports the perioperative incidence of death to be 1: 13,000-15000 however the incidence of death exclusively related to anesthesia is rare (>1:100000). In spite of this *Death is the leading cause of claims* as per American Society of Anesthesiologists (ASA) claim studies. Major factors responsible for perioperative death are increased age of the patient (odds ratio of death for >80 years vs. < 60 is 3.29), ASA status of the patient (odds ratio for ASA III-V vs. I-II is 10.65), sex (female less prone for mortality, odds ratio as compared to males is 0.77), nature of surgery (odds ratio for major vs. minor surgery is 3.82).

RESPIRATORY COMPLICATIONS

HYPOXIA

The common causes of hypoxemia seen in perioperative period are:

Failure to Intubate/Ventilate

Failure to intubate and not even able to ventilate is the worst nightmare for an anesthetist. A proper assessment of airway and readiness to face and handle such situation (*See Chapter 5*) can prevent this catastrophe.

Pulmonary Aspiration of Gastric Contents

Aspiration can occur any time in perioperative period. Although it is not always possible to prevent aspiration however it is still *considered as preventable complication of anesthesia.* Pulmonary aspiration is one of a major cause of death associated with anesthesia. Mortality after aspiration is 5-70% depending on the volume and pH of aspirated material and time interval between detection and management.

Incidence: 1 in 3,000.

Hydrodynamics of Regurgitation

Normal intragastric pressure is 5–7 cm H_2O and regurgitation is prevented by the tone of lower esophageal sphincter (LES).

A pressure of >20 cm H_2O is required to overcome the competency of LES (below 20 cm H_2O increase in intragastric pressure reflexly increases the tone of LES) which can lead to regurgitation but in conditions like pregnancy, hiatus hernia which distorts the anatomy of LES, a pressure > 15 cm H_2O can cause regurgitation of gastric contents. During anesthesia tone of cricopharyngeal sphincter is also decreased which can lead to aspiration.

Predisposing factors

1. *Full stomach*: It is single most important factor
2. Depressed level of consciousness.
3. Conditions decreasing the tone of LES:
    - Pregnancy (Acid aspiration in late pregnancy was described by Mendelson and is called it as Mendelson syndrome). The gravid uterus compresses the stomach leading to distortion of gastro-esophageal angle making LES to become incompetent.
    - Abdominal tumors, abdominal obesity, ascites, laparoscopy—increase intra-abdominal pressure distorts gastro-esophageal angle.
    - Hiatus hernia—LES is impaired in Hiatus hernia patient
    - Presence of nasogastric (Ryle's) tube
    Ryle's tube increases the chances of aspiration because of the following reasons:
    - i. Presence of Ryle's tube decreases the tone of lower esophageal sphincter (which is the main protective mechanism).
    - ii. Presence of Ryle's tube in pharynx stimulates vomiting.
    - iii. It is impossible to completely evacuate the stomach with Ryles tube
4. Drugs
    - Atropine/Glycopyrrolate
    - Opioids
    - Thiopentone
    - Sodium nitroprusside
    - Dopamine
    - Halothane
    - Ganglion blockers

5. Conditions delaying gastric emptying:
    - Diabetes
    - Hypothyroidism
    - Narcotics
    - Pain
    - Anxiety
    - Anticholinergics.

Risk Factors

- *Volume > 25 mL is the most important risk factor*
- pH < 2.5.
- Solid particles.
    Therefore acidic solid particles in large quantity (> 25 mL) will produce the most fulminant reaction.

Signs and Symptoms

- Tachypnea, cough due to laryngospasm/bronchospasm (in conscious patient)
- Tachycardia.
- Wheezing and crepitations.
- *Cyanosis/hypoxia*: During general anesthesia aspiration is usually diagnosed by persistent hypoxia.
- X-ray chest shows infiltrates.

Pathology

Chemical trauma to bronchial and alveolar mucosa and injury to vascular endothelium can cause exudative pneumonitis or pulmonary edema (ARDS).

Segments of Lungs Involved in Aspiration

See Chapter 1, page no. 4.

Management

Prevention

- Keep the patient nil orally as per recommendations.
- Inhibition of gastric acid secretion by H_2 antagonists like ranitidine, famotidine night before surgery in patients who are at high risk of aspiration.
- *Metoclopramide*: It fastens gastric emptying and increases the tone of LES.
- Neutralization of gastric content (to increase the pH) by antacids like sodium citrate.

Anesthetic management

- Full stomach or other high risk cases of aspiration posted for emergency surgery should be managed in the following way to prevent aspiration:
  - All high risk patients for aspiration must be premedicated with metoclopramide and ranitidine and/or sodium citrate.
  - Regional anesthesia is preferred over general anesthesia.
  - If there is slightest doubt of difficult intubation and situation permits (not life threatening emergency) then awake intubation with topical analgesia of upper airways is highly recommended
  - If general anesthesia is to be given, *rapid sequence induction* technique must be employed in the following manner:

Preoxygenation with 100% oxygen for 3–4 minutes is mandatory (in case of emergency 4 deep breaths with 100% O_2 can be used as an alternative to preoxygenation).

After preoxygenation induction is accomplished with ketamine or thiopentone. Theoretically ketamine is preferred because it maximally preserves pharyngeal and laryngeal reflexes but because of its side effects it is hardly used. Propofol maximally inhibit upper airway reflexes therefore not an optimal selection in patients vulnerable for aspiration. Succinylcholine (suxamethonium) is given immediately after the induction agent [if suxamethonium is absolutely contraindicated then rocuronium can be used as an alternative agent]. Succinylcholine and ketamine do increase the intragastric pressure but not above critical (20 cm H_2O) therefore can be safely used.

As soon as the patient becomes unconscious the assistant applies the backward and downward pressure of 30–40 Newtons (which is equivalent to 8–9 pounds) on cricoid cartilage (called as *Sellick's maneuver*) which compresses esophagus between assistant finger and vertebral column preventing aspiration as well as air leak into esophagus. Although the efficacy of cricoid pressure has been doubted by number of clinicians however its use is still recommended strongly.

Ventilation with bag and mask is absolutely contraindicated because mask ventilation will lead to air leak into stomach to achieve intragastric pressure above critical (> 20 cm H_2O).

Since ventilation with mask is contraindicated therefore intubation should be done at the earliest.

Cricoid pressure should be released only once cuff is inflated and the position of endotracheal tube is confirmed.

Modified rapid sequence induction: It is the technique in which gentle positive pressure ventilation (inspiratory pressure <20 cm H_2O) with mask is given along with the cricoid pressure. It is required in the situations where delayed intubation can put the patient at the risk of hypoxemia.

Treatment of aspiration

- Immediately turn the patient to one side with head low position.
- Do suction to prevent further aspiration. Tracheal suction may be sufficient in mild cases.
- Oxygen and continuous positive airway pressure (CPAP) in conscious patient till the patient is maintaining the oxygen saturation. If saturation is not maintained on CPAP then patient is put on mechanical ventilation.
- Antibiotics, bronchodilators, steroids (doubtful and empirical role only).

Decrease Inspired Concentration (FiO$_2$)

Decrease delivery of oxygen may be due to exhausted stores, leaks in central supply pipelines, machine and circuit, disconnections and malpositioned tubes. Use of oxygen analyzers (showing final delivered concentration of oxygen to patient) can prevent hypoxia due to decreased FiO$_2$. In fact, use of oxygen analyzers is mandatory as per ASA task force guidelines.

Hypoventilation

Causes

The usual cause of hypoventilation in intraoperative period is inappropriate ventilatory setting or leaks in machine and circuit while in postoperative period the usual cause of hypoventilation is the residual effect of anesthetic agents or muscle relaxants (inadequate reversal). Pain and splints in thoracic and upper abdominal surgeries can cause significant hypoventilation.

Ventilation Perfusion (V/Q) Mismatch

Ventilation perfusion abnormalities may occur because of atelectasis, pulmonary edema, pneumothorax or pulmonary embolism. *Atelectasis is the most common postoperative pulmonary complication*. The most common cause of atelectasis is the secretions. *V/Q mismatch caused by atelectasis is the most common cause of postoperative hypoxia*.

Early mobilization of the patient, physiotherapy, incentive spirometry, and positive airway pressure by facemask are the effective strategies in treating atelectasis.

Upper Airway Obstruction

This may occur at induction or in postoperative period.

Causes

- *Tongue fall:* This is due to abolition of tone of genioglossus muscle during anesthesia.
  Treatment
  - Jaw is lifted upwards and forwards and head is extended.
  - Oropharyngeal (Gudel)/nasopharyngeal airways.
  - Intubation.
- *Secretions:* Blood, mucous can irritate larynx producing *laryngospasm* (glottic closure) and desaturation. *Secretions are the most common cause of laryngospasm in anesthesia.*
  Treatment
  - Remove the secretions by suction.
  - IPPV with bag and mask may relieve the laryngospasm in significant number of cases.
  - If not relieved with bag and mask ventilation, a small doses of succinylcholine (25–50 mg IV) should be given.
  - Intravenous Xylocard should be given to prevent further laryngospasm.
- *Kinking or blockage of endotracheal tube* by secretions.
  Treatment: Remove secretions through suction or change the tube.

Bronchospasm

Light anesthesia (particularly in asthmatics), secretions and noxious stimuli can induce bronchospasm.

Treatment

- Good depth of anesthesia.
- Bronchodilators.

Light anesthesia during Lord's (anal) stretching and cervical dilatation can initiate parasympathetic over activity causing laryngospasm, bronchospasm, bradycardia and even cardiac arrest. This reflex is called as *Breuer Lockhart reflex.*

Pulmonary Edema

The causes of pulmonary edema in perioperative period may be cardiac failure, fluid overload (particularly in pediatric patients), transfusion related, aspiration, sepsis or *negative pressure pulmonary edema due to upper airway obstruction (particularly laryngospasm).*

The management of pulmonary edema includes continuing mechanical ventilation, diuretics, steroids, opioids, antibiotics and the treatment of the cause.

Pulmonary Embolism

Usually present in second week but can present with sudden onset from 2nd to 4th postoperative day.

Signs and Symptoms

- Dyspnea, substernal discomfort/chest pain, pleural pain, hemoptysis, tachycardia, increased CVP, hypotension, and Gallop rhythm.
  X-ray chest may show linear shadow, effusion or oligaemia if embolus is large.
  ECG shows findings of right ventricular strain.
- Massive embolus may present as cardiac arrest.

Treatment

- Prevention of deep vein thrombosis (DVT) by:
  - Early ambulation.
  - Pneumatic compression of calf muscles.
  - Leg movements in bed.
  - Low dose heparin.
- For small embolus, anticoagulant may be sufficient.
- For large embolus, streptokinase therapy should be instituted.
- For massive embolus, resuscitation followed by surgical embolectomy may be considered.

Pneumothorax

This is a dangerous complication requiring immediate treatment. It is usually due to surgical causes like rib resection, renal surgery however can occur after supraclavicular block.

Other Causes

Other rare causes of hypoxemia seen in perioperative period may be carbon monoxide poisoning (desiccated soda lime with desflurane), methemoglobinemia (Nitroglycerine infusion), cyanide poisoning (Sodium nitroprusside infusion), diffusion hypoxia (nitrous oxide) and shock.

HYPERCARBIA

Causes

- Hypoventilation
- Increased airway resistance (bronchospasm).
- Exhausted sodalime.
- Increased production like in malignant hyperthermia and thyrotoxicosis.

Treatment

Rectify the cause.

HYPOCAPNIA

It is almost always due to hyperventilation.

COUGH/HICCUPS

Usually occurs due to light anesthesia.

CARDIOVASCULAR COMPLICATIONS

HYPERTENSION

Interestingly, it has been observed that *postoperative hypertension and tachycardia are more responsible for unplanned ICU admission and carries higher morbidity and mortality than hypotension and bradycardia.*

Causes of hypertension:
In intraoperative period the usual causes are:
- Light anesthesia.
- Response to laryngoscopy and intubation.
- Hypercapnia.
- Drugs like ketamine.
- Undiagnosed pheochromocytoma.

In postoperative period the usual causes are:
- Pain.

- Hypercapnia.
- Full bladder.
- Emergence delirium.

CARDIAC ARRHYTHMIAS

Although, any arrhythmia ranging from sinus arrest to ventricular fibrillation may occur in perioperative period however the *most common arrhythmia seen in perioperative period is tachycardia.* The most common cause of tachycardia in intraoperative period is inadequate depth of anesthesia and in postoperative period is pain and anxiety.

Treatment

Increasing the depth or treating the pain should settle the tachycardia. If not (or is due to other cause) then it should be treated with *esmolol.* If esmolol is not available then labetalol is used. Other drugs which can be used are metoprolol, propranolol (usually avoided because it is not beta1 selective and can have S/E like bronchospasm however is recommended for specific cases), verapamil (can cause hypotension and conduction block with inhalational agents but these concerns are only theoretical).

HYPOTENSION

The most common cause of hypotension in perioperative period is intravascular volume depletion which could be because of excessive blood and fluid loss (particularly in major GI surgeries) or inadequate volume replacement. Other causes may be (but not limited to) third space (extravascular) fluid transfer occurs as a response to surgery and anesthesia, effect of anesthetic drugs (majority of anesthetic agents are vasodilators), anesthetic techniques (spinal and epidural), cardiac event/arrhythmias, transfusion reaction and sepsis or anaphylactic reactions.

Prevention

- Surgeon to achieve adequate hemostasis
- *Controlled hypotension:* Controlled hypotension is the technique of deliberately reducing the blood pressure to decrease intraoperative bleeding. Controlled hypotension is usually employed for the surgeries where excessive blood loss is expected or when

blood is not available or cannot be given due to religious reasons like Jehovah's convention.

- *Definition:* In a person with normal blood pressure no organ dysfunction occurs if blood pressure is maintained within the limits of autoregulation, i.e. if mean arterial pressure is maintained between 50–65 mm Hg. Therefore, for a patient with normal BP *controlled hypotension means reduction of mean arterial pressure to 50–65 mm Hg* however reducing BP to such low levels may not be tolerated by hypertensive patients. That's why the best clinical definition of controlled hypotension is to reduce the blood pressure by one-third of preoperative value. Continuous measurement of BP by invasive BP monitoring is mandatory.

- *Techniques:* Although agents used in GA (inhalational agents, propofol, opioids), technique, i.e. positive pressure ventilation (by decreasing the venous return) or spinal/epidural causes hypotension however up to a certain limits. Therefore, *to produce controlled hypotension short acting vasodilator especially nitroglycerin as continuous infusion is the most commonly used to produce controlled hypotension.* The concern to produce methemoglobinemia by nitroglycerine is very rare and can be treated with methylene blue. Sodium nitroprusside (SNP) used in past in not preferred now a days due to the possibility of *cyanide toxicity.*

- Others agents which can be used to produce controlled hypotension are α-blockers, β-blockers (however α + β-blocker, i.e. *labetalol is most preferred now a day*), calcium channel blockers (nicardipine, clevidipine) and Dexmedetomidine.

Contraindications: Patients suffering from cerebrovascular disease, coronary artery disease, and severe anemia may not be able to tolerate hypotension.

Risks: Usually if BP is maintained within the limit of autoregulation there should not be any organ ischemia however controlled hypotension can produce devastating complications like myocardial ischemia, cerebral infarct, cord ischemia leading to paraplegia, hepatic and renal necrosis or even blindness. In fact, due to the possibility of these complications many anesthesiologists avoid controlled hypotension as far as possible.

Treatment

- Adequate fluid infusion.
- Vasopressors and inotropes.
- Treatment of the cause.

MYOCARDIAL ISCHEMIA

Surgery and anesthesia are stressful conditions which can precipitate MI in susceptible individuals. The lifetime risk of re-infarction in a known patient of MI is 6%.

Treatment includes oxygen, morphine, nitroglycerine, inotropes, thrombolytic therapy and intra-aortic balloon counterpulsations.

CARDIAC ARREST

More than 80% of cardiac arrest occurs at the time of induction. The common causes of cardiac arrest are inability to ventilate, side effects of anesthetic agents like severe hypotension with inhalational agents or bradycardia proceeding to asystole after succinylcholine and anaphylaxis.

NEUROLOGICAL COMPLICATIONS

CONVULSIONS

May occur due to:

- Hypoxia.
- Drugs like *local anesthetics, methohexitone, enflurane, sevoflurane and atracurium/cisatracurium*
- Cerebrovascular accidents.

Treatment

Maintain airway and anticonvulsants.

DELAYED RECOVERY

Delayed recovery (which means patient not regaining consciousness within 30–60 minutes after discontinuing anesthesia) *is the most common CNS complication* and is usually due to the residual effect of anesthetic agents. Most often the patient recovers spontaneously however if the patient does not exhibit the signs of recovery after considerable time he/she should be investigated for other causes of delayed recovery like electrolyte imbalance, acid base abnormalities, metabolic abnormalities like *hypoglycemia or cerebrovascular accident.*

AWARENESS (INADEQUATE AMNESIA)

Incidence is < 1% however very important from medico legal point of view. Most common type is auditory.

Methods to Prevent Awareness and Recall of Events

- Premedication with benzodiazepines (produce anterograde amnesia).
- Inhalational agents (all inhalational agents are very good amnestic agents except nitrous oxide)

Therefore awareness usually occurs when oxygen, nitrous oxide and opioids are used for maintenance of anesthesia.

AGITATION, DELIRIUM AND EMERGENCE EXCITEMENT

The common causes of agitation are pain and full bladder. *Emergence excitement* is a transient confusional state usually seen in children at the emergence from general anesthesia. It should not be confused with Delirium which is often because of the side effect of drugs like ketamine.

Treatment

- Treat the cause.
- Midazolam.

POSTOPERATIVE COGNITIVE DYSFUNCTION

The incidence of postoperative cognitive dysfunction (POCD) at 1 year after cardiac surgery is 20% to 40% and 4–10% after noncardiac surgery. It is more common in old age. The possible causes may be cerebral microemboli (atheroma, fat, platelet aggregates, and air), brain cell damage caused by toxic substances (like general anesthesia drugs) or hypoxia or surgery-induced release of hormones and inflammatory mediators.

PERMANENT BRAIN DAMAGE

Due to prolonged hypoxia following cardiac arrest, prolonged hypotension, cerebrovascular accidents, raised ICT.

CRANIAL NERVE PALSIES

If trielene is used with closed circuit.

EXTRAPYRAMIDAL SIDE EFFECTS

Seen with neuroleptanalgesia (droperidol + fentanyl).

PERIPHERAL NEUROPATHIES

Although the overall incidence of neuropathies is less (<1%) but they represent the *2nd most common cause of claims* as per American Society of Anesthesiologists (ASA) Closed Claims studies. As per the recent close claim studies *Brachial plexus injuries are the most common postoperative nerve injury associated with general anesthesia* followed by ulnar nerve. However *after regional anesthesia lumbosacral nerve roots are most commonly involved nerves* followed by spinal cord injury. *When combined (GA+RA) spinal cord injury becomes the most common injury* followed by brachial plexus.

Causes

- Faulty position leading to compression of nerve
- Direct injection of drug in nerves during blocks.
- Prolonged hypotension leading to nerve ischemia
- Direct neurotoxicity of local anesthetics
- *Tourniquet palsies*: Pressure in tourniquet should not exceed more than 100 mm Hg above systolic pressure (maximum 250 mm Hg) and duration as per current recommendations should not exceed more than 2 hours for both upper and lower limb.

GASTROINTESTINAL COMPLICATIONS

POSTOPERATIVE NAUSEA AND VOMITING

The incidence of postoperative nausea and vomiting (PONV) is 20% to 30% making it as the *second most common complain* after pain in postoperative period.

Risk Factors

- *Female gender*: Three times more vulnerable than males
- *General anesthesia*: Patient given GA has 4 times more incidence of PONV than patients who received regional anesthesia. The most common reason may be opioids.
- *Type of the surgery*: Surgeries like middle ear surgeries, strabismus surgery, laparoscopies and adenotonsillectomies can have incidence of nausea, vomiting as high as 30–40%.
- *Young age*: The incidence of PONV is much higher in adults as compared to old age
- *Nonsmokers*: For unknown reasons nonsmokers are 1.8 times more vulnerable than smokers to have PONV.

Treatment

- *Serotonin antagonists* (Ondansetron, granisetron) *remains the drugs of choice for treatment as well as prophylaxis for PONV.* Interestingly all are equally effective at equipotent doses.
- *Metoclopramide*: *It is the preferred antiemetic for the conditions associated with high incidence of aspiration.*
- *Dexamethasone*: Dexamethasone is long acting and studies suggest its efficacy similar to ondansetron
- *Aprepitant*: It is a neurokinin receptor antagonists. It is very effective antiemetic however its cost restricts its use.
- *Transdermal scopolamine*: Useful for preventing nausea and vomiting in high risk patients if applied a night before or early in the morning on the day of surgery.
- *Droperidol*: The serious side effect, i.e. QT prolongation which can precipitate torsade pointes has not only lead to withdrawal of this drug from use but also has put Droperidol in black box warning by FDA.

Usually one antiemetic is sufficient to treat PONV, however if patient is not responding then as a rule antiemetic from another class should be chosen.

RENAL COMPLICATIONS

Renal function may be impaired due to hypotension or nephrotoxic anesthetics like methoxyflurane.

HEPATIC COMPLICATIONS

Hepatic functions may be impaired due to hypotension or hepatotoxic anesthetics like halothane.

PAIN

As per the recent close claim studies *pain is the most common complication is postoperative period. For details of postoperative pain management see Chapter 39, page no. 270.*

THERMAL PERTURBATIONS

HYPOTHERMIA AND SHIVERING

Hypothermia is the most common thermal perturbation seen in anesthesia. *For details of hypothermia see Chapter 6, page no. 66.*

Shivering occurs as a protective mechanism to hypothermia. O_2 consumption may increase to 4 times (400%) [100 to 600% depending on heat loss during surgery] during shivering. Therefore, oxygen supplementation during shivering is mandatory.

Shivering can be abolished by inhibition of hypothalamus. Most commonly shivering is seen after halothane.

Treatment of Shivering

- *Pethidine is the drug of choice.*
- Tramadol is 2nd drug of choice after pethidine
  Other drugs which can be also be used are alpha 2 agonist (clonidine, dexmedetomidine), butorphanol, chlorpromazine, physostigmine, magnesium sulfate, ketanserin and propofol.

HYPERTHERMIA

Causes of Hyperthermia in Anesthesia

- Hypermetabolic states like thyrotoxicosis and pheochromocytoma.

- Neuroleptic malignant syndrome due to phenothiazines.
- Drug induced like atropine, pethidine, MAO inhibitors, tricyclic antidepressants and amphetamines.
- Injury to hypothalamic temperature regulatory centers.
- Malignant hyperthermia (MH).

MALIGNANT HYPERTHERMIA

Malignant hyperthermia (MH) is the clinical syndrome associated with high mortality (4%), seen during general anesthesia in which there is rapid rise in temperature, as high as 1°C/5 min.

Etiology

It is due to abnormality of type I Ryanodine receptor (RYR1) which is calcium releasing channel of sarcoplasmic reticulum. The abnormality leads to excessive accumulation of calcium in sarcoplasmic retinaculum which causes sustained contraction of muscle. It is a genetic disease usually autosomal dominant but can be recessive also.

Associated risk factors:
- Conditions like Duchenne muscle dystrophy, arthrogryposis multiplex congenita, osteogenesis imperfecta, congenital strabismus, central core diseases.
- Patient with history of neuroleptic malignant syndrome are susceptible of MH (but not vice versa)
- Children are more prone as compared to adults
- Positive family history of malignant hyperthermia
- Patients who develop masseter spasm after succinylcholine are more prone to develop malignant hyperthermia. Although the correlation is not absolute but has strong association therefore these patients must be observed carefully for signs of malignant hyperthermia.

Incidence

1 in 15,000 for pediatric and 1 in 40,000 for adults patients given GA with volatile anesthetics and succinylcholine. It is more common in males as compared to females.

Causative Agents

Muscle relaxant: *Succinylcholine is the most commonly implicated drug.*

Inhalational agents:
- *Halothane is the most commonly implicated inhalational agent.* Others are:
  - Isoflurane
  - Enflurane
  - Desflurane
  - Sevoflurane
  - Methoxyflurane
  - Cyclopropane
  - Ether

Other drugs (probable triggering agents):
- Tricyclic antidepressants, Monoamine oxidase (MAO) inhibitors and phenothiazines.
- Lignocaine, which used to be considered as weak triggering agent, is now a days not considered as triggering agent
- Exercise, heat-stroke, excessive excitement and statins as potential triggers for malignant hyperthermia episode continues to be debated. Malignant hyperthermia induced by these factors is called as *non-anesthetic or awake malignant hyperthermia.*

Clinical Features

Due to increase muscle metabolism and activity
- *Hyperthermia* (temperature may rise to more than 109°F). *Hyperthermia is the most important sign in diagnosing MH but unfortunately it is a late sign.* The heat production is due to increased muscle metabolism (both aerobic and anaerobic), glycolysis and hydrolysis of high energy phosphates involved in the process of contraction-relaxation.
- Increased end tidal CO_2 ($ETCO_2$): This may rise to more than 100 mm Hg (normal 32–42 mm Hg). *Rapid increase in end tidal CO_2 is the most sensitive early sign of malignant hyperthermia.*
- Hypoxia, cyanosis and decrease in mixed venous oxygen saturation (due to increased oxygen consumption)
- Severe metabolic acidosis (pH < 7.0).
- Masseter spasm
- Hyperkalemia, muscle rigidity, increased creatinine phosphokinase, increased myoglobin, myoglobinuria

- Renal failure, DIC, pulmonary and cerebral edema.
- Death: *Hyperkalemia induced ventricular fibrillation is the most common cause of death in malignant hyperthermia.*

Due to sympathetic stimulation
- Tachycardia, hypertension, cardiac arrhythmias.

Treatment
Specific: *Dantrolene*, 2 mg/kg to be repeated every 5 minutes to a maximum of 10 mg/kg. Dantrolene should be continued 1 mg/kg every 6 hourly for next 24 hours as chances of recurrence is 50%. Dantrolene directly binds to ryanodine receptor inhibiting calcium release.

General measures:
- Stop the triggering anesthetic (inhalational agent) immediately and change the circuit as some residual agent may be present in circuit.
- Hyperventilation with 100% oxygen to wash out CO_2.
- Control temperature by:
  - Ice cooling.
  - Ice cold saline.
- Correct acidosis
- Because ventricular fibrillation is the most common cause of death therefore correction of hyperkalemia should be done on priority.
- Myoglobin by blocking renal tubules may cause renal failure therefore maintain urine output from the beginning.

Screening/Evaluation of Suspected Individuals
The patients who have associated risk factors (described above) should be evaluated by the following protocol:

All high risk patients (particularly with history of malignant hyperthermia in close relative) must undergo *blood creatinine kinase (CK) levels*. Patients with elevated CK levels in normal resting conditions should be managed as susceptible and do not require further testing.

Patients with normal CK levels should undergo *muscle contracture test*. In this test a muscle biopsy is taken and subjected to Halothane and caffeine to see the pathological changes of malignant hyperthermia. If muscle biopsy studies are negative then only the patient can be considered non-susceptible. *Muscle contracture test is considered as gold standard test for diagnosing susceptibility to malignant hyperthermia.*

Anesthesia for Patients Susceptible for Malignant Hyperthermia
- Local or regional anesthesia is preferred over general anesthesia.
- Safe drugs for general anesthesia are barbiturates, *propofol* (propofol can delay or prevent malignant hyperthermia), narcotics, benzodiazepines, nitrous oxide, *nondepolarizing muscle relaxants* (can delay or prevent malignant hyperthermia).
- Mild hypothermia is beneficial
- Must be kept in recovery room for 4–6 hours
- Must be instructed to avoid heat as these patients are very prone for heat stroke.

Differential Diagnosis of Malignant Hyperthermia
- Neurolept malignant syndrome (NMS)
  The important differentiating features are:
  - History of intake of antidopaminergic drugs (like phenothiazines or metoclopramide) or missing the intake of levodopa in Parkinson patient
  - Rise in CO_2 and muscle rigidity are slow and in proportion to rise in temperature. (While in MH, CO_2 rise is disproportionate and very rapid)
  - As neuromuscular junction is normal, muscle rigidity can be reversed with nondepolarizing muscle relaxants while in malignant hyperthermia due to abnormality at neuromuscular junction it is not possible to reverse muscle rigidity by nondepolarizers.
- *Thyrotoxicosis:* Other than history of hyperthyroidism and proportionate rise in CO_2, *hypokalemia* is the most important distinguishing feature.
- Other differential diagnoses are pheochromocytoma, sepsis or drug induced hyperthermia.

ANAPHYLACTIC/ANAPHYLACTOID REACTIONS

Incidence: 1 in 10,000.

Anaphylactic reaction can occur with any of the drug used in perioperative period except inhalational agents.

The most common cause of anaphylaxis is muscle relaxants (60–70%) followed by latex allergy (12%) and then antibiotics (8–10%). Among muscle relaxants, maximum incidence is with *rocuronium* to be followed by suxamethonium.

During anesthesia cardiovascular signs (tachycardia, hypotension) and cutaneous (rash, angioedema) are more important than respiratory manifestations (laryngospasm, bronchospasm) in the diagnosis of anaphylactic reactions.

Treatment

- Maintenance of airway (if laryngeal edema or bronchospasm develops).
- *Adrenaline* is the mainstay of treatment.
  Doses: 0.5–1 mg of 1: 1000 intramuscularly or subcutaneously (less preferred due to poor absorption). In life-threatening situations, 1:10,000 adrenaline can be given by intravenous route in doses of 1 microgram/kg to a maximum of 1 mg (usually 50–100 mcg for adult). If IV route is not accessible than it can be given through intra-tracheal or Intraosseous route.
- Steroids (hydrocortisone).
- Histamine antagonist like diphenhydramine.

COMPLICATIONS OF DIFFERENT POSITIONS

LITHOTOMY

- Functional residual capacity and vital capacity decreases by approx. 20% increasing the V/Q mismatch.
- Nerve injuries:
  - Common peroneal nerve (compressed between head of fibula and bar)— *Common peroneal neuropathy is the most common neuropathy of the lower limb*
  - Saphenous nerve (pressure over medial condyle)
  - Femoral nerve (Due to angulation of thigh)
  - Obturator nerve
- Muscle injury:
  - Compartment syndrome (due to extreme tightening of straps).
- Increased cardiac load due to increased venous return.

TRENDELENBURG

- Increased central venous pressure and increased cardiac load due to increased venous return.
- Decreased vital capacity and function residual capacity (FRC) by 15–20%.
- Increased intraocular and intracranial pressure, venous congestion of face and cerebral hemorrhage due to decrease venous return from head and neck area.
- Lingual and buccal neuropathy.

SITTING

- Spinal cord ischemia and quadriplegia can occur due to extreme flexion of neck.
- *Brachial plexus injury:* Weight of arm during general anesthesia can stretch the brachial plexus.
- Femoral and obturator nerve injury due to extreme angulation at thigh.
- Venous air embolism (*for details see Chapter 27, page no. 226*).

LATERAL AND PRONE

- Transient Horner syndrome.
- Brachial plexus injury.
- Compartment syndrome of hand.
- Spinal cord ischemia (due to extreme flexion of neck).
- Breast injury.
- Genitalia injury.
- Radial and ulnar nerve injuries.
- Ischemic optic neuropathy.

OCULAR COMPLICATIONS

Exposure keratitis (Corneal abrasion) is a common complication of general anesthesia if eyes remain open (because of loss of blinking reflex). To prevent keratitis artificial tears/eye ointment should be instilled and eyes should be covered with eye pads.

Ischemic optic neuropathy (due to severe hypotension or pressure on eyes in prone position) is rare but dreadful complication leading to blindness.

FIRES AND ELECTRIC HAZARDS IN OPERATION THEATER

There are three prerequisites for a fire (the triad of fire): Ignition source, fuel and an oxidizer (gas supporting combustion).

1. *Ignition source:* The ignition source may be
   - *Cautery—Responsible for 68% of fires.*
   - Laser—Another important source for fires.
   - Electric sparks and short circuits. Maximum leakage allowed in operation theater is 10 µA. These may occur through plugs, monitors, suction machines, etc.
   - *Static electricity:* This can be a cause of fire hazard in anesthesia. Static current is produced when two dissimilar surfaces come in contact and get separated, so walking, movement of machine and trolleys can produce static current. Gas flow (especially oxygen) through circuits and machine can generate static current and if there is short circuit explosions can occur. Nylon and woolen clothing of patient can produce static current.
   - Other sources like fiberoptic illuminators, defibrillators, etc.
2. *Fuel:* Anything which catches fire like endotracheal tubes, laryngeal airway, antiseptic solutions, etc. Silicone is most resistant to fire followed by PVC while red rubber tubes are most vulnerable to catch fire.
3. *Oxidizer:* Both oxygen and nitrous oxide support combustion.

The fire and explosion can take very bad shape if an *inflammable agent like Ether and Cyclopropane* is used. Although these agents are no more used however if used then cautery should be avoided and if that is not possible then cautery should be at least 25 cm away from the agent.

PRECAUTIONS TO PREVENT FIRE AND BURNS

- *Earthing (grounding):* Proper grounding of all electrical equipment is mandatory.
- Electric wiring of Operation Theater should be leak proof.
- Use of isolation transformers.
- *Grounding (patient plate) of diathermy:* Proper use of diathermy plate is must to prevent burns to patient. It should be applied over large muscle mass (like gluteus muscle), as near as to surgical site and away from ECG electrodes. It should not be applied over bony prominences, scar tissue or metal prosthesis and do not reuse the pad.
- Prefer bipolar cautery wherever possible
- *Precautions during laser surgery:*
  - Use laser resistant tubes or apply protective covering like aluminum or copper tapes over tubes
  - Fill the cuff of endotracheal tube with water instead of air and use minimum concentration of oxygen
  - Everyone in OT should wear protective eye shield during laser surgery.
- *Measures to decrease static current:*
  - Conductive flooring.
  - Every person in theater should wear rubber soled shoes.
  - Tyres of anesthesia machines, trolleys, OT tables should be made up of antistatic rubber.
  - Breathing circuits, face mask (can cause facial burns) should be made up of antistatic rubber (which is made antistatic by addition of carbon).
  - Silk, nylon and woolen clothing of patient is not permitted in OT.
  - Humidity should be more than 50% (static current is generated more in dry air).
- Smoking, lighters should not be allowed in and around operation theater.
- Over heating of bulbs, endoscopes should not be allowed.

OCCUPATIONAL HAZARDS

The additional occupational hazards to anesthetists are—
- Higher risk of exposure to anesthetic agents
- Increase chances of acquiring infectious diseases like HIV, hepatitis B and C
- More vulnerability to substance abuse (due to easy availability, work stress and more

adventurous nature)—Drug related death odds ratio of anesthetists as compared to physicians is 2.87.

DISCHARGE CRITERIA FROM POSTANESTHESIA CARE UNIT

The criteria vary depending whether patient is discharged to ICU, ward or home. Although there are many recovery scores but the most popular are ALDRETE score (which includes color, respiration, consciousness level, circulation and activity level) and postanesthesia discharge scoring system (PADS).

KEY POINTS

- Maximum complications are reported in maintenance period however more than 80% of cardiac arrest occurs at the time of induction.
- Postoperative respiratory depression has been cited as the most common cause of anesthesia related death in perioperative period.
- Death is the leading cause of claims as per American Society of Anesthesiologists (ASA) claim studies.
- Aspiration is considered as preventable complication of anesthesia.
- Full stomach is the single most important predisposing factor for aspiration.
- Rapid sequence induction technique must be employed for giving GA to the patients who are at high risk of aspiration.
- Atelectasis is the most common postoperative pulmonary complication and the most common cause of atelectasis is secretions.
- Use of oxygen analyzers is mandatory as per ASA task force guidelines.
- Secretions is the most common cause of laryngospasm in anesthesia.
- Postoperative hypertension and tachycardia are more responsible for unplanned ICU admission and carries higher morbidity and mortality than hypotension and bradycardia.
- Tachycardia is the most common arrhythmia seen in perioperative period.
- The most common cause of hypotension in perioperative period is intravascular volume depletion.
- Nitroglycerin as continuous infusion is the most commonly used agent to produce controlled hypotension.
- Anesthetic drugs which can cause convulsion are—Local anesthetics, methohexitone, enflurane, sevoflurane and atracurium/cisatracurium.
- Delayed recovery is the most common CNS complication.
- Brachial plexus injuries are the most common postoperative nerve injury associated with general anesthesia followed by ulnar nerve. However after regional anesthesia lumbosacral nerve roots are most commonly involved nerves.
- Ondansetron/Granisetron remains the drugs of choice for treatment as well as prophylaxis for postoperative nausea and vomiting.
- Pain is the most common complication is postoperative period.
- Hypothermia is the most common thermal perturbation seen in anesthesia.
- Succinylcholine is the most commonly implicated drug while halothane is the most commonly implicated inhalational agent for causing malignant hyperthermia.
- Hyperkalemia induced ventricular fibrillation is the most common cause of death in malignant hyperthermia.
- Propofol and non-depolarizing muscle relaxants can delay or prevent malignant hyperthermia.
- Muscle relaxants are the most common cause of anaphylaxis followed by latex allergy.
- Cautery is responsible for 68% of fires seen in OT.

Regional Anesthesia

CHAPTER **15**

Local Anesthetics

First local anesthetic (LA) used in clinical practice was cocaine by Carl Koller for anesthetizing the cornea.

CLASSIFICATION

Local anesthetics are classified on the basis of chemical structure and duration of action.

Based on Chemical Structure

Chemically local anesthetics consist of a benzene ring separated from tertiary amide either by ester or amide linkage. Based on this intermediate chain they are classified as aminoesters and aminoamides.

Aminoesters	Aminoamides
• Procaine	• Lignocaine
• Chloroprocaine	• Mepivacaine
• Tetracaine (Amethocaine)	• Prilocaine
• Benzocaine	• Bupivacaine
• Cocaine	• Etidocaine • Ropivacaine
• Esters are metabolized by pseudocholinesterase (except cocaine which is metabolized in liver)	• Amides are metabolized primarily in liver
• High incidence of allergic reactions due to para aminobenzoic acid.	• Low incidence of allergic reactions
• Solutions are not stable	• Solutions are so stable that not destroyed even by autoclaving

Based on Duration of Action

Short duration (15–30 minutes)
- *Chloroprocaine: Shortest acting local anesthetic*
- Procaine

Intermediate duration (30–90 minutes)
- Lignocaine
- Mepivacaine
- Prilocaine
- Cocaine

Long duration (2–3 hours)
- Bupivacaine.
- Levobupivacaine
- Ropivacaine.
- Tetracaine (Amethocaine).
- Etidocaine.
- Dibucaine: *Longest acting local anesthetic.*

Other Drugs with Local Anesthetic Properties

Opioids

Pethidine: Patients hypersensitive to local anesthetics can be given pethidine in place of local anesthetics.

Buprenorphine: Because of its local anesthetic properties it is frequently used to supplement the effect of local anesthetics for nerve blocks.

Tramadol: Although weak but tramadol do have local anesthetic properties.

Methoxyflurane

The droplets of methoxyflurane has got local anesthetic properties.

Newer Formulations/Formulation Under Research

- Synera (S-Caine) is a combination of Lignocaine and Tetracaine that has heating element to enhance the onset
- *Depot formulations:* Depot formulations have been synthesized to prolong the duration of local anesthetics. *Exparel* has recently been approved in U.S. for infiltration analgesia (but not for nerve block). *Posidur*, another lipid depot formulation is still under clinical trials
- Liposomal encapsulation of the local anesthetics can prolong the block.

MECHANISM OF ACTION OF LOCAL ANESTHETICS (FIG. 15.1)

Local anesthetics are deposited all around the nerve. Drug in undissociated (nonionized) form penetrates the axonal membrane. Once inside it gets dissociated (ionized). It is this dissociated (ionized, protonated, cationic or uncharged) form which binds to *sodium channel* (alpha subunit) from inner side, blocking the channel, preventing depolarization and action potential. Although local anesthetics can block sodium channel in any state however activated channels (positive resting

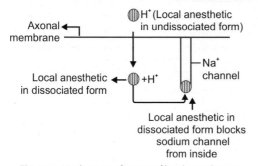

Fig. 15.1: Mechanism of action of local anesthetics

membrane potential) are more easily blocked as compared to inactivated channels (zero resting membrane potential) which in turn are more sensitive than resting state channel (negative resting membrane potential).

Recent studies have proven that local anesthetics not only act on sodium channels, but also block potassium and calcium channels in a manner that hypokalemia and hypercalcemia can antagonize the effect of local anesthetics. They are also found to block N-methyl-D-asparate (NMDA) receptors.

GENERAL CONSIDERATIONS IN ACTION OF LOCAL ANESTHETICS

Sensitivity of Nerve Fiber to Local Anesthetics

Based on fiber diameter the nerve fibers are classified as type A, B and C; A being the thickest and C the thinnest **(Table 15.1)**.

Two major factors which determine the sensitivity of nerve fibers to local anesthetics are fiber diameter and myelination. *Thin diameter fibers are more sensitive than thick diameter fibers.* As myelinated fibers are covered by nerve sheath and local anesthetics need to block nodes of ranvier only therefore *myelinated fibers are more sensitive than nonmyelinated.* Considering both factors (and other also like physiological and anatomic considerations) together it has been seen that *small myelinated fibers (A gamma and A delta) are the most sensitive* to local anesthetic block followed by large myelinated (A alpha and A beta) and then B (mixed, myelinated + nonmyelinated). *Non-myelinated C fibers are most resistant* to the actions of local anesthetics. Therefore, it can be concluded that sequence of blockade is—*A (Aγ > Aδ > Aα = Aβ) > B >C. The traditional notion that thin fibers are most sensitive to the action of local anesthetics does not hold true in present day practice.*

■ **Table 15.1:** Classification of nerve fibers

Fiber	Subclass	Myelin	Diameter	Function
A	α	+	6–22 μ	Motor, proprioception
	β	+	6–22 μ	Motor, proprioception
	γ	+	3–6 μ	Muscle tone
	δ	+	1–4 μ	Pain, touch, temperature
B	–	Mixed	< 3 μ	Preganglionic autonomic
C	C (sympathetic)	–	0.3–1.3 μ	Postganglionic autonomic
	C (dorsal root)	–	0.4–1.2 μ	Pain, touch, temperature

In functional terms, in peripheral nerve blocks motor function is blocked earliest followed by sensory and then autonomic (*motor > sensory > autonomic*). However in central neuraxial blocks (spinal/epidural) due to anatomical variations of mixed spinal nerve (autonomic on most outer side and motor on most inner side) the sequence of blockade is *autonomic > sensory > motor. Sequence of recovery is in reverse order of blockade.*

Among sensory sensations sequence of blockade is pain > temperature (cold before hot) > touch > deep pressure > proprioception (except for central neuraxial blocks where temperature is blocked earlier than pain).

Onset of Action

Depends on number of factors like:

- *Dose and concentration:* Higher dose or higher concentration facilitates onset.
- *pKa:* It is the pH at which a local anesthetic is 50% ionized and 50% nonionized. Since local anesthetics are weak bases, agents with pKa closer to physiologic pH will have more drugs in nonionized form which can diffuse through axonal membrane enhancing the onset. That is why lignocaine with lower pKa of 7.8 has fast onset as compared to bupivacaine with higher pKa of 8.1.
- *Addition of sodabicarbonate:* As local anesthetics are bases, adding sodabicarbonate will prevent ionization making more drug to be available in nonionized form to cross the axonal membrane. On the other hand in ischemic tissue (like abscess) acidic pH will ionize the drug, delaying the onset of action
- *Type of nerve fiber:* A fibers are blocked earlier than B which are blocked earlier than C
- *Frequency of nerve stimulation:* Since activated channels are blocked more easily, a stimulated nerve will be blocked earlier as compared to nonstimulated nerve. This kind of block by local anesthetics is called as *use-dependent block.*

Duration of Action

It depends on:

- *Dose:* Increased dose increases the duration.
- *Pharmacokinetic profile of drug:* It includes:
  - *Potency (lipid solubility):* Potency, which correlates with lipid solubility, is directly proportional to duration; *more the potency, longer is the duration* with the exception of chloroprocaine which in spite of having intermediate potency is shortest acting.
  - *Plasma protein binding (α1 acid glycoprotein):* Agents with high protein binding like bupivacaine have prolonged action.
  - *Metabolism:* Esters are metabolized by pseudocholinesterase and amides are metabolized in liver by microsomal enzymes therefore esters have shorter duration of action than amides.
- *Addition of vasoconstrictors:* Vasoconstrictors by decreasing the systemic absorption increases the duration of action. The most commonly used vasoconstrictor is *adrenaline* in a concentration of *1 in 2,00,000* (1 in 2 lakhs). Adrenaline when added to Lignocaine increases the duration of both sensory and motor blockade while with bupivacaine only sensory block is prolonged. Other vasoconstrictors which can be used are phenylephrine (1 in 20,000), noradrenaline and felypressin (octapressin), a synthetic derivative of vasopressin.
- *Sodium bicarbonate:* Addition of sodium bicarbonate not only enhances the onset but also increases the duration as carbon dioxide released from sodium bicarbonate metabolism enters intracellularly making the pH to become more acidic favoring more drug to be available in ionized form to bind to sodium channel. Interestingly addition of sodium bicarbonate by unknown mechanism decreases the pain of injection.

Systemic Absorption

It depends on:

- *Site of injection:* It is proportionate to the vascularity of the site of injection. *Maximum systemic absorption has been seen after intercostal nerve block.*
- *Addition of vasoconstrictors:* Addition of vasoconstrictor decreases the systemic absorption.

Potency

Potency directly correlates with Lipid Solubility.

Concentration minimum (Cm) is the minimum concentration of local anesthetic that will block nerve impulse conduction. It depends on number of factors like:

- Fiber type and myelination
- *pH:* Acidic pH by causing ionization increases the Cm
- *Frequency of nerve stimulation:* As stimulated nerve will have more activated channels therefore will need less Cm.
- *Electrolyte:* Hypokalemia and hypercalcemia antagonize the block.
- *Adjuvants:* Adjuvants like opioids (pethidine, buprenorphine, and tramadol) and α 2 agonist enhances the effect of LA. Sodium channel blocker, neosaxitoxin, as an adjuvant is under clinical trials.
- Progesterone increases the susceptibility of nerves to local anesthetics therefore doses of local anesthetics should be decreased in pregnancy.

Differential Block

It depends on *concentration.* A drug at lower concentration will produce only sensory block while at higher concentration can produce motor block.

Metabolism

Esters are metabolized by plasma pseudo-cholinesterase (except cocaine which is metabolized in liver) and amide by hepatic microsomal enzymes (except articaine, a local anesthetic used in dentistry, is metabolized in plasma). Lungs can also extract significant amount of local anesthetics like *prilocaine*, lignocaine and bupivacaine. Due to poor water solubility of local anesthetics renal excretion of unchanged drug is only less than 5%.

SYSTEMIC EFFECTS AND TOXICITY

Toxicity is proportional to potency. *Due to diversion of blood central nervous system (CNS) and cardiovascular system (CVS) toxicity of local anesthetics gets increased in shock.*

Central Nervous System

The CNS: CVS dose ratio for lignocaine is 1:7 and for bupivacaine is 1:3 that means CNS is involved at much lower doses as compared to CVS.

As central nervous system is the first system involved in local anesthetic toxicity therefore initial signs and symptoms of local anesthetic toxicity are related to CNS. Typical sequence is excitation followed by depression of cerebral tissue (inhibitory neurons are more sensitive than excitatory neurons). The common signs and symptoms are circumoral numbness, dizziness, tongue paresthesia, visual and auditory disturbances, muscle twitching, tremors, convulsions followed by coma and death. Convulsions as first presentation are quite common in local anesthetic toxicity.

Treatment includes maintenance of adequate ventilation and oxygenation. Convulsion can be controlled by diazepam/midazolam or thiopentone.

Cardiovascular System

Electrophysiological effects of local anesthetics on cardiac tissue are decrease in rate of depolarization (main effect), effective refractory period and duration of action potential.

All local anesthetics have negative inotropic action on myocardium, causes depression of conduction system (prolonged PR interval and increased duration of QRS complex). At very high doses they may block conduction of sinus node producing bradycardia or even sinus arrest. In addition to the above effects bupivacaine (and to lesser effect levobupivacaine and ropivacaine) can also produce ventricular arrhythmias. Therefore, either the isolated or combined actions like bradycardia, decreased myocardial contractility, ventricular arrhythmias, hypotension can produce cardiac arrest with local anesthetics. Management of cardiac arrest is immediate CPCR.

At lower doses local anesthetics may act as vasoconstrictors by directly inhibiting nitric oxide but at *clinically used doses all local anesthetics are vasodilators except cocaine, levobupivacaine and Ropivacaine* which are vasoconstrictor at all doses.

Respiratory System

Lignocaine depresses hypoxic drive. Direct depression of medullary respiratory centre can occur at high dose.

Immunologic: *Allergic reactions are common with esters but rare with amides.* The reaction with amides is because of the *preservative* (methyl paraben) it contains. Cross sensitivity *does not exist between classes* (i.e. esters and amides) *but exist between agents of same class.*

Methemoglobinemia: Usually seen with *Prilocaine however benzocaine can also cause methemoglobinemia.*

Treatment: IV methylene blue.

Coagulation: Lignocaine can inhibit coagulation.

Local toxicity: When directly injected into nerve any local anesthetics can damage the nerve. However local neurotoxicity can occur even without direct injection into nerve. The classical example of local anesthetic induced local neurotoxicity is *cauda equina syndrome seen with lignocaine and tetracaine* if used through small bore continuous spinal catheters. *Transient neurologic symptoms* (dysesthesia, radicular pain in lower extremities) is another example of local neurotoxicity *seen with lignocaine and mepivacaine.* However, *overall maximum local neurotoxicity has been reported with chloroprocaine.*
- When directly injected into muscle they are myotoxic
- Local anesthetics with *adrenaline can cause necrosis and gangrene if used for ring block of fingers, toes, penis or pinna because these structures have end arteries*

Combination of two local anesthetics: The use of two local anesthetics is quite common in clinical practice (usually lignocaine for rapid onset and bupivacaine/ropivacaine for long duration). *The toxicity of two local anesthetics should be considered additive,* not independent and therefore maximum safe doses should be reduced accordingly.

COMMERCIAL PREPARATIONS

Local anesthetics are weak bases however their commercial preparations are made acidic (pH to around 6) to enhance their chemical stability so they are available as hydrochloride salts. Local anesthetics containing adrenaline are made even more acidic (pH around 4) because adrenaline can become unstable at alkaline pH. Antimicrobial preservative (methylparaben) is added to multi dose vials. *For spinal and epidural anesthesia preservative free preparations should be used.*

INDIVIDUAL AGENTS

Esters

Cocaine

Cocaine was the first local anesthetic used by Carl Koller for anesthetizing cornea. It is extracted from the leaves of *Erythroxylum coca.* Cocaine is not preferred because it is a very *potent vasoconstrictor,* stimulates sympathetic system and can cause CNS excitement leading to euphoria, agitation, violence, convulsions, apnea and death.

It is the only ester which is not metabolized by pseudocholinesterase. It is metabolized in liver. One metabolite ecgonine is also CNS stimulant.

Procaine

- Like other esters it is metabolized by pseudocholinesterase.
- It is the *agent of choice in patients with history of malignant hyperthermia.* In fact, historically it had been used for the treatment of malignant hyperthermia.

Chloroprocaine

Chloroprocaine is the shortest acting local anesthetic (Duration of effect 15–25 minutes). As the preservative, sodium bisulfite used with chloroprocaine, caused high incidence of neurotoxicity, chloroprocaine became almost obsolete from clinical practice and became contraindicated for spinal. However, recently preservative free preparation of chloroprocaine has been launched and is gaining popularity as short duration spinal anesthetic for day care surgery in some countries. Maximum safe dose is 1,000 mg.

Amethocaine (Tetracaine)

It is only used as lozenges for bronchoscopies.

Benzocaine

Used as lozenges for stomatitis, sore throat. *Benzocaine can cause dangerous levels of methemoglobinemia.*

Amides

Lignocaine (Xylocaine, Lidocaine)

It is the most commonly used local anesthetic.
- First synthesized by Lofgren and first used by Gordh.

- Solution is very stable, not even decomposed by boiling.
- Contains preservative, methyl paraben.
- pKa = 7.8.

Concentration used

Surface (topical) analgesia	:	4% and 10%
Nerve blocks	:	1–2%
Urethral procedures (as jelly)	:	2%
Spinal	:	5% (heavy)
Epidural	:	1–2%
Intravenous regional analgesia (Bier's block)	:	0.5%
Infiltration block	:	1–2%

Metabolism

Metabolized in liver, excreted by kidney. t½: 1.6 hrs.

Duration of Effect

Without adrenaline	:	*45–60 minutes.*
With adrenaline	:	*2–3 hours.*

Maximum Safe Dose

Without adrenaline	:	*4.5 mg/kg (maximum 300 mg)*
With adrenaline	:	*7 mg/kg (maximum 500 mg)*

Toxicity

- Systemic toxicity (especially cardiotoxicity) is less than bupivacaine, levobupivacaine and ropivacaine.
- Can cause *cauda equina syndrome or transient neurological symptoms* after spinal anesthesia therefore, not preferred for spinal anesthesia in current day practice.

Other Uses

- *Used for treating ventricular tachycardia: Preservative free lignocaine (available as xylocard 2%) is used intravenously in dose of 2 mg/kg.*
- Intravenous xylocard is used for blunting cardiovascular response to laryngoscopy and intubation.
- Lignocaine infusion is used for the treatment of neuropathic pain.

Mepivacaine

Pharmacology is similar to lignocaine except duration of action slightly longer than lignocaine.

Prilocaine

Pharmacology is similar to lignocaine. Other than liver it also has *extrahepatic metabolism* in kidneys, lungs and by amidase making it as *safest local anesthetic.* Methemoglobinemia seen with prilocaine usually occurs at high doses. Methemoglobinemia occurs because of the accumulation of its metabolite orthotoluidine which can convert hemoglobin to methHb.

Bupivacaine (Sensorcaine, Marcaine)

Bupivacaine is very commonly used drug in anesthetic practice. Chemically bupivacaine is a racemic mixture of S (levo) and R (dextro) isomers. It is 4 times more potent than lignocaine.

Metabolized in liver, t ½ : 3.5 hours.

Concentration Used

For nerve block	:	0.5%
Spinal	:	0.5% (heavy)
Epidural	:	0.125–0.5% (depending whether used for sensory block or motor block)

The very unique property of bupivacaine is *wide differential sensory and motor blockade* which means motor block will occur only at high concentrations making it a local anesthetic of choice for *postoperative pain relief and painless labor.*

Maximum Safe Dose

Without adrenaline	:	*2.5 mg/kg (maximum 175 mg)*
With adrenaline	:	*3 mg/kg (maximum 225 mg)*

Duration of Effect

Without adrenaline	:	*2–3 hours.*
With adrenaline	:	*3–5 hours.*

Addition of adrenaline only prolongs the duration of sensory block.

Toxicity

Cardiotoxicity of bupivacaine deserves special attention due to many reasons:

- It is far more cardiotoxic than lignocaine
- R component contributes more than S component in causing cardiotoxicity
- Cardiotoxicity increases in pregnancy, hypoxia and acidosis.

- Cardiotoxicity of bupivacaine may manifest as bradyarrhythmias, conduction blocks, ventricular arrhythmias or cardiac arrest. Its high tissue binding (slow reversal of sodium channels) and high degree of protein binding makes *resuscitation after cardiac arrest prolonged and very difficult*. Therefore, it is *absolutely contraindicated for Bier's block*.

Management of cardiac arrest includes CPR along with the rapid bolus of *Intralipid 20%*, 1.5 mL/kg followed by infusion if required. Intralipid binds the active form of bupivacaine. Contrary to the previous recommendation of bretylium as a drug of choice for ventricular tachycardia induced by local anesthetics, *amiodarone nowadays is considered as drug of choice for the treatment of bupivacaine (and other local anesthetic) induced ventricular tachycardia*. In fact, bretylium is not recommended to be used in such cases. For ventricular tachycardia not responding to drugs defibrillation should be done immediately.

Levobupivacaine

Levobupivacaine is the S isomer of bupivacaine. As it does not contain R isomer therefore cardiotoxicity of levobupivacaine is less than bupivacaine. Studies have shown that not only cardiotoxicity, neurotoxicity of levobupivacaine is also slightly lesser than bupivacaine. Maximum safe dose of levobupivacaine are similar to bupivacaine, i.e. 2.5 mg/kg (maximum 175 mg).

As far as anesthetic properties are concerned it is less potent (1:1.3) than bupivacaine therefore duration (which is directly proportional to potency) and density of block of block is also proportionately less. However clinically this difference is not significant.

Ropivacaine

To further reduce the cardiotoxicity of levobupivacaine its butyl groups were replaced by propyl group producing the drug called as Ropivacaine.

Systemic Effects

Cardiotoxicity and CNS toxicity of ropivacaine is less as compared to bupivacaine and even lesser than levobupivacaine (but still higher than lignocaine). Since cardiotoxicity of ropivacaine is less it can be given in higher doses. *Maximum safe dose is 3 mg/kg (maximum 225 mg).*

Clinically more important than absolute decrease in cardiotoxicity is *better prognosis of cardiac arrest* after ropivacaine as compared to bupivacaine for two reasons—Rapid reversal of sodium channel and rapid clearance from circulation.

Another advantage of ropivacaine is that its *cardio toxic potential is same in pregnant versus non pregnant females* making it a safer option for pregnant ladies.

Anesthetic Properties

As it is also less potent than bupivacaine therefore its duration and intensity of motor block will also be proportionately less however as clinically this difference is insignificant therefore *ropivacaine is always preferred over bupivacaine for postoperative analgesia and painless labor.*

Etidocaine

Chemically similar to lignocaine but duration of action is similar to bupivacaine and less cardiotoxic than bupivacaine.

Dibucaine (Cinchocaine)

Longest acting, most potent and *most toxic* local anesthetic.

METHODS OF LOCAL ANESTHESIA

Topical (Surface Anesthesia)

Mepivacaine, bupivacaine, levobupivacaine and ropivacaine do not have any absorption from skin on mucous membranes therefore *cannot be used for topical anesthesia*. The absorption of procaine and chloroprocaine is so poor that they *should not be used for surface anesthesia*.

Common preparations used for surface analgesia include:

EMLA cream: EMLA stands for eutectic (easily melted) mixture of local anesthetics. It is a combination of 5% *prilocaine* and *5% lignocaine* in equal amount (1:1 ratio). It is used for intravenous cannulation in children or sensitive individuals, small skin procedures like skin grafting, biopsy or removal of mole. *As half strength EMLA cream (2.5%) allows higher doses to be used therefore, more commonly used in clinical practice is 2.5% EMLA cream.* It should not be used on broken skin, mucous membranes, and infants less than 1 month. The major limitation of EMLA cream is its slow onset (30–60 min.)

TAC (Tetracaine, adrenaline and cocaine) and LET (lidocaine, epinephrine and tetracaine): Useful for producing local anesthesia on cut skin

Xylocaine spray 4%, tetracaine and benzocaine lozenges: Used for mucous membranes of mouth, pharynx and larynx.

Xylocaine (lignocaine) jelly 2%: Used for urinary catheterization and proctoscopies.

Cocaine drops and tetracaine ointment: Used for eye in past

Lignocaine 4%, dibucaine 1% and benzocaine 5% ointment: Used for anal fissure and painful piles.

Oxethazaine (mucaine gel) 0.2%—Used for gastritis

Infiltration Anesthesia

Local anesthetic is infiltrated at operation site. Most commonly used for infiltration is lignocaine, 1–2%.

Nerve Blocks

Drug is injected around the nerve supplying the operation site. Most commonly are lignocaine 1–2% and bupivacaine 0.125%–0.5%

Intravenous Regional Anesthesia (Bier's Block)

0.5% lignocaine is used for Biers block.

Central Neuraxial Blocks

Central neuraxial blocks include spinal and epidural anesthesia.

Refrigeration Analgesia

Nerve conduction is blocked by cooling the nerves using cryoprobes which deliver CO_2 or nitrous oxide at –5 to –20°C.

Tumescent Anesthesia

It is a technique used by plastic surgeons during liposuction where dilute combination of lignocaine with adrenaline is injected subcutaneously in large quantities in the area from where liposuction has to be done. Peak concentration may even occur in postoperative periods producing toxicity.

CAUSES OF FAILURE OF LOCAL ANESTHESIA

The usual cause of failure are inappropriate technique, inadequate volume or concentration of local anesthetic however certain factors like infection (acidosis), genetic variation or drug tolerance and tachyphylaxis can also contribute in failure.

For summary of properties of local anesthetics see **Table 15.2**.

■ **Table 15.2:** Summary of properties of local anesthetics

Drug	Potency	t1/2	Duration of action		pKa	Maximum safe dose (mg/kg)	Comments
			Without adrenaline	With adrenaline			
Esters							
Procaine	+		15–30 minutes	30–90 minutes	8.9	12 mg/kg	
Chloroprocaine	+		15–25 minutes	30–90 minutes	9.0	12 mg/kg	Shortest acting
Cocaine	++		–	–	8.7	3 mg/kg	Potent vasoconstrictor
Tetracaine	++++		2–3 hours	3–5 hours	8.2	3 mg/kg	
Amides							
Lignocaine (300 mg) (Xylocaine)	++	1.6 hours	45–60 minutes	2–3 hours	7.8	4.5 mg/kg without adrenaline	Most commonly used local anesthetic
						7 mg/kg (500 mg) with adrenaline	

Contd...

Contd…

Drug	Potency	t1/2	Duration of action		pKa	Maximum safe dose (mg/kg)	Comments
			Without adrenaline	With adrenaline			
Prilocaine	++		45–60 minutes	2–3 hours	7.8	8 mg/kg	Can cause methemoglobinemia
Mepivacaine	++		45–60 minutes	2–3 hours	7.6	4.5 mg/kg	
Etidocaine	++++		2–3 hours	3–5 hours	7.7	4 mg/kg	
Bupivacaine (Sensorcaine, Marcaine))	++++	3.5 hours	2–3 hours	3–5 hours	8.1	2.5 mg/kg (175 mg) without adrenaline, 3 mg/kg (225 mg) with Adrenaline	Very commonly used local anesthetic in anesthesia
Levobupivacaine	+++		2–3 hours	3–5 hours	8.1	2.5 mg/kg (175 mg) without Adrenaline	Less cardiotoxic than bupivacaine
Ropivacaine	++++		2–3 hours	3–5 hours	8.1	3 mg/kg (225 mg) without adrenaline	Less cardiotoxic than bupivacaine and Levobupivacaine
Dibucaine	++++	4 hours	2.5–3.5 hours	3.5–5.5 hours	8.8	1 mg/kg	Longest acting, most potent, most toxic

KEY POINTS

- Local anesthetics are classified on the basis of chemical structure and duration of action.
- Chloroprocaine is the shortest acting and dibucaine is the longest acting local anesthetic.
- Recent studies have proven that local anesthetics not only act on sodium channels, but also block potassium and calcium channels.
- Sequence of blockade of nerve fibers is A > B> C. The traditional notion that thin fibers are most sensitive to the action of local anesthetics does not hold true in present day practice.
- Potency is proportional to the duration of action.
- Maximum systemic absorption has been seen after intercostal nerve block.
- Central nervous system is the first system involved in local anesthetic toxicity.
- At clinically used doses all local anesthetics are vasodilators except cocaine, levobupivacaine and ropivacaine.
- Allergic reactions are common with esters but rare with amides.
- Methemoglobinemia is usually seen with prilocaine however benzocaine can also cause methemoglobinemia.
- Maximum local neurotoxicity has been reported with chloroprocaine.
- Local anesthetics with adrenaline can cause necrosis and gangrene if used for ring block of fingers, toes, penis or pinna because these structures have end arteries.
- For spinal and epidural anesthesia preservative free preparations should be used.
- Maximum safe dose of lignocaine without adrenaline is 4.5 mg/kg (maximum 300 mg) while with adrenaline it is 7 mg/kg (maximum 500 mg).
- Wide differential blockade of bupivacaine and ropivacaine makes them local anesthetic of choice for postoperative pain relief and painless labor.
- Prilocaine has significant extrahepatic metabolism.
- Because of high cardiotoxicity bupivacaine is absolutely contraindicated for bier's block.
- Amiodarone now a days is considered as drug of choice for the treatment of bupivacaine (and other local anesthetic) induced ventricular tachycardia.
- Cardiotoxicity and CNS toxicity of ropivacaine is far lesser than bupivacaine and lesser than levobupivacaine (but still higher than lignocaine).
- Mepivacaine, bupivacaine, levobupivacaine and ropivacaine cannot be used while procaine and chloroprocaine should not be used for surface anesthesia.

CHAPTER 16

Peripheral Nerve Blocks

Nerve blocks may be classified as central neuraxial blocks (spinal and epidural) and peripheral nerve blocks. Nerve blocks are given either for regional anesthesia or for acute and chronic pain relief. (*For pain relief blocks see Chapter 39, page no. 273*).

TECHNIQUE

The conventional method of giving a nerve block is by eliciting paresthesia and/or using the nerve stimulator. However, the *use of ultrasound has revolutionized the practice of nerve block in modern day anesthetic practice*.

BLOCKS OF UPPER LIMB

Brachial Plexus Block

This is the second most commonly performed block (after central neuraxial block). It is used for surgery of upper limb and shoulder. Brachial plexus can be blocked by 4 approaches—interscalene, supraclavicular, infraclavicular and axillary approach.

Interscalene Approach

The usual indication for interscalene block is surgery on the shoulder or upper arm. In this technique brachial plexus is blocked *between anterior and middle scalene* at the level of cricoid. Blockade occurs at the level of the superior and middle trunks. *Ulnar nerve is usually spared with this approach* making it unsuitable for hand surgeries.

Complications:
- *Phrenic nerve block:* Phrenic nerve block occurs in almost all patients but unilateral phrenic nerve block has no clinically

significant consequences in a normal individual (pulmonary functions are only reduced by 20–25%).
- Horner syndrome (due to block of stellate ganglion).
- Epidural and intrathecal injection can be dreadful complication.
- Pneumothorax if the needle insertion is too low.
- General complications like nerve injury, neuritis, intravascular injection, bleeding and hematoma formation, infection or injury to a nearby structure and systemic toxicity of local anesthetic.

Supraclavicular Approach

This is very commonly used approach. This approach is usually employed for surgeries on lower arm, elbow, forearm and hand. Distal trunk and proximal division of brachial plexus is blocked by this approach.

Technique: Patient lies supine with a small wedge under the shoulder. The arm is extended and adducted; needle is inserted at a point 1 cm superior to midpoint of clavicle after palpating the subclavian artery. The needle is inserted *lateral* to subclavian vessels **(Fig. 16.1)**. The needle is inserted in downward and backward direction till paresthesia is elicited. After eliciting paresthesia 20–30 mL of 1–1.5% xylocaine alone or mixed with bupivacaine is injected.

Complications:
- *Pneumothorax:* Dome of pleura can be punctured. Incidence is *1–6%* but fortunately in more than 98% of the cases pneumothorax

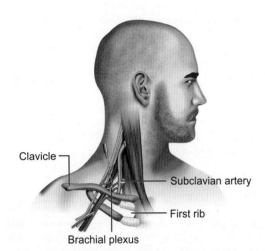

Fig. 16.1: Supraclavicular approach to brachial plexus block (needle is inserted just lateral to subclavian artery)

is small enough to require any intervention. As the dome of pleura is on medial side therefore *best way to avoid pneumothorax is to keep the direction of needle laterally.*

- Phrenic nerve block (incidence is 40–60%). Unilateral block does not cause any problem.
- Horner syndrome.
- General complications.

Axillary Approach

Axillary approach is also commonly used approach. The drug is injected around axillary artery in axilla. Blockade occurs at the level of the terminal nerves.

Advantage over supraclavicular approach: Complications like pneumothorax, phrenic nerve block and Horner syndrome can be avoided.

Disadvantage: *Musculocutaneous and inter-costobrachial nerves are spared* therefore axillary block is not suitable for arm surgery. Musculocutaneous and intercostobrachial nerves have to be blocked separately with axillary approach (musculocutaneous is blocked in the substance of coracobrachialis muscle while intercostobrachial in subcutaneous tissue over axillary artery). The chances of intravascular injection and hematoma formation are also high with axillary approach.

Infraclavicular Approach

In this approach brachial plexus is blocked either just below the midpoint of clavicle (classical approach) or just medial to coracoid process (coracoid approach). The theoretical advantage is that musculocutaneous and axillary nerve can be blocked.

Due to high failure rate in coracoid approach and increased incidence of pneumothorax and hemothorax in classical approach infraclavicular route for blocking brachial plexus is not utilized routinely.

Individual Nerve Blocks

Radial, ulnar and median nerves can be blocked separately at elbow and wrist.

Wrist block is used for hand surgeries where ulnar nerve is blocked just lateral to flexor carpi ulnaris tendon, median nerve is blocked between tendons of Palmaris longus and flexor carpi radialis and radial nerve is blocked by 8–10 mL subcutaneous injection of local anesthetic extending from radial artery anteriorly to extensor carpi radialis tendon posteriorly.

Intravenous Regional Block (Bier Block)

Intravenous regional anesthesia (IVRA) is also called as Bier block as it was first time given by August Bier.

Technique

After applying tourniquet (which prevents systemic absorption of drug) 30–40 mL of *0.5% lignocaine (xylocard) or prilocaine* is injected into a peripheral vein. Adequate tourniquet functioning is most vital in Bier block. Deflation or leak can cause drug toxicity and death therefore toxic drug like *bupivacaine is absolutely contraindicated for Bier block.* As tourniquet has already compromised the vascular supply therefore lignocaine with adrenaline should not be used.

Advantages
- Easy procedure.
- Almost no chances of failure.
- Rapid onset (within 5 minutes).
- Good muscle relaxation.

Disadvantages
- Tourniquet discomfort or compartment syndrome.

- Venous engorgement caused by venodilatation creates difficulty in providing bloodless field.
- As duration of action of lignocaine without adrenaline is 30–60 minutes, it can be utilized only for short duration procedures.
- *Accidental deflation or leak of tourniquet can cause severe drug toxicity and even death.*
- Tourniquet cannot be released before 30 minutes (even if the surgery finishes before it).

Contraindications
- The old recommendation of not giving intravenous regional anesthesia (Bier's block) to sickle cell patients does not hold true in current day practice.
- Raynaud's disease and scleroderma (tourniquet is contraindicated due to compromised vascular supply.

BLOCKS OF LOWER LIMB
Blocks of lower limb are rarely used for providing anesthesia as majority of the lower limb surgeries can be performed under spinal and epidural anesthesia. The nerve blocks which are sometimes utilized are:
- *Psoas compartment block:* To block lumbar plexus.
- *Perivascular block (3 in 1 block):* Drug injected in femoral canal while maintaining distal pressure will result in upward spread of drug, blocking femoral, sciatic and obturator nerves simultaneously (that is why called as 3 in 1 block).
- *Femoral nerve, sciatic nerve and obturator nerve block:* These nerves can be blocked separately depending on which part of the lower limb surgery is to be performed.
- *Fascia iliaca nerve (modified femoral) block:* A large volume of drug is injected just below the fascia iliaca to block femoral nerve as it traverses the fascia iliaca. Usually performed under ultrasound guidance however can be performed blindly with double pop technique; first pop of fascia lata followed by second pop of fascia iliaca.
- *Ankle block:* Performed for foot surgeries. In ankle block deep peroneal, superficial peroneal and saphenous nerve are blocked with subcutaneous infiltration at the dorsum of foot, posterior tibial posterior to medial malleolus and sural laterally between lateral malleolus and achilles tendon. As it requires multiple injection ankle block can be a painful. Lignocaine with adrenaline should not be used for ankle block.
- *Bier's block for lower limb:* Not commonly performed as it requires very large volumes (60–80 mL).

BLOCKS OF THE HEAD AND NECK, THORACIC AND ABDOMINAL AREA

Cervical Plexus Block
As patient's awake state is the best monitor to assess the neurologic status, cervical plexus block is best utilized for carotid endarterectomy. In selected cases, it is possible to do tracheostomy and thyroidectomy with bilateral cervical plexus block.

Airway Block
Airway block (glossopharyngeal at the base of posterior tonsillar pillar, superior laryngeal below the tip of greater cornu of hyoid bone and recurrent laryngeal by topical application through cricothyroid membrane) was popular in the past for awake intubation. However, in current day practice awake intubation is invariably done with fiberoptic bronchoscopy under topical analgesia of airways.

Phrenic Nerve Block
Sometimes performed for intractable hiccups; nerve is blocked 3 cm above the clavicle just lateral to the posterior border of sternocleidomastoid.

Ilioinguinal and Iliohypogastric Nerve Block
Performed for hernia repair, these are blocked at a point 3 cm medial to anterior superior iliac spine.

Penile Block
Pudendal nerve is blocked by injection of 10–15 mL of local anesthetic at the base of penis. Xylocaine with adrenaline is contraindicated for penile block.

Paravertebral Block
In paravertebral block, each spinal nerve is blocked just after it exit from intervertebral foramen.

Can be utilized for breast, thoracic or abdominal surgeries in patients where general anesthesia is contraindicated.

If large volumes are used then drug may spread laterally into superior and inferior paravertebral spaces, superior and inferior intercostal spaces and medially along with the nerve sheath into epidural space.

Intercostal Nerve Block

Most often performed for pain relief for rib fractures and post-herpetic neuropathies however can be used for chest tube insertion or doing thoracoscopies. Block is given at the lower border of rib, usually at the posterior angle of rib.

The most bothersome complications may be pneumothorax and risk of systemic local anesthetic toxicity (maximum systemic absorption occurs after intercostal nerve block).

CONTRAINDICATIONS FOR PERIPHERAL NERVE BLOCKS

- Patient suffering from coagulopathy or on anticoagulants (except aspirin)
- Infection at the site of needle placement
- Known case of drug allergy to local anesthetics
- Pre-existing neuropathy—Avoid regional anesthesia to avoid medicolegal issues.

KEY POINTS

- The use of ultrasound has not only made the nerve blocks technically easy but also has improved the precision.
- Ulnar nerve is usually spared with interscalene approach while musculocutaneous is usually spared with axillary approach.
- The most bothersome complication of supraclavicular block is pneumothorax. Keeping the direction of needle lateral to the Subclavian artery is the best way to avoid pneumothorax.
- Only safe local anesthetics, i.e. lignocaine and prilocaine are permitted for Bier block. Drug with high toxicity like bupivacaine is absolutely contraindicated.
- Cervical plexus block is best utilized for carotid endarterectomy.
- Maximum systemic absorption of local anesthetic occurs after intercostal nerve block.
- Associated coagulopathy and infection at needle site are the absolute contraindication for nerve blocks.

CHAPTER 17

Central Neuraxial Blocks (Spinal and Epidural Anesthesia)

APPLIED ANATOMY

Vertebral column consist of 33 vertebrae: 7 cervical, 12 thoracic, 5 lumbar, 5 fused sacral and 4 fused coccygeal. Vertebral column has 4 curves: Thoracic and sacral spine are convex posteriorly (kyphotic) while cervical and lumbar spine are convex anteriorly (lordotic).

Vertebral canal is bounded anteriorly by vertebral bodies and intervertebral disc, laterally by pedicles, posteriorly by lamina, ligamentum flavum and roots of vertebral spines. In vertebral canal lies the spinal cord with meninges.

Structures encountered during spinal anesthesia.

Structures encountered while giving spinal anesthesia (Fig. 17.1)—from posterior to anterior.

- Skin.
- Subcutaneous tissue.
- *Supraspinous ligament:* Connecting the tips of spinous processes.
- *Interspinous ligament:* Joins the spinous processes together.
- *Ligamentum flavum:* Running from lamina to lamina. Composed of yellow elastic fibers therefore also called *yellow ligament* (flava in Latin means yellow)
- Dura.
- Arachnoid.

The tips of spinous processes are such that epidural/spinal needle should be inserted obliquely (cephalad) in thoracic region and almost straight in lumbar region.

Surface landmarks which are important while giving spinal or epidural anesthesia are:

C7: Spinous process of 7th cervical vertebrae is very prominent and easily palpable.

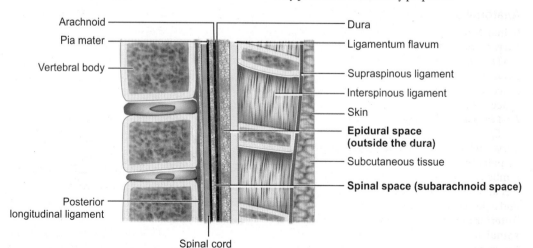

Fig. 17.1: Structures encountered during spinal anesthesia

T7: T7 lies opposite to inferior angle of scapula.

The line joining the highest point on iliac crest (intercristal line, also called as Tuffier's line) corresponds to L4 and L5 interspace or L4 spine: It is very important to identity this intervertebral space while choosing the space for giving spinal or epidural anesthesia.

Epidural Space (Extradural or Peridural Space)

It lies outside the duramater, i.e. between dura and ligamentum flavum. It extends from foramen magnum to sacral hiatus. Epidural anesthesia is given in this space. Epidural space is triangular in shape with apex dorsomedial.

Contents of Epidural Space

- Anterior and posterior nerve roots
- Epidural veins
- Spinal arteries
- Lymphatics
- Fat.

The epidural veins forms a plexus in epidural space called as *plexus of Batson*. These veins are very important from clinical point of view because they directly drain into inferior vena cava. Any pressure on inferior vena cava (as in pregnancy, abdominal tumors, ascites) lead these veins to becomes engorged, pushing the dura medially which reduces the subarachnoid space leading to higher spread of local anesthetic.

Anatomy of Spinal Cord

Spinal cord extends from medulla oblongata to *lower border of L1 in adults and L3 in infants (Adult level is achieved by the age of 2 years).* Therefore in infancy spinal anesthesia should be given in L4-5 space while in adults it can be given in L3-4 or L4-5 space (or even in L2-3) however *usually given in L3-4 interspace.*

Spinal cord is divided into segments by spinal nerves which arise from it. The spinal nerves are 31 pairs in number, i.e. 8 cervical, 12 thoracic, 5 lumbar, 5 sacral and 1 coccygeal. Each spinal nerve has an anterior root which is efferent and motor and a posterior root which is afferent and sensory. Anterior and posterior roots join to form mixed spinal nerve which exists from intervertebral foramina. As spinal cord ends at L1 therefore lumbar, sacral and coccygeal nerve has to run downwards to exit from intervertebral foramina forming cauda equina (horse tail).

Blood Supply of Spinal Cord

It is supplied by 2 posterior spinal arteries which arise from posterior inferior cerebellar arteries and 1 anterior spinal artery which is formed by branch of vertebral artery of each side.

Anterior spinal artery is reinforced by many arteries of which *artery of Adamkiewicz (arteria radicularis magna)* is very important which can enter anywhere between T5 and L2 and usually (75%) it enters from left side. Damage/vasoconstriction to this artery can lead to cord ischemia and paraplegia.

Meninges

Spinal cord is enveloped from *inside to outside* by piamater, arachnoid mater and duramater. *Duramater extends up to S2 in adults and S3 in children while piamater, as filum terminale, extend up to coccyx.*

Cerebrospinal Fluid

Cerebrospinal fluid (CSF) is present between pia and arachnoid mater (i.e. subarachnoid space). As spinal anesthesia is given in subarachnoid space it is also called as *subarachnoid block or intrathecal (inside the meninges) block.*

The CSF is secreted by choroid plexus of third, fourth and lateral ventricles and is absorbed into venous sinuses via arachnoid villi. 500 mL is secreted in 24 hours. Volume of CSF at one time is 140 ml, half of which is present in cranium and half in spinal canal. Specific gravity = 1.003–1.009 (Average 1.004) and pH is 7.35.

CSF pressure: It is same in cranium and spinal canal in lying position which is *100–150 mmH$_2$O* (10–15 cmH$_2$O) while in sitting position the CSF pressure at lumbar level may increase to 180–240 mmH$_2$O.

ADVANTAGES OF CENTRAL NEURAXIAL BLOCKS (CNB) OVER GENERAL ANESTHESIA (GA)

- Cheaper.
- Lessens the risk of respiratory complications like pulmonary aspiration, bronchospasm, laryngospasm, postoperative atelectasis.

- Avoids serious consequences of intubation like cardiovascular response or failed intubation.
- Avoids the systemic side effects of GA drugs
- Bleeding is less (because of low mean arterial pressure). Studies have shown significant reduction in blood requirement in total knee replacement done in central neuraxial blocks as compared to general anesthesia.
- Decreased incidence of thromboembolism due to increased vascularity of lower limbs.
- By alleviating the surgical stress response central neuraxial blocks decreases the chances of infarction as well as arrhythmias.
- Reduction in overall morbidity and mortality. For the reasons mentioned above several meta-analyses have shown a *reduced risk in overall mortality and morbidity as high as 30%* in patients who underwent surgeries under CNB as compared to general anesthesia (GA).

SYSTEMIC EFFECTS (PHYSIOLOGICAL ALTERATIONS) OF CENTRAL NEURAXIAL BLOCKS

Cardiovascular System

The *most prominent effect is hypotension* which occurs due to of the following reasons:

1. *Sympathetic block*: The sympathetic block lead to venodilatation, venous pooling, decreased venous return and hence decrease cardiac output and hypotension.
2. *Bradycardia*: Bradycardia can further decrease the cardiac output. The reasons for bradycardia are:
   - Decreased atrial pressure because of decreased venous return *(Bainbridge reflex)*
   - Parasympathetic over dominance due to sympathetic block
   - Direct inhibition of cardioaccelerator fibres (T1 to T4).
3. Blockage of nerve supply to adrenal glands with consequently decreased catecholamine release.
4. Direct absorption of drug into systemic circulation.
5. Compression of inferior vena cava and aorta by pregnant uterus, abdominal tumors (*supine hypotension syndrome*).

Nervous System

Due to the anatomy of spinal nerve, central neuraxial blocks do not follow the block sequence of peripheral nerves (motor > sensory > autonomic). In spinal nerve autonomic fibers are on most outer (posterior) side while motor on most inner (anterior) side therefore first function to be blocked is autonomic followed by sensory and then motor, i.e. the sequence of blockade is *autonomic > sensory > motor*. The recovery occurs in reverse order however few studies have suggested return of autonomic activity before sensory.

Due to this different sensitivity of nerve fibers to local anesthetics, *autonomic level is 2 segments higher than sensory which is 2 segments higher than motor*. This is called as *differential blockade* and the segments where one modality is blocked and another is not, forms the *zones of differential blockade*.

Autonomic level is tested by temperature (cold), sensory by pin prick (by non-pricking needles) and motor by toe movement.

Respiratory System

Tidal volume, minute volume, arterial oxygen tension are well maintained in normal individuals however in COPD/Asthma patients whose expiration is dependent on abdominal muscles or respiratory compromised patients who cannot bear the blockage of intercostals, there can be severe impairment of respiratory function *(Dyspnea)* if block is high enough to block abdominal and intercostal muscles.

Apnea after spinal anesthesia is usually due to severe hypotension causing medullary ischemia. Other causes of apnea are:

- *High spinal:* High enough to block phrenic nerve (C3, 4, 5) which is rare.
- *Total spinal:* When the drug reaches up to cranium, it is considered as total spinal. It usually happens due to accidental intrathecal injection of large volume of drug during epidural anesthesia.
- *Intravascular injection and systemic toxicity:* Usually seen after epidural anesthesia because large volume of drug is used.

Gastrointestinal System

- Sympathetic block leads to parasympathetic over activity producing *contracted gut with relaxed sphincters; Peristalsis* is increased.

- *Nausea and vomiting:* The most common cause of nausea and vomiting is hypotension leading to central hypoxia and nausea/vomiting. Other causes may be bile in stomach (due to relaxed pyloric sphincter) or increased peristalsis due to parasympathetic over activity. Nausea, vomiting due to these causes (parasympathetic over dominance) is treated by atropine.

Liver

Hypotension can decrease liver blood flow but impairment is minimal.

Genitourinary System

- Renal functions are not impaired unless mean arterial pressure falls below *critical pressure of kidney for autoregulation (MAP- 55 mm Hg).*
- *Urinary retention is the most common postoperative complication of central neuraxial blocks in present day practice.* It is due to blockade of sacral parasympathetic fibers (S2, 3, 4).
- Flaccid (paralysis of nervi erigentes) and engorged penis is one of the signs of successful block.

Endocrinal System

- Central neuraxial blocks by blocking the sympathetic nerves and adrenals blocks the stress response to surgery.
- The response to insulin is augmented and there can be hypoglycemia.

Thermoregulation

Vasodilatation causes heat loss which is compensated by vasoconstriction above the block and *shivering* which is a very common occurrence after spinal anesthesia.

SPINAL ANESTHESIA (SUBARACHNOID BLOCK, INTRATHECAL BLOCK)

It is the most commonly used anesthetic technique. It can be well utilized for almost all open gynecology and obstetrics surgeries, orthopedic and plastic surgeries of lower limb and pelvis, general surgeries of pelvis and lower abdomen and majority of urology procedures.

Procedure

- Spinal anesthesia is usually given in lateral position or sitting position (possible in prone position also) with body in flexion position (*fetal position).*
- Approach may be midline (most commonly used), lateral (paramedian) and lumbosacral (Taylor) (In this approach point of insertion is 1 cm medial and 1 cm caudal to posterior superior iliac spine).
- After cleaning and draping lumbar puncture is done in desired space (*usually L3-4)* and the local anesthetic drug is injected after confirming the free flow of CSF.

Site of Action of Local Anesthetic

Local anesthetic mainly acts on *spinal nerves* and dorsal ganglia but a small concentration can be detected in substance of spinal cord.

Drugs used for Spinal Anesthesia

1. *Local anesthetics (Table 17.1):* Lignocaine and bupivacaine are the two local anesthetics which are mainly used for spinal in India.
   - *Lignocaine: Concentration used is 5%.* The drug used for spinal is *hyperbaric* (or heavy) that means its specific gravity is more than that of CSF therefore it tries to settle down. The solution is made hyperbaric by *addition of 7.5% dextrose.* Due to the possibility of transient neurological symptoms (TNS) and cauda equina syndrome lignocaine is rarely used in current day clinical practice.
   - *Bupivacaine: Bupivacaine is the most commonly used drug for spinal. The concentration used* is 0.5% and it is *made hyperbaric by* addition of *8% dextrose.*
   - *Ropivacaine and levobupivacaine:* The newer drugs like ropivacaine or levobupivacaine offer no considerable

■ Table 17.1: Local anesthetics for spinal anesthesia

Drug	Concentration	Specific gravity
Lignocaine	5% in 7.5% dextrose	1.0333
Bupivacaine	0.5% in 8% dextrose	1.0278
Tetracaine	1%	
Chloroprocaine	3%	
Levobupivacaine	0.5%	
Ropivacaine	0.5–1%	

advantage over bupivacaine for spinal (due to low amount of bupivacaine used for spinal, the risk of cardiotoxicity seen with bupivacaine is negligible) rather disadvantage is that due to less potency duration and quality of motor block is less.

- *Chloroprocaine:* Recently a preservative free preparation of chloroprocaine has been introduced in the market for short duration procedures.
- Other drugs like *tetracaine, mepivacaine* or *procaine* are hardly used in current day practice

2. *Opioids:* A small dose of fentanyl (20–25 mcg) is usually added as supplement to local anesthetics. Preservative-free morphine can provide analgesia for up to 24 hours however with the risk of delayed respiratory depression.

3. *α2-Agonists:* Clonidine and dexmedetomidine by decreasing the neurotransmitter release and causing hyperpolarization of membrane can prolong the duration of spinal block therefore can be used as an adjuvant to local anesthetics.

4. *Vasoconstrictors (epinephrine, phenylephrine):* Although no human study has suggested that vasoconstrictors used with local anesthetics can compromise the vascular supply of spinal cord but still majority of the clinicians do not use vasoconstrictors for spinal anesthesia.

5. *Neostigmine:* Neostigmine by increasing the concentration of acetylcholine can prolong the analgesic effect of spinal therefore can be used as an adjuvant to local anesthetics.

6. Others drugs like midazolam, ketamine, tramadol or even nonsteroidal anti-inflammatory drugs (NSAIDS) have been tried intrathecally but with variable results.

Spinal Needles

Spinal needles are of two types; dura cutting and dura separating.

Dura cutting: Standard *Quincke-Babcock*, Greene and Pitkin needle are the examples of dura cutting needles. As these needles causes more damage to dural fibers the incidence of postspinal headache is high however cost wise they are far cheaper than dura separating needles.

Dura separating: These have *pencil tip point end.* The commonly available types are Whitacre and Sportte. As these needles only separates the dural fibers, damage to dural fibers and hence incidence of postspinal headache is less but these needles are expensive.

Factors Affecting the Height (Level) of Block

Factors which Significantly Affect the Level of Block

- *Dosage of drug:* Greater the dose, higher the level of block attained.
- *Baricity:* Baricity is the ratio of specific gravity of an agent at a specific temperature (body temperature) to specific gravity of CSF at same temperature. This is very important factor in determining the migration and eventual extent of block.
  - *Hyperbaric technique:* Hyperbaric solutions are most often used for spinal anesthesia. As hyperbaric solutions tends to settle downwards the level achieved by hyperbaric solutions is governed by the position of the patient during spinal anesthesia and after injection till drug gets fixed to neuronal tissue, *which normally takes 10–15 minutes for xylocaine and 20–30 minutes for bupivacaine.*
  - *Hypobaric:* Local anesthetics are made hypobaric by addition of sterile water. As hypobaric solutions ascend higher they are very rarely used for colorectal surgery where head is lower than buttocks (Jack-knife position). The drug will migrate caudally to block sacral dermatomes.
  - *Isobaric:* The local anesthetic settles at the same level at which it is injected.
- *Position of the patient:* It is an important factor. Spinal given in lateral position (with hyperbaric solution) will attain higher level as compared to spinal given in sitting. Similarly Trendelenburg position will produce higher level of block as compared to supine position.
- *Site (intervertebral space) of injection:* Higher the space chosen, higher is the level of block achieved.
- *CSF volume:* CSF volume has *inverse relation with the level of block;* decreased CSF volume

will lead to higher spread of drug while increased CSF volume will lead to attainment of lower levels.

- *Pregnancy:* Pregnant women attains higher level of blocks in comparison to non-pregnant due to number of reasons like decreased subarachnoid space (due to engorgement of epidural veins), change in spine curvature (lumbar lordosis of pregnancy), progesterone induced increased sensitivity to neuronal tissues.
- *Age:* Old age people achieve higher levels due to reduced subarachnoid space (because of dural fibrosis), reduced CSF volume and age related increased sensitivity to local anesthetics.
- *Epidural after spinal*: The bolus or infusion of local anesthetic in epidural space after giving spinal during combined spinal epidural compresses the dural sac increasing the block height. This technique is called as *epidural volume extension.*

Factors which Affect the Level of Block but not very Significantly

- *Height:* At a normal range, height is not an important factor however at extremes it is an important factor having inverse relation with the level of block; taller individuals will attain a lower level while short statured will achieve higher level with the same volume of drug.
- *Spinal curvature:* Severe kyphosis (or kypho-scoliosis) may reduce the subarachnoid space leading to higher spread of drug.
- *Intra-abdominal pressure:* Increase in intra-abdominal pressure by ascites, pregnancy, abdominal tumors, obesity decreases the volume of subarachnoid space due to engorgement of epidural veins, producing higher block.
- *Direction of needle:* If the orifice of needle points cephalad, the level of block achieved is comparatively higher to when it points downwards.
- *Volume and concentration of local anesthetic*: Dose is a very important factor while volume and concentration are less important determinants of level of block.

Factors not Affecting the Level of Block

- *Sex:* Despite the difference in density of CSF in males and females there is no significant difference in block height has been observed.
- *Speed of injection:* Contrary to general belief rapid injection does not increases the level of block
- *Increased CSF pressure:* Increase CSF pressure produced by Barbotage (It is the technique in which repeatedly CSF is taken out and drug is injected), coughing or straining does not affect the level of block.
- Addition of vasoconstrictor.
- Additives other than opioids

Factors Affecting the Duration of Block

- Dose.
- Increased concentration.
- Pharmacological profile of drug like protein binding, metabolism.
- *Added vasoconstrictors:* Vasoconstrictors increase the duration of spinal anesthesia by 10–50% but they should not be used for spinal anesthesia as there is a theoretical concern that vasoconstrictors can cause spinal cord ischemia.

Complications of Spinal Anesthesia

Intraoperative

- *Hypotension: Hypotension is the most common complication of spinal anesthesia. Mild hypotension do occur in almost all patients and significant hypotension (systolic BP < 90 mm Hg) may be seen in up to 1/3rd of the patients. Mild hypotension is beneficial in reducing the blood loss.*
  Treatment
  Prophylactic: Although preloading with 1 to 1.5 liters of crystalloid is still practiced by many anesthesiologists however has not been proven to prevent hypotension therefore is *no longer recommended.*
  Curative
  – *Head low position (Trendelenburg position):* It is done to increase the venous return from legs and pelvic area. A head low position of 15–20° has not been found to significantly increase the level of block. Therefore, Trendelenburg

up to 15–20° still remains the very vital part of management of spinal hypotension.

- *Fluids:* Crystalloids preferred however if there is indication colloids can be used safely.
- *Vasopressors (sympathomimetics):* If hypotension does not responds to Trendelenburg and fluids or if it is severe than vasopressors should be used. As *Ephedrine* not only produces vasoconstriction (α agonist) but also increases the cardiac output and heart rate by its β adrenergic properties, it is the *most preferred vasopressor for the treatment of spinal hypotension.* However, *Mephentermine* is more frequently used in India. Other vasopressors which can be used are methoxamine, phenylephrine, metaraminol and epinephrine as a vasopressor of last resort.
- *Inotropes (dopamine, dobutamine):* Hypotension after spinal is because of sympathetic blockade therefore sympathomimetic drugs are used for treatment. The inotropes only benefit indirectly by improving the cardiac output therefore are hardly ever used.
- Oxygen inhalation to prevent hypoxia from hypotension.

- *Bradycardia:* Bradycardia after spinal anesthesia is quite common (incidence around 10%) for the reasons already stated above. *Treatment:* Intravenous atropine.
- *Dyspnea:* Mild respiratory difficulty due to lower intercostal paralysis is treated by oxygenation and assurance.
- *High spinal/total spinal:* High spinal is an arbitrary term. In general, high spinal means spinal above desired level which is causing problems to the patient however in strict terms high spinal refers to level high enough to block phrenic nerve causing diaphragmatic paralysis and apnea. If the drug reaches cranium and involve cranial nerves it is called as *Total spinal.*
  Management: Management depends on level of block. If it is involving only intercostals then oxygenation and assurance may be enough. High spinal involving diaphragm and total spinal will require intubation. *Severe*

bradycardia and hypotension seen in high spinal will require atropine and vasopressors.

- *Respiratory paralysis (apnea):* It is usually because of hypotension, therefore treat hypotension and maintain positive pressure ventilation till spontaneous breathing returns. If it is because of high or total spinal then patient will require immediate intubation.
- *Nausea and vomiting:* This is most commonly because of hypotension causing central hypoxia therefore treating oxygenation and treating hypotension should alleviate nausea and vomiting. If not then antiemetics may be used.
- *Difficulty in phonation:* This is because of high spinal extending up to cervical level.
  Treatment: IPPV
- *Shivering:* Shivering is one of the very common complication of spinal anesthesia seen in almost half of the patients. Oxygen consumption can increase by 4–5 times in shivering therefore the patient who is shivering must receive oxygen and shivering should be treated by warm air, covering the patient by warm blankets and by giving anti-shivering drugs. *The drug of choice for treatment of shivering is pethidine* followed by tramadol.
- *Restlessness, anxiety and apprehension:* Hypoxia should be ruled out otherwise sedate and assure the patient.
- *Local anesthetic toxicity:* Happens due to intravascular injection. Treat symptomatically. If convulsions occur give diazepam, oxygenate and manage any cardiac arrhythmia.
- *Local anesthetic anaphylaxis:* It is rare.
- *Cardiac arrest:* It can be because of:
  - Severe hypotension
  - Severe bradycardia proceeding to asystole.
  - Total spinal/very high spinal.
  - Local anesthetic toxicity/anaphylaxis.
  Immediately start the cardiopulmonary resuscitation.
- *Broken needle:* Attempt the removal at once. If not possible get a portable X-ray and call for neurosurgeon.
- *Pain during injection:* Can be decreased by local anesthetic infiltration before giving spinal.

- *Bloody tap:* Bleeding after spinal usually occurs due to puncture of epidural vein. The needle should be withdrawn and reinserted.

Postoperative

Urinary retention: *Blockade* of sacral para-sympathetic fibers (S2, 3, 4) is responsible for causing urinary retention. Due to significant decrease in postspinal headache *urinary retention has now become the most common postoperative complication of spinal anesthesia.* It can occur in as much as one-third of the patients. Concurrent administration of intrathecal opioids especially morphine is strongly associated with higher incidence of urinary retention. Catheterization may be required.

Neurological complications

1. *Post-spinal headache*: It is *low pressure headache* due to seepage of CSF from dural rent (hole) created by spinal needle. CSF leakage results in decreased intracranial pressure leading to traction of pain sensitive structures like dura, vessels and tentorium producing pain.

The CSF loss around *10 mL/hr.* is considered as significant loss to cause post-spinal headache.

Clinical features:
- Patient can present with headache anytime between 12–72 hours depending when he/she starts sitting or ambulation.
- The pain in throbbing in nature and is usually *occipital* however can occur in any part of the brain. Headache may be associated with nausea, vomiting, dizziness, tinnitus, diplopia or even seizures.
- As there is meningeal stretching the pain may be associated with stiffness and pain in neck; in that case it has to be differently diagnosed from meningitis. As the CSF pressure at lumbar level become double in sitting position leading to more loss of CSF, the typical symptomatology of post spinal headache is that *patient will complain of pain in sitting and standing position while pain gets relived in lying down* whereas the headache due to meningitis will remain same in all positions.
- *Incidence:* Due to the use of smaller gauge needles incidence has been significantly reduced now a days, overall it is around *1 to 5%.*

- *In majority of the cases the headache gets resolved in 7 to 10 days.*

Etiological factors
- *Needle size:* Needle size is the single most important factor; incidence with 16G needle may be 75% while with 26G needle it is 1 to 3%.
- *Type of needle:* Incidence is significantly less with dura separating (pencil tip point) needle.
- *Altitude:* High incidence at high altitude.
- *Type of the patient:* Patient with history of headaches is more prone for spinal headache.
- Inadequate hydration.
- Pregnancy, female gender and young patients have more incidence of postspinal headache
- Incidence is less (statistically significant) with paramedian approach and low glucose concentration of the drug.

Treatment
Preventive:
- *Use of small gauge and dura separating needles are the most important preventive measures.*
- Adequate hydration so that CSF production exceeds loss.
- Avoiding spinal in patient with history of headache.
- It is now proven that *early ambulation does not increase the incidence of post-spinal headache* if other factors like needle size, needle type are taken care of.

Curative:
1st Line: First line of management is conservative and it includes:
- Ask the patient to lie supine in slight Trendelenburg position as far as possible.
- Analgesics.
- Intravenous fluids (15 mL/kg/hr) or oral fluids 3 liters/day. The aim of adequate hydration is to increase CSF production.
- *Oral or intravenous caffeine:* 500 mg of caffeine in 1 liter of ringer lactate inhibits the vasospasm cycle in cerebral vessels.
Most often headache is relieved by conservative measures.

2nd Line: 2nd line may include abdominal binders, desmopressin (retains fluid), inhalation of 5–6% CO_2 in oxygen (CO_2 by cerebral vasodilation will promote CSF production), triptans (sumatriptan, zolmitriptan) and xanithol.

3rd Line: Third line of management is although interventional but definitive method of treatment. It includes *autologous Epidural blood patch.* In this technique 10–20 mL of the patient's own blood is given in the same or just caudal epidural space in which spinal was given. Blood will clot and seal the rent. 1st blood patch is effective in treating headache in 95% patients and 2nd blood patch in 99%. 15–20 mL of blood is not likely to cause significant hematoma however can cause transient radiculopathy.

The current recommendation favors the early application of epidural blood patch if headache is compromising the quality of life and not responding to conservative management for 24 hours or in other words there is a very limited role left for 2nd line management.

Other causes of headache after spinal anesthesia:

- *Meningeal irritation:* It is because of chemical meningitis or bacterial meningitis. Headache produced by meningitis is *high pressure headache* and is not related to postural changes.
- *Queckenstedt's test* is employed to differentiate between high pressure and low pressure headache. In this test applying pressure on jugular veins increases the headache in meningitis while relieves in post-spinal headache.

2. *Paralysis of cranial nerves:* All cranial nerves except 1st, 9th and 10th can be involved after spinal anesthesia. *Most commonly (90%) 6th nerve is involved* (because of the longest intracranial course of 6th nerve).

Cause: As a result of low CSF pressure, descent of pons and medulla can cause stretching of 6th nerve at the apex of petrous temporal bone.

Clinical features: Paralysis appears after 3rd to 12th postoperative day. Blurred vision, double vision, headache, photophobia are the usual symptoms.

Treatment
Prophylactic:
- Vigorous hydration.
- Use of small bore needles.

Curative:
- Dark glasses with outer 1/3rd of glass to be made opaque.
- Ocular muscle exercise.
- Adequate fluids.

Recovery: 50% cases recover in 1 month and most of the cases in 2 years. If recovery is not seen after 2 years surgical correction should be done.

3. *Meningitis*
- *Aseptic:* Aseptic meningitis was seen in past because of the chemical detergents used in antiseptic solutions. It is no longer a concern in modern day practice because antiseptic solutions used now a days are preservative free. Aseptic meningitis responds to symptomatic treatment
- *Infective:* Infective meningitis although rare (incidence is 0.3 per 10,000 spinals and almost double after epidural) but is the matter of serious concern therefore highest degree of asepsis should be maintained during the procedure. Chlorhexidine in an alcohol base is the most effective antiseptic.

Interestingly *Streptococcus viridans (an oral flora) has been cited as the most common organism responsible for meningitis after spinal* emphasizing the mandatory requirement of facemask to be worn by clinicians throughout the procedure. However *after epidural, meningitis most often occurs because of Staphylococcus epidermidis* which can contaminate the epidural catheter to reach the meninges.

Treatment: Intravenous antibiotics.

4. *Transient neurological symptoms:* Transient neurological symptoms (TNS), previously used be called as transient radicular irritation, theoretically can occur with any local anesthetic used in clinical practice however *most often it is seen with lignocaine.* The incidence with lignocaine can be as high as 10–11% (that is why lignocaine is hardly used for spinal).

Patients may complain of pain in buttocks radiating to legs without any neurological deficit. The symptoms resolve themselves with in few days (< 1 week).

5. *Cauda equina syndrome:* Cauda equina syndrome (CES) is one of the classical examples of neurotoxicity caused by local anesthetic.

It is usually seen with lignocaine when given as continuous spinal with small bore catheters however there has been case reports of CES reported with single shot spinal with lignocaine. Although, *it most often occurs with spinal but there has been case reports of CES with epidural too.*

Clinical features: Retention of urine, incontinence of feces, loss of sexual function and loss of sensation in perineal region.

Pathological lesion: Vacuolation of nerve fibers.
Most of these cases recover spontaneously.

6. *Neuropathies:* Neuropathies may be caused by:
   - *Direct trauma to nerve by needle:* Fortunately majority of neuropathies caused by needle trauma resolves spontaneously
   - Neurotoxicity by local anesthetics like TNS and cauda equina by lignocaine. *The preservative used with chloroprocaine has caused severe neurological deficits in past.*

7. *Paraplegia:* Paraplegia is one of the most fearsome complications of neuraxial blocks. It may be due to:
   - *Epidural hematoma:* Although bleeding during spinal is quite common but the incidence of epidural hematoma leading to paraplegia is rare (1:200000). Epidural hematoma large enough to cause paraplegia occurs in patients on anticoagulants therapy or suffering from coagulopathies.
   The presentation is sharp back pain with motor weakness and/or bladder/bowel dysfunction. The diagnosis should be confirmed by MRI and management includes immediate neurosurgical intervention to drain the hematoma.
   - *Epidural abscess:* Strict asepsis should be maintained to prevent this devastating complication. The diagnosis should be confirmed by MRI and management includes immediate neurosurgical intervention to drain the abscess.
   - *Arachnoiditis:* Inflammation of arachnoid can compromise the vascular supply of spinal cord leading to ischemia and permanent paraplegia. Arachnoiditis can be infective or non-infective. Cases of non-infective arachnoiditis occurred in the past when procaine was used with its preservative. Therefore *any drug given through meninges as rule must be preservative free.* Non-infective arachnoiditis has also been reported with subarachnoid steroids.
   - *Spinal cord ischemia:* Ischemia of spinal cord can cause permanent paraplegia. The cause of ischemia may be severe prolonged hypotension, use of vasoconstrictors (only theoretical concern) and arachnoiditis.
   - *Direct trauma to spinal cord:* To avoid this complication spinal in adults should be given below L1 and in children up to 2 years below L3.

8. *Anterior spinal artery syndrome:* Epidural hematoma, abscess, epidermoid tumor (skin tissue carried with needle can cause epidermoid tumor), can lead to compression of anterior spinal artery causing anterior spinal artery syndrome manifested by motor deficit without involving posterior columns.

9. *Intracranial complications:* Sudden changes in hydrodynamics of CSF can cause intracranial complications like subdural hematoma, brain herniation especially uncus or intracranial hemorrhage.

Pruritus: Pruritis is the most common side effect of intrathecal opioids. It can be treated with opioid antagonists.

Backache: Many patients report backache after spinal anesthesia however neuraxial blocks do not cause chronic back pain therefore patient must be reassured.

SPINAL ANESTHESIA IN CHILDREN
- Should be given in lower space (L4-5).
- Children *less than 8 years* are virtually free of hemodynamic side effects.
- Due to more CSF volume (4 mL/kg vs. 2 mL/kg for adult) dose of local anesthetic required is more and duration of block is less.
- Use of narcotics is contraindicated.
- Chances of systemic toxicity is high.

SADDLE BLOCK
It is the *spinal given in sitting position and the patient remains seated for 5–10 minutes till drug get fixed.* As only sacral segments are blocked it can be utilized only for perianal surgeries. The advantage is that hemodynamic fluctuations are minimal and there is no possibility of high spinal.

EPIDURAL (EXTRADURAL) ANESTHESIA (ALSO CALLED AS PERIDURAL BLOCK)

Indications

All surgeries which can be performed under spinal anesthesia can be performed under epidural block. In addition, epidural can be utilized for upper abdominal, thoracic (under thoracic epidural) and even neck surgeries (under cervical epidural). However in clinical practice epidural is mainly used for postoperative pain management and painless labor (by continuous infusion through a catheter). Epidural is also used in chronic pain management.

Epidural Needles

The most commonly used needle for epidural is *Tuohy needle*. It has blunt bevel with curve of 15 to 30 degree at tip **(Fig. 17.2)**. This curved tip is called as Huber tip. Other needles which can be used for epidural are Weiss (it is winged) and Crawford (straight blunt bevel with no curve).

Technique

Like spinal it can be given in sitting and lateral position. Usually epidural space is encountered at *4–5 cm* from skin and has *negative pressure* in 80% individuals.

Most commonly used method to locate epidural space is by *loss of resistance technique*. Once the needle pierces the ligamentum flavum there is sudden loss of resistance and the syringe filled with air or saline will be felt literally sucked in epidural space.

Another popular technique of past, *hanging drop technique* (Gutierrez's sign) {If a drop of saline is placed on the hub of needle it will be sucked in due to negative pressure once the needle is in epidural space} is hardly used in current day practice.

Once the needle is confirmed in epidural space, a test dose of 2–3 ml of hyperbaric lignocaine with adrenaline (except for obstetric patient where epinephrine should not be used) is given and if in 5 minutes there is no evidence of either spinal block (inability to move foot) or intravascular injection

(tachycardia by adrenaline), further doses can be given.

Epidural catheter is passed through the needle. 3–4 cm of catheter should be in epidural space. A microfilter is attached to catheter to prevent contamination.

Onset of effect takes place in 15–20 minutes.

Site of Action of Drug

- Anterior and posterior nerve roots (main site of action).
- Mixed spinal nerves.
- Drug diffuses through dura and arachnoid and inhibits descending pathways in spinal cord.

Drugs used for Epidural Anesthesia

Local Anesthetics (Table 17.2)

Usually 2–3 mL of local anesthetic is required for blocking 1 segment; therefore normally 15 to 20 mL of drug is required.

- Lignocaine (with or without adrenaline): 1–2% concentration is used.
- Bupivacaine 0.625–0.5%, Ropivacaine 0.1–1.0% and Levobupivacaine 0.125–0.75% depending whether used for sensory or motor block. *Ropivacaine because of if high safety profile is most preferred.*

Other drugs like prilocaine, chloroprocaine or mepivacaine are seldom used now a day. However, a new preservative free preparation of chloroprocaine has been recently launched for central neuraxial blocks.

Opioids

Morphine: 4–6 mg (diluted in 10 mL saline). Onset within 30 minutes. Effect lasts for 12–16 hours. Depodur is an extended-release liposomal formulation of morphine which can provide analgesia for 48 hours.

Fentanyl: 100 mcg (diluted in 10 mL saline). Onset within 10 minutes. Effect lasts for 2–3 hours.

■ **Table 17.2:** Local anesthetics for epidural anesthesia

Drugs	Concentration
Lignocaine	1–2%
Levobupivacaine	0.125–0.75%
Ropivacaine	0.1–1%
Bupivacaine	0.625–0.5%

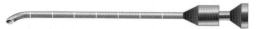

Fig. 17.2: Tuohy needle (for epidural anesthesia)

Fentanyl (2–4 µg/mL) + *bupivacaine* (0.125%) *or ropivacaine* (0.2%) *(ropivacaine preferred)* as continuous infusion given by syringe pump through epidural catheter is the *most commonly used combination for postoperative analgesia and painless labor.*

Site of action of opioids after epidural administration: Opioids after diffusion through meninges reaches the spinal cord where they bind to opioid receptors present in substantia gelatinosa of dorsal horn cells.

The *advantages* of epidural opioids over local anesthetics:
- Only *sensory block is produced* while with local anesthetics there are chances of motor blockade if high concentration is used.
- The effect of single dose (especially morphine) lasts long (12–16 hrs) obviating the need for frequent injections.
- No sympathetic block.

Disadvantages:
- *Respiratory depression:* Respiratory depression is more profound with less lipid soluble opioids like morphine than with more lipid soluble (fentanyl, alfentanil, sufentanil). The less lipid soluble agents because of prolonged stay in CSF mixes with CSF to reaches brain to inhibit respiratory medullary centers producing *delayed respiratory depression after 6–12 hours.*
- Urinary retention.
- Pruritus.
- Nausea and vomiting.
- Sedation.

Adjuvant Drugs

Adjuvant drugs like clonidine, dexmedetomidine, neostigmine and ketamine has been tried to enhance the onset, augment analgesic effect and improve quality of block but with variable results.

Liposomal Bupivacaine

Liposomal bupivacaine which can produce longer lasting analgesia is currently under investigation.

Factors Affecting the Spread (Level) of Block

- *Volume of the drug:* It is the most important factor.
- *Age:* Old requiring less dose because volume of epidural space is less.

- *Gravity (Patient's position):* Does not affect level too much as in case of spinal.
- *Intra-abdominal tumors, pregnancy:* Less dose is required.
- Level of injection.
- *Length of vertebral column:* Taller individuals require higher dose.
- *Concentration of local anesthetic:* High the concentration, higher is the spread

Factor Effecting Onset and Duration of Block

The same factors which govern the onset and duration of local anesthetics (*Refer to Chapter 15, page no. 153*).

Advantages of Epidural over Spinal

- *Less hypotension:* As the onset of action of epidural is slow body gets sufficient time to compensate for hypotension making epidural a better choice than spinal for cardiac compromised patients.
- *No postspinal headache* however headache can occur if dura is punctured accidentally.
- By giving top up doses through catheter *level of block* and *duration of anesthesia can be changed.*

Disadvantages Over Spinal

- *Inadequate (patchy) block/block failure rate is high:* Epidural space has fibrous bands and other tissues leading to unequal distribution of drug producing patchy block/failed block. Because of the large size and anatomy *L5 and S1 segments are most vulnerable to spared.*
  Another reason for failed block is *subdural block.* It is rare complication when drug enters the subdural space. The presentation is extremely variable. There may occur very high unilateral block or there may be block with sparing of one modality.
- *Higher chances of total spinal:* Total spinal is one of the most feared complication of epidural. It occurs, if accidently dura is punctured during drug injection and whole volume (10–20 mL) of drug is injected in subarachnoid space. As plain bupivacaine and lignocaine are slightly hypobaric this volume will reach cranium producing total spinal *manifested as marked hypotension,*

bradycardia, apnea, dilated pupils and unconsciousness.

Prevention
- Always confirm the position of needle or catheter by giving a test dose with lignocaine with adrenaline
- Never inject as a bolus, always give drug in increments of 3–5 mL and confirm negative aspiration of CSF before injecting next increment of the drug.

Treatment
- Intubate and IPPV with 100% oxygen.
- Vasopressors.
- Atropine.

- *Accidental dural puncture:* Although the incidence is <1% but if dura gets punctured with epidural needle the incidence of postspinal headache is very high as epidural needles have broader gauge as compared to spinal; most often 18 or 19 G epidural needle is used to pass 19 or 20G catheter.

  If dura is punctured with epidural needle, there are two alternatives:
  - Give hyperbaric local anesthetic through this needle, i.e., convert it to spinal.
  - Remove the needle and give epidural in higher space.

- *More chances of epidural hematoma and intravascular injection:* As the needle or catheter is near to epidural venous plexus chances of bleeding, hematoma formation and intravascular injection are more. *The possibility of hematoma formation can be 10 fold higher than spinal.* As the veins are denser laterally the epidural should be given in midline. To prevent intravascular injection inject the drug only after confirming negative aspiration of blood.

- *Higher chances of infectious complications:* The presence of catheter for many days increases the chances of infectious complications like meningitis, epidural abscess. Although there are no study to exactly confirm the maximum safe time for which an epidural catheter can be kept however majority of the clinicians recommended a *maximum period of 4 days.*

- *Higher incidence of local anesthetic toxicity:* Higher volumes used in epidural increases the chances of local anesthetic toxicity.

- *Higher incidence of neuropathies:* Studies have shown higher incidence of radiculopathies with epidural as compared to spinal.

- *Intraocular hemorrhage:* Rapid injection of drug can raise intraocular pressure causing subhyaloid bleeding.

- Higher incidence of acute back pain as compared to spinal.

- Catheter related complications like broken catheter. If the catheter gets broken in epidural space and is not infected, it can be left in situ (a retained catheter is no more reactive than a suture) and reassure the patient however if it gets broken in subcutaneous tissue then it should be removed.

- Compare to spinal epidural sets are *more expensive.*

- Technically epidural is more difficult as compared to spinal.

COMBINED SPINAL EPIDURAL ANESTHESIA

Combined spinal epidural (CSE) is now very commonly performed technique where spinal is used for surgery and epidural is utilized if surgery gets prolonged or surgeon want to extend the incision. Later epidural catheter can be used for postoperative analgesia.

Technique

Epidural needle is placed in epidural space. Through this needle special spinal needle (longer ones, 120 mm while normal spinal needle is 90 mm) is passed and once CSF flows out hyperbaric local analgesic is injected, spinal needle is taken out and epidural catheter is passed through epidural needle.

CAUDAL BLOCK (EPIDURAL SACRAL BLOCK)

It is a type of epidural block commonly utilized in children where drug is injected in sacral hiatus after piercing sacrococcygeal membrane. Most often utilized to produce analgesia for perianal surgeries, genital surgeries like circumcision, urethral surgeries like urethroplasties or lower abdominal surgeries like herniotomies. *In children, it is easy to perform caudal block because sacral hiatus can be easily identified.*

Complications and contraindications are same as for epidural. In addition any infection in perianal region is a contraindication for caudal.

Contraindications for Central Neuraxial Blocks

Absolute

- *Raised intracranial tension:* Medullary coning can cause death if spinal is given to patients with raised ICT. Like spinal, epidural should not be given to patients with raised ICT as there is always a possibility of accidental dural puncture. Moreover, large volume of drug in epidural space can increase CSF pressure.
- Patient refusal.
- Severe hypovolemia and hypotension.
- *Patients on anticoagulants*:* Patients on anticoagulants can bleed significantly to cause epidural hematoma and paraplegia.
  - *Patients on thrombolytic/fibrinolytic therapy:* As there is no clear cut data available therefore the traditional approach of withholding CNB for 10 days after last dose of thrombolytic/fibrinolytic therapy still holds valid.
  - *Patients on oral anticoagulants:* Central neuraxial blocks can be given only when prothrombin time becomes normal and INR becomes less than 1.5. Warfarin can be restarted 2 hours after central neuraxial blocks or epidural catheter removal.
  - Patients on *heparin*
    - *Standard (unfractioned) heparin:*
      - If the dose is < 10,000 units/day subcutaneously, central neuraxial blocks (CNB) can be given without any delay. However, if the dose is >10,000 units/day then CNB should be given only *8 hours* after last dose of heparin.
      - Heparin can be restarted safely after 1 hour of CNB.
      - Epidural catheter should be removed 4 hours after last dose of heparin and heparin can be restarted 1 hour after catheter removal.
- *Low molecular weight heparin (LMWH) {unfractioned}.*
  - *It is considered safe to give central neuraxial block 12 hours after last dose of LMWH if the dose is prophylactic* (dose of enoxaparin < 40 mg) however if doses are therapeutic then central neuraxial blocks should be given only after 24 hours.
  - *LMWH can be safely given 6 hours after central neuraxial blocks* however if the CNB was traumatic (bloody) then LMWH (and unfractionated heparin also) should be delayed for 24 hours.
  - It is safe to start prophylactic dose of LMWH with epidural catheter in situ however if LMWH is required in therapeutic dose then catheter has to be removed before starting LMWH.
  - *Epidural catheter should be removed 10 hours after last of LMWH and LMWH can be restarted 2 hours after removal of catheter.*
  - *Patients on new anticoagulants*
    - CNB should be delayed for 48 hours after fondaparinux, 72 hours after rivaroxaban (Xarelto) and 5 days after dabigatran (Pradaxa). They can be given safely 6 hours after CNB or epidural catheter removal.
    - *Patients on antiplatelets: Patients on aspirin and NSAIDs can be safely given central neuraxial blocks* while for other antiplatelets CNB should be delayed for *7 days after clopidogrel,* dipyridamol, and prasugrel, 14 days after eticlopidine, 2 days after abciximab and 8 hours after eptifibatide. Antiplatelets can

---

*Different countries (and even different societies within a country) follows different guidelines however the most acceptable guidelines are the guidelines prescribed by American Society of Regional Anesthesia and Pain Medicine (ASRA). Recommendations mentioned here are based on most recent (3rd and 4th) editions of ASRA.

be restarted 6 hours after CNB or epidural catheter removal.

- Bleeding disorders/coagulopathy. In Patients suffering from bleeding diathesis there are very high chances of epidural hematoma and paraplegia.
- Infection at local site.
- Severe fixed cardiac output lesions (aortic and mitral stenosis, constrictive pericarditis, coarctation of aorta): These patients can not compensate for decrease in cardiac output and cannot tolerate fluid overload, therefore should not receive CNB.

Relative

- *Mild to moderate fixed cardiac output lesions:* Mild to moderate cases can be given central neuraxial block if necessary. Epidural because of less hypotension is preferred over spinal.
- Mild to moderate hypotension and hypovolemia.

- *Uncontrolled hypertension:* Uncontrolled hypertensives may develop sudden hypotension after spinal. Controlled hypertensives can safely receive central neuraxial blocks.
- Severe ischemic heart disease especially history of recent MI.
- *Thrombocytopenia:* Patients with platelet count more than 80,000/cubic mm can be safely given central neuraxial blocks. Platelet count between 50,000–80,000/cubic mm is a relative contraindication while count less than 50000 becomes an absolute contraindication.
- *Heart blocks and patient on β blockers:* Severe bradycardia can occur.
- *Spinal deformity and previous spinal surgery:* Due to distorted anatomy CNB not only becomes technically difficult there are also increased chances of traumatic nerve injury especially in patient with spina bifida or in patient underwent multiple levels of laminectomies.

■ **Table 17.3:** Comparison between spinal and epidural anesthesia

	Spinal	*Epidural*
Cost	Cheap	Expensive
Onset	Fast	Slow (15–20 minutes)
Duration	Less (45 minutes to 1 hour with lignocaine and 2–3 hours with bupivacaine	Prolonged and with epidural catheter longer duration surgery can be performed by giving top up doses.
Technically	Easy	Difficult
Quality of block	More dense	Patchy block is common
Change of level of block	Not possible once drug gets fixed	Can be changed by giving top of doses through catheter
Block failure rate	Less	More
Uses	For surgeries	Mainly for analgesia
Level	Given at lumbar level	Can be given at sacral, lumbar, thoracic or even cervical level
Complications		
1. Hypotension	More	Less
2. Postspinal headache	Yes	No (can happen with accidental dural puncture)
3. Epidural hematoma	Less	More
4. Infectious complications	Less	More
5. Neuropathies	Less	More
6. Intravascular injection and drug toxicity	Less	More
7. Total spinal	Very rare	More chances
8. Catheter related complications	Not seen (can happen with spinal catheters but they are hardly used)	Seen

- *Psychiatric and uncooperative patients:* These patient will not cooperate during positioning.
- *History of headache:* For unknown reasons patients with history of headache are more vulnerable for post spinal headache.
- *GIT perforation:* Theoretically parasympathetic over activity increases the peristalsis and can open the seal.
- *Myelopathy and peripheral neuropathies:* The evidence that CNB (and other peripheral blocks also) exaggerates an existing neuropathy is lacking. Nerve blocks should be avoided in these patients for medicolegal reasons. If a nerve block has to be given in such patients it is mandatory to mention all the deficits in pre-anesthetic sheet to avoid any litigation.
- *CNS disorders:*
  - *Multiple sclerosis:* Due to increased sensitivity of local anesthetics patients of multiple sclerosis exhibit a prolonged block however, the evidence proving the exacerbation of multiple sclerosis symptoms by central neuraxial blocks is lacking.
  - *Spinal stenosis:* These patients may be at increased risk of neurologic complications after neuraxial blocks

- Resistant surgeon
- *Chronic backache:* Chronic low back pain without neurologic deficit is not a contraindication for CNB. Moreover CNB does not causes the exacerbation of back pain however many clinicians avoid CNB in such patients to avoid medicolegal hassles.
- Septicemia and bacteremia.

LEVEL OF BLOCK REQUIRED FOR COMMON SURGERIES

When deciding the level of block it is important to block nerve supply of all the organs involved during surgery, not only the level of skin incision. For example, Skin incision level for cesarean section is at T11 level but since intestine and peritoneum are also handled, block required is up to T4. Level of block required for some common surgeries:

Cesarean section	:	Up to T4.
Prostate	:	Up to T10.
Testicular surgeries	:	Up to T10.
Hernia	:	Up to T10.
Appendix	:	Up to T8.
Hysterectomies	:	Up to T6.
Perianal surgeries	:	Sacral segments.

For comparison between spinal and epidural anesthesia see **Table 17.3**.

KEY POINTS

- The line joining the highest point on iliac crest corresponds to L4 and L5 interspace or L4 spine.
- Spinal cord extends from medulla oblongata to lower border of L1 in adults and L3 in infants.
- The sequence of blockade after CNB is autonomic > sensory > motor.
- Several meta-analyses have shown a reduced risk as high as 30% in overall mortality and morbidity in patients who underwent surgeries under CNB as compared to GA.
- Apnea after spinal anesthesia is usually due to severe hypotension.
- The most common cause of nausea and vomiting is hypotension.
- Hypotension is the most common complication of spinal anesthesia.
- Urinary retention is the most common postoperative complication of central neuraxial blocks in present day practice.
- Hyperbaric bupivacaine is the most commonly used drug for spinal.
- Dose and Baricity are 2 very important determinants of level of block.
- Ephedrine is the most preferred vasopressor for the treatment of spinal hypotension.
- High spinal is associated with bradycardia and hypotension.
- The drug of choice for treatment of shivering is pethidine.
- Postspinal headache is low pressure, meningovascular headache.
- Postural relation, i.e. pain in sitting and standing position and getting relived in lying down is diagnostic of postspinal headache.

Contd...

Contd...

- Use of small gauge and dura separating needles are the most important preventive measures to prevent post spinal headache.
- 6th is most commonly involved cranial nerve after spinal anesthesia.
- *Streptococcus viridans* has been cited as the most common organism responsible for meningitis after spinal while *Staphylococcus epidermidis* is the most common organism responsible for meningitis after epidural.
- Transient neurological symptoms and cauda equina syndrome lead to almost elimination of lignocaine for spinal.
- The most commonly used needle for epidural is Tuohy needle and most commonly used method to locate epidural space is by loss of resistance technique.
- Fentanyl + bupivacaine or ropivacaine as continuous infusion is the most commonly used combination for postoperative analgesia and painless labor.
- There is less hypotension in epidural as compared to spinal.
- Chances of infectious complications, epidural hematoma and neurotoxicity is more with epidural as compared to spinal.
- It is considered safe to give central neuraxial block 12 hours after last dose of LMWH and LMWH can be given safely given 6 hours after central neuraxial blocks.
- Patients on aspirin and NSAIDs can be safely given central neuraxial blocks while CNB should be delayed for 7 days after clopidogrel.
- Patients with platelet count more than 80,000/cubic mm can be safely given central neuraxial blocks.

Anesthesia for Coexisting Diseases

CHAPTER 18

Anesthesia for Cardiovascular Diseases (For Noncardiac Surgeries)

ISCHEMIC HEART DISEASE

The patients coming for surgery with ischemic heart diseases (IHD) have been on constant rise.

Preoperative Evaluation

Preoperative evaluation should be done in detail with special emphasis on *assessing the effort tolerance. Effort tolerance > 4 METS is generally associated with lesser complications*. A very important part of the preoperative evaluation of cardiac patients is to stratify their cardiac risk based on Lee revised cardiac risk index which includes the following 6 parameters:

1. High risk surgery like aortic surgery or thoracotomies.
2. History of ischemic heart disease
3. History of cerebrovascular disease
4. History of congestive heart failure
5. Insulin dependent diabetes mellitus
6. Preoperative serum creatinine > 2 mg/dL.

Investigations: Special investigations like Holter, exercise electrocardiography (Treadmill test), echocardiography or dobutamine stress echocardiography (DSE), myocardial perfusion scan or coronary angiography should be done based on the medical condition of the patient after consultation with cardiologist.

Management of existing drug therapy:

- *β-blockers:* β-blockers must not be stopped at any cost if the patient is on β-blockers (stopping β-blockers can significantly increase morbidity and mortality) however they should not be started afresh in a patient who is not on β-blockers unless they can be started at least 1 week before surgery.

- *Antiplatelets: Aspirin should be continued, Clopidogrel to be stopped 5 days before* (however central neuraxial block can be given only after 7 days) and prasugrel to be stopped 7 days before surgery.
- Rest all antianginal drugs (nitrates, calcium channel blockers, ACE inhibitors) should be continued.

Timing of surgery:

- *Elective surgery must be deferred for 6 weeks* (preferably 3 months) after an episode of ischemia/infarct if the patient was treated without stenting.
- If the patient was treated with stent then *elective surgery must be deferred for 6 weeks* (preferably 3 months) *if bare metal stent was used and for 6 months with new generation drug eluting stents and 1 year with conventional drug eluting stents.*
- If the patient was treated by coronary artery pass graft (CABG) then elective surgery should be deferred for *6 weeks* (preferably 3 months).

Monitoring

- *ECG:* Other than routine monitoring, *ECG is mandatory. Lead V5* is the best to diagnose left ventricle infarction and lead II for arrhythmia (as well as inferior wall MI) therefore a combination of lead II and V5 can detect majority (94–95%) of intraoperative ischemic events. Monitors with facility of ST analysis are ideal for these patients.
- Invasive monitoring like central venous pressure (CVP) or invasive BP monitoring should be considered only if large intravascular fluid shifts are expected. Similarly, pulmonary

artery catheterization is reserved for extreme situations only.

- *Transesophageal echocardiography (TEE):* TEE is *the earliest and most sensitive monitor to detect intraoperative infarction* (can detect more than 99% of ischemic events) however it limitations like cost, extensive training in interpretation and application only in intubated patients (while ischemic events do occur more commonly during intubation) limits its use as a routine monitor.

Anesthetic Management

The most important goal of anesthetic management for patients of ischemic heart disease is to *avoid a imbalance between myocardial oxygen demand and supply* therefore anything which decreases myocardial oxygen supply like anemia, hypotension, hypocapnia (by causing coronary vasoconstriction), tachycardia (by decreasing diastole time) or increasing oxygen demand like tachycardia, hypertension (by increasing after load), stress, sympathetic stimulation are not permitted.

Choice of anesthesia: Although central neuraxial blocks (CNB) are not absolutely contraindicated but hypotension associated with spinal can be deleterious therefore general anesthesia is preferred over CNB.

Premedication: As stress can precipitate MI, pre-medication with anxiolytics like benzodiazepines is *must.*

Induction: Cardiovascular stability of *etomidate makes it an induction agent of choice for cardiac patients.* Other IV agents like thiopentone and propofol can be used if hypotension can be avoided however *ketamine must not be used* because it can stimulate sympathetic system.

As *tachycardia and hypertension can precipitate MI they are not acceptable at any cost* therefore sympathetic stimulation seen during laryngoscopy and intubation must be blunted by lignocaine, β-blockers or opioids.

Maintenance:

- Although inhalational agents decrease the cardiac output however *inhalational agents can be safely used if patient's left ventricular function is normal.* The concern of isoflurane

induced coronary steal is only theoretical therefore if necessary it can also be used safely for IHD patients.

- *Patients with compromised left ventricular function* cannot receive inhalational agents therefore *anesthesia is best maintained with opioids.*
- Nitrous oxide should be avoided for two reasons. First, it may cause mild sympathetic stimulation and second, it is a pulmonary vasoconstrictor.
- *Vecuronium* is the most cardiac stable muscle relaxant therefore muscle relaxant of choice for cardiac patients.
- *Reversal:* Only glycopyrrolate (no atropine) should be used along with neostigmine.

Postoperative period: Interestingly *majority of MI occur in postoperative period (within 48 hours)* therefore all the events which can cause misbalance between myocardial oxygen demand and supply (especially pain) should be avoided in postoperative period.

Treatment of Intraoperative Myocardial Infarction

- If the patient is hemodynamically unstable
  - Intravenous nitroglycerine (mainstay of treatment)
  - β-blockers
- If the patient is hemodynamically unstable
  - Treat arrhythmia as per advanced cardiac life support (ACLS) protocol
  - Intra-aortic balloon pump
  - Inotrope for circulatory support
  - Percutaneous intervention (PCI) angiography and/or angioplasty as early as possible in postoperative period.

Emergency Surgery in Patients with Stents

As stated earlier that elective surgery should be deferred for 6 weeks in patients with bare metal stents and for 1 year in patients with drug eluting stents however patients with stents do come for emergency surgery.

As these patients are on dual antiplatelet therapy (Aspirin+ Clopidogrel) decision has to be taken as whether to continue or stop antiplatelet therapy. Stopping antiplatelet therapy carries the risk of thrombotic complications (including coronary or cerebral thrombosis) while continuing therapy carries the risk of bleeding. Thrombotic complications are more devastating and are not in the control of surgeon and anesthetist whereas bleeding complications are controllable (by pressure or platelet therapy) therefore *continuing antiplatelet therapy is always preferred* except for few situations, like major vascular surgeries or neurosurgeries, where bleeding may not be acceptable/controllable.

VALVULAR DISEASES

- The most important goal of preoperative assessment is to assess the severity of valvular lesion.
- Invasive monitoring (pulmonary artery catheterization or transesophageal echocardiography) is only reserved for severe cases of valvular lesions.

Mitral Stenosis

Mitral stenosis (MS) is considered to be severe if transvalvular pressure gradient is > 10 mm Hg (normal < 5 mm Hg).

Anesthetic Management

- *Avoid tachycardia:* Tachycardia by decreasing the diastole will decrease the left ventricular filling and hence stroke volume and cardiac output.
- *Avoid hypotension:* As these patients have already low cardiac output, hypotension can be detrimental.
- *Avoid sudden increase is blood volume:* MS patients if given volume overload may develop pulmonary edema.
- *Avoid hypoxia, hypercarbia:* Hypoxia and hypercarbia by causing pulmonary vasoconstriction can worsen already existing pulmonary hypertension.

Choice of Anesthesia

Central neuraxial blocks (CNB) should be avoided as hypotension is not acceptable in already low cardiac output state and moreover fluid infusion can precipitate pulmonary edema however CNB can be considered for mild to moderate lesion by ensuring that significant hypotension is avoided.

As atrial fibrillation is seen in one-third of the patients with MS, a significant number of MS patients will be on oral anticoagulants contraindicating the use of CNB.

General Anesthesia

Induction: Etomidate being the most cardiac stable is the agent of choice.

Maintenance: Isoflurane being most cardiac stable is most preferred however sevoflurane and desflurane in lower concentrations can be safely used. Nitrous oxide can cause mild pulmonary vasoconstriction therefore should be avoided.

Relaxant: As vecuronium is the most cardiac stable, it is the muscle relaxant of choice.

Reversal: As tachycardia is not acceptable atropine should not be used with neostigmine.

Mitral Regurgitation

Mitral regurgitation (MR) is said to be severe if regurgitant fraction is > 0.6.

Anesthetic Management

- Avoid *bradycardia:* Bradycardia by increasing the diastole will increase the regurgitation.
- Avoid *hypertension:* Hypertension by increasing the afterload increases the regurgitation.

Choice of Anesthesia

As decrease in afterload decreases the regurgitation Central neuraxial blocks appears to be a good selection however excessive hypotension should be avoided.

General Anesthesia

- *Induction:* Etomidate
- *Maintenance:* Isoflurane
- *Muscle relaxant:* Vecuronium

Mitral Valve Prolapse

Generally mitral valve prolapse (MVP) is a benign condition however can become clinically significant if associated with mitral regurgitation (MR). The hemodynamic principles of management of MVP without MR and with MR are different. For example, increasing left ventricular volume by giving fluids, by causing bradycardia and hypertension decreases the degree of prolapse while on the other hand the same interventions are detrimental if there is associated MR. Therefore it is very important *to assess in preoperative period whether MVP is associated with MR or not.*

Majority of the MVP cases have normal left ventricular function therefore can be given CNB or GA. If GA is to be given then cardiac stable drugs (Etomidate, Isoflurane and Vecuronium) should be preferred.

Aortic Stenosis

Among the valvular lesions aortic stenosis (AS) have most devastating complications like infarction, arrhythmia or even sudden death. 75% of the symptomatic patients with severe AS (transvalvular gradient > 50 mm Hg or aortic valve orifice is less than 0.8 cm^2) may die within 3 years without valve replacement.

Anesthetic Management

- *Maintain normal sinus rhythm;* neither bradycardia nor tachycardia is acceptable. Bradycardia can cause over distension of already hypertrophied left ventricle while tachycardia by decreasing the ventricular filling can further decrease the cardiac output.
- *Maintain normal blood pressure.* Hypertension by increasing the afterload can further deteriorate left ventricular function. Hypotension is not acceptable at any cost; severe hypotension by reducing the coronary blood flow can precipitate myocardial ischemia or even cardiac arrest. Unfortunately patients with severe AS may not be able to generate adequate stroke making *CPR to be ineffective.* Therefore hypotension should be managed very aggressively. *As phenylephrine does not causes tachycardia it is the vasopressor of choice for patients with AS.*

Choice of Anesthesia

As central neuraxial blocks can cause hypotension therefore *anesthetic technique of choice is GA.*

General Anesthesia

Induction: Etomidate.

Maintenance: O_2 + N_2O and isoflurane if LV function is not significantly compromised however if LV function is compromised then opioids are selected over inhalational agent.

Muscle relaxant: Vecuronium.

Aortic Regurgitation (AR)

- *Avoid bradycardia and hypertension.* Bradycardia by increasing diastole and hypertension by increasing the afterload can increase the regurgitant fraction.
- As decrease in afterload decreases the regurgitation central neuraxial blocks appears to be a good selection however excessive hypotension should be avoided.

General Anesthesia

Induction: Etomidate

Maintenance: O_2 + N_2O and isoflurane if LV function is normal otherwise opioids.

Muscle relaxant: Vecuronium.

Considerations for Patients on Prosthetic Heart Valves

Prosthetic heart valves may be mechanical (more prone for thromboembolism but have long life of 20–30 years) or bioprosthetic (less prone for thromboembolism but have shorter life of 10–15 years). The two most important considerations for patients on prosthetic heart valves are:

- They are on *oral anticoagulants: As discussed in Chapter 4, page no. 48* stop Warfarin 5 days before and start heparin which is stopped 12–24 hours before surgery.
- They need *antibiotic prophylaxis to prevent infective endocarditis:* There has been drastic change in guidelines for antibiotic prophylaxis for patient with prosthetic heart valve. Contrary to the previous recommendation of antibiotic prophylaxis to all patients undergoing any procedure the new guidelines recommends antibiotics prophylaxis *only for the following conditions*:
  - The dental procedures which involves gingiva, oral mucosa and periapical region of teeth.
  - Invasive procedure that involve incision on infective tissue.

CONGENITAL HEART DISEASES

Left to Right Shunts [Ventricular Septal Defect (VSD), Atrial Septal Defect (ASD) and Patent Ductus Arteriosus (PDA)]

Anesthetic Management

- Increase in systemic vascular resistance (SVR) or decrease in pulmonary vascular resistance (PVR) increases the shunt fraction in left to right shunts, therefore the basic *aim of anesthetic management is to maintain low vascular resistance (hypotension) and high pulmonary vascular resistance.*
- Antibiotic prophylaxis to prevent infective endocarditis is recommended for VSD and PDA however for ASD only if there is concomitant valvular abnormality (mitral valve prolapses may be associated with ASD)

Choice of Anesthesia

As central neuraxial blocks can cause hypotension therefore will be beneficial however excessive hypotension may not be acceptable in already low cardiac output state.

General Anesthesia

Induction: Propofol or thiopentone (causes hypotension). Although increase in pulmonary blood flow causes dilution of IV agents however this has no clinical implication.

Maintenance: O_2 + N_2O and isoflurane (sevoflurane, halothane or desflurane <6% can also be safely used) + positive pressure ventilation (IPPV). Inhalational agents are beneficial by decreasing SVR while nitrous oxide and IPPV are beneficial by increasing the PVR.

Muscle relaxant: Vecuronium.

Right to Left Shunts (Cyanotic Heart Diseases) [Tetralogy of Fallot (TOF), Eisenmenger Syndrome, Transposition of Great Vessels]

Anesthetic Management

- Decrease in systemic vascular resistance (SVR) or increase in pulmonary vascular pulmonary vascular resistance (PVR) increases the shunt fraction therefore the *aim of anesthetic management is to maintain high vascular resistance (hypertension) or decrease pulmonary vascular resistance.*
- Antibiotic prophylaxis to prevent infective endocarditis is must
- As there is compensatory erythrocytosis there are *very high chances of thromboembolism.*
- *Paradoxical embolism* can be disastrous complication therefore avoid even minute volume of air through IV lines.

Choice of Anesthesia

As central neuraxial blocks cause hypotension therefore should be avoided; *GA is the anesthetic technique of choice.*

General Anesthesia

Induction: As *ketamine* increases the systemic vascular resistance it *is agent of choice for induction in right to left shunts.* As pulmonary circulation is bypassed the induction with IV agents will be rapid.

Maintenance: O_2 (50%) + N_2O (50%) + Ketamine infusion (or desflurane >6% if LV function is normal).

Induction with inhalational agents is delayed due to dilutional effect of shunted blood which does not contain inhalational agent. Although nitrous oxide increases the pulmonary vascular resistance but this disadvantage is offset by increase in systemic vascular resistance produced by nitrous oxide due to sympathetic stimulation. As high FiO_2 (delivered oxygen) decreases the PVR therefore the concentration of oxygen used is 50% (not 33%). Positive pressure ventilation and acidosis can increase PVR therefore avoid excessive airway pressure and treat acidosis promptly.

Muscle relaxant: As pancuronium causes hypertension it is the muscle relaxant of choice.

Coarctation of Aorta

Majority of the coarctation are post ductal (distal to subclavian artery). The patient is at risk of ischemia to spine, gut, kidney and lower limbs therefore blood pressure monitoring in lower limbs is must in these patients and ensure that mean arterial pressure of lower limb remains at least >40 mm Hg.

HEART FAILURE

The patient in heart failure carries very high risk of perioperative morbidity and mortality therefore *elective surgery is contraindicated in patient with heart failure.*

The most common cause of right heart failure is left heart failure.

The activation of renin-angiotensin-aldosterone system (RAAS) plays a very important role in pathophysiology of heart failure. Therefore, inhibitors of RAAS, i.e. angiotensin converting enzyme (ACE) inhibitors, angiotensin II receptor blockers (ARB) and aldosterone antagonist remains the primary drugs for the treatment of chronic heart failure.

Anesthetic Management

The basic anesthetic principle of management lies in accordance with the 3 basic principles of management of heart failure, i.e. decrease preload, improve myocardial contractility and decrease afterload.

Medications:
- Digitalis and β-blockers are continued.
- ACE inhibitors and ARB are stopped 1 day before if exclusively used for the treatment of heart failure however if used for coexisting hypertension then they are continued, omitting the morning dose on the day of surgery.
- Diuretics should be withheld on the day of surgery.

As these patients are on diuretics and digitalis *checking preoperative electrolytes (especially potassium) is must.*

Choice of Anesthesia

Central neuraxial blocks are beneficial by decreasing preload (venous return) and afterload (systemic vascular resistance) however excessive hypotension should be avoided.

General Anesthesia

Induction: Etomidate is the induction agent of choice. Ketamine appears to be beneficial by its positive inotropic effect however tachycardia produced by ketamine may negate this effect by decreasing the diastolic filling time.

Maintenance: O_2 + N_2O and *opioids*. Inhalational agents can be used if LV function is not very significantly compromised.

Muscle relaxant: Vecuronium.

Inotropic support with dopamine or dobutamine may be required intraoperatively.

Positive pressure ventilation is beneficial by decreasing the venous return.

CARDIOMYOPATHIES

Hypertrophic Cardiomyopathy

Hypertrophic cardiomyopathy (HCM), also called as subaortic stenosis is the most common genetic cardiovascular disease. Dynamic left ventricular outflow obstruction (LVOT) is the most important feature of HCM. Anything which increases the myocardial contractility (sympathetic stimulation, β agonists) or decreases the left ventricular volume [decrease preload (hypovolemia, venodilatation) or decrease afterload (hypotension, vasodilators)] promotes the left ventricular outflow obstruction.

Anesthetic Management

The most basic principle of management of HCM is to *avoid any factor which increases LVOT.*

Choice of Anesthesia

Central neuraxial blocks (especially spinal) can increase LVOT by decreasing preload and afterload therefore *should be avoided.*

General Anesthesia

Induction: Etomidate is the induction agent of choice. Drug like ketamine which stimulate sympathetic system are contraindicated. Sympathetic stimulation caused by intubation must be blunted.

Maintenance: *Opioids* are preferred however inhalational agents can be used if hypotension can be well controlled. Positive pressure ventilation can increase LVOT by decreasing the venous return therefore low tidal volumes should be used.

Muscle relaxant: Vecuronium is the preferred muscle relaxant. Pancuronium is contraindicated because it can cause sympathetic stimulation.

Pulmonary edema in these patients can not be treated by diuretics (decreases preload), nitrates (decreases afterload) and digitalis (increases myocardial contractility). Therefore is treated by vasopressors (phenylephrine) and β-blockers (Esmolol).

Other Cardiomyopathies

Dilated cardiomyopathy is the most common cardiomyopathy. It may be primary (idiopathic) or secondary like alcoholic or peripartum cardiomyopathy. The anesthetic management principles are exactly same for heart failure.

Considerations in Cardiac Transplant Patients

- They are immunocompromised so strict asepsis should be maintained during procedures.
- Transplant heart is denervated therefore bradycardia will not respond to atropine; it should be treated by direct β agonist like isoproterenol.
- Transplant heart can increase cardiac output by increasing the stroke volume therefore adequate preload (intravascular volume) is must.

PERICARDIAL DISEASES (CONSTRICTIVE PERICARDITIS/CARDIAC TAMPONADE)

Patients with pericardial diseases are in low cardiac output state therefore *central neuraxial blocks (spinal/epidural) are contraindicated.*

Pericardiocentesis should be done under local anesthesia before proceeding to GA.

General Anesthesia

Induction: *Ketamine* by stimulating sympathetic system will increase the cardiac output.

Maintenance: *Opioids.*

Muscle relaxant: *Pancuronium* by stimulating sympathetic system will increase the cardiac output.

CONSIDERATIONS IN PATIENTS ON CARDIAC IMPLANTED ELECTRONIC DEVICES (PACEMAKERS)

Patients with cardiac implanted electronic devices (CIED) are seen more frequently in current day practice. CIED are used for treating:

- Bradyarrhythmias—sick sinus syndrome being the most common indication
- Tachyarrhythmias—Ventricular as well atrial

- *Ventricular dysfunction:* Cardiac resynchronization therapy (CRT) [also called as biventricular pacing] is used if LV ejection fraction is <35% or QRS > 120 ms
- Ventricular assist devices are used for terminal stages of heart failure patients
- Defibrillate or cardiovert in susceptible individuals—The patients susceptible for ventricular tachycardia/fibrillation are fitted with implantable cardioverter—defibrillator (ICD).

Anesthetic Considerations

The electromagnetic interference (EMI) seen during surgery can cause malfunction or even complete failure of device which can produce life threatening complications. *The most common source of EMI is cautery* followed by radiofrequency devices and MRI (MRI is contraindicated for patients with CIED). Hemodynamic alterations or even electrolyte imbalance can cause interference.

To prevent complications related to EMI the following precautions should be taken:

- *CIED should be programmed to asynchronous mode before surgery.* In asynchronous mode pacemakers delivers a fixed rate (70–72 beats/minute) irrespective of the patient's own rate avoiding the risk of CIED to be effected by interference. It can be done by placing a magnet over the CIED however preferably this should be done by company engineer by their special programmed devices.
- *Turn off the permanently implanted cardioverter-defibrillator (ICD) before surgery.* If they are kept on then any interference in ECG (by cautery or improper earthing) may be read as ventricular fibrillation by ICD devices which may deliver shock.
- External defibrillators and pacing devices must be kept ready.
- Always prefer bipolar cautery in these patients.
- *CIED should be reset to their original settings as soon as the surgery is over.*

HYPERTENSION

Hypertension is defined as blood pressure >140/90 on at least 2 occasions 1–2 weeks apart while hypertensive crisis is defined as BP> 180/120.

Anesthetic Management

- All hypertensive patients should be considered to be having ischemic heart disease until proved otherwise.
- Ideally elective surgery should be deferred till the patient becomes normotensive however most often this is not practically feasible and in fact, not desirable also because autoregulation range of BP (particularly cerebral autoregulation) get reset at higher level in hypertensives. Although there is no universal standard cut off limit of BP to delay surgery however a general consensus is to *delay elective surgery if diastolic blood pressure is > 110 mm Hg.*
- *Antihypertensives should be continued except ACE inhibitors and angiotensin II receptor antagonist which are stopped on the day of surgery.* Studies have shown that patient continued on ACE inhibitors and angiotensin II receptor antagonist are more vulnerable to develop profound hypotension in intra-operative period.

Choice of Anesthesia

Uncontrolled hypertensives are more vulnerable for hypotension therefore central neuraxial blocks (especially spinal) should be avoided for uncontrolled hypertensives.

General Anesthesia

Induction: *Etomidate* being most cardiovascular stable *is the ideal agent.* When using propofol and thiopentone one should keep in mind that these patients are more sensitive to hypotensive effects of propofol and thiopentone. Drug like ketamine which stimulate sympathetic system should not be used. Sympathetic stimulation caused by intubation must be blunted.

Maintenance: All inhalational agents can be used safely if hypotension is well controlled. Selection of inhalational agent is based on associated comorbidities in hypertensives like cardiac, renal or cerebral disease.

Muscle relaxant: *Vecuronium.* Pancuronium is contraindicated because it can cause sympathetic stimulation.

HYPOTENSION (ANESTHESIA FOR SHOCK PATIENTS)

Patient must be resuscitated to at least mean arterial pressure > 65 mm Hg or systolic pressure > 90 mm Hg before considering for anesthesia.

Choice of Anesthesia

Central neuraxial blocks are absolutely contraindicated for severely hypovolemic and relatively contraindicated for mild to moderate hypovolemic patient. Other blocks are safe however *CNS and CVS toxicity of local anesthetics is increased in shock due to relatively more perfusion to brain and heart.*

General Anesthesia

The general rule of shock is—whichever drug is used, it should be given in small incremental doses.

Induction: *ketamine is the induction agent of choice for shock* however in chronic/severe shock due to sympathetic depletion its direct myocardial depressant effect may predominate. Due to contracted intravascular volume the effects of IV agents are exaggerated.

Maintenance: O_2 + N_2O + *Desflurane* > 6%. Desflurane > 6% stimulates sympathetic system. As there occurs concomitant rise in ventilation as compensation to metabolic acidosis, the rate of rise of alveolar concentration of inhalational agents becomes rapid.

Muscle relaxants: *Pancuronium* stimulates sympathetic system therefore is the muscle relaxant preferred for shock patients.

KEY POINTS

- Effort tolerance > 4 METS is generally associated with lesser complications.
- Beta blockers should not be started afresh in a patient who is not on beta blockers unless they can be started at least 1 week before surgery.

Contd...

Contd...

- Aspirin should be continued while Clopidogrel should be stopped 5 days before surgery.
- If a patient had myocardial infarction/ischemia then elective surgery must be deferred for 6 weeks if the patient was treated without stenting, for 6 weeks if bare metal stent was used, for 6 months if new generation drug eluting stent was used, for 1 year if conventional drug eluting stent was used and for 6 weeks if treated with coronary artery pass graft (CABG).
- If a patient with drug eluted stent has to undergo emergency surgery then continuing antiplatelet therapy is always preferred.
- Transesophageal echocardiography(TEE) is the earliest and most sensitive monitor to detect intra-operative infarction.
- The most important goal of anesthetic management for patients of ischemic heart disease is to avoid a imbalance between myocardial oxygen demand and supply.
- Etomidate is the induction agent of choice for cardiac patients.
- Cardiac patients with normal left ventricular function can safely receive inhalational agents however if left ventricular function is compromised then anaesthesia should preferably be maintained with opioids.
- Vecuronium is the muscle relaxant of choice for cardiac patients.
- Central neuraxial blocks (CNB) should be avoided for fixed cardiac output lesions like mitral or aortic stenosis.
- CPR may be ineffective in patients with severe aortic stenosis.
- Contrary to the previous recommendation of antibiotic prophylaxis to all patients of prosthetic heart valves undergoing any procedure the new guidelines recommends antibiotics prophylaxis only for dental procedures which involves gingiva, oral mucosa and periapical region of teeth and invasive procedure that involve incision on infective tissue.
- The basic aim of anesthetic management of patients with Left to Right Shunts is to maintain low vascular resistance (hypotension) and maintain high pulmonary vascular resistance while for Right to Left Shunts is to maintain high vascular resistance (hypertension) or decrease pulmonary vascular resistance.
- As ketamine increases the systemic vascular resistance it is agent of choice for induction in right to left shunts.
- Elective surgery is contraindicated in patient with heart failure.
- Cardiac implanted electronic devices (CIED) should be programmed to asynchronous mode before surgery and reset to their original settings as soon as the surgery is over.
- Permanently implanted cardioverter-defibrillator (ICD) must be turned off before surgery.
- Although there is no universal standard cut off limit of BP to delay surgery however a general consensus is to delay elective surgery if diastolic blood pressure is > 110 mm Hg.
- All Antihypertensives should be continued except ACE inhibitors and angiotensin II receptor antagonist which are stopped on the day of surgery.
- Patient in shock must be resuscitated to at least mean arterial pressure > 65 mm Hg or systolic pressure > 90 mm Hg before considering for anesthesia.
- Central neuraxial blocks are absolutely contraindicated for severely hypovolemic and relatively contraindicated for mild to moderate hypovolemic patient.
- Ketamine is the induction agent of choice for shock.

CHAPTER 19

Anesthesia for Respiratory Diseases

Pulmonary diseases are broadly classified as obstructive (asthma and COPD) or restrictive.

GENERAL CONSIDERATIONS IN MANAGEMENT OF PATIENT WITH PULMONARY DISEASE

Preoperative Considerations

- One of the very important parts of preoperative evaluation is to determine the *major risk factors* which predispose the patient to post-operative pulmonary complications. The following factors have been cited as the major risk factors:
  - Age > 60 years
  - Severity of pulmonary disease (Dyspnea at minimal activity)
  - ASA grade > 2
  - Congestive heart failure
  - Heavy smoker
  - Surgery under general anesthesia
  - Surgical factors like site of surgery (thoracic and upper abdominal), nature (major) and duration (> 3 hours)
  - Serum albumin < 3.5 g/dL

  Dyspnea at minimal activity and site of surgery are the two most important predictors of postoperative complications.
- Always rule out associated cor pulmonale in patients with pulmonary disease.
- Ideally smoking should be stopped *8 weeks before surgery* however stopping smoking 12 hours before may be beneficial by reducing carboxyhemoglobin levels.
- Although pulmonary function test (PFT) do determine the severity of disease but are not always predictors of complications therefore *routine use of PFT is not recommended.*

- Patients with pulmonary diseases should be given chest physiotherapy, antibiotics, bronchodilators and steroids in preoperative period to improve their respiratory status.
- Patients who are on steroids at present or have taken steroid earlier should receive supplemental steroid (*for details see Chapter 4, page no. 49*).
- Any infection must be treated before taking the patient for surgery.
- *Bronchodilators should be continued* as instructed; however, there is no role of prophylactic nebulization in asymptomatic patient. The patient should bring his/her inhalers with him/her in operation theater (OT).
- *Premedication*: Premedication with benzodiazepines should be avoided as these patients are more sensitive to respiratory depression. Theoretically premedication with anticholinergic is beneficial by causing bronchodilatation, however, clinical advantage has not been seen. Premedication with H_2 blockers (Ranitidine) should be avoided because H_2 blockade leads to unopposed H_1 activation and bronchospasm.

Intraoperative Considerations

Hypoxia, hypercarbia, acidosis and sepsis are not acceptable.

Choice of Anesthesia

- *Regional anesthesia is always preferred over general anesthesia.* Central neuraxial blocks are excellent choice if the level of block required is below T6. Level above T6 can cause paralysis of abdominal muscles causing significant distress (particularly in COPD patients) because these patients have active expiration dependent on abdominal muscles.

- If general anesthesia is to be given following should be given due consideration:
    - Gases must be humidified. Dry gases can inhibit ciliary function causing atelectasis in postoperative period. Moreover, all inhalational agents (except ether) also inhibit ciliary activity.
    - General anesthesia increases the dead space and V/Q mismatch (*for details see Chapter 1, page no. 7*).
    - Ventilatory responses to hypoxia and hypercarbia are blunted by inhalational agents, barbiturates and opioids and this can be deleterious in a patient on spontaneous ventilation.
    - Ventilation principle includes *low tidal volume* (6–8 mL/kg) to avoid barotrauma, *low I: E ratio* and *slow respiratory rate* of (6–10 breaths/min.) to allow adequate exhalation and prevent air trapping.

Postoperative Considerations

Pulmonary patients are prone to develop atelectasis and hypoxia in postoperative period. Not only they require respiratory monitoring and supplemental oxygen but lung expansion measures (incentive spirometry, chest physiotherapy, deep breathing exercises) should also be instituted as early as possible. Ideally the improvement in pulmonary functions should be guided by functional residual capacity (FRC).

Pain can significantly compromise the pulmonary functions especially in thoracic and upper abdominal surgeries therefore *pain management is most vital for thoracic and upper abdominal surgeries in respiratory compromised patients. Thoracic epidural is the most preferred, most safe, most effective and most commonly used approach to achieve analgesia for thoracic and upper abdominal surgeries.* Other techniques which can be used are intercostal block, local infiltration (2 levels above and below the thoracotomy incision site), intrapleural analgesia and cryoanalgesia with special probes which freezes intercostal nerves. Cryoanalgesia, although produces effective pain relief, however, not used commonly due to delayed onset, nonavailability of probes and very long lasting effect (nerve recovery may even take 1–6 months). *Parenteral*

opioids can causes respiratory depression therefore should be avoided as far as possible.

ASTHMA

To consider for elective surgery the patient must not have active asthma (no wheeze or rhonchi) and ideally should have 80% of predicted value of peak expiratory flow rate.

Anesthetic Management

Choice of Anesthesia

As discussed *regional anesthesia is preferred* over general anesthesia. Avoid central neuraxial block if the level of block required is above T6. The other concern of spinal that sympathetic block leads to parasympathetic stimulation and consequent bronchospasm has not been found to be clinically relevant.

General Anesthesia

Induction

- Ketamine in spite of its best bronchodilator property is generally avoided due to its side effect (especially vivid reactions) and propensity to increase tracheobronchial secretions. The use of ketamine in present day practice is restricted to *patients in active asthma (wheezing) undergoing life threatening emergency surgeries.* Ketamine in patient taking theophylline can precipitate seizures.
- *Propofol* is a reasonable bronchodilator devoid of side effects seen with ketamine therefore, is *more preferred for asthma patients in present day anesthesia practice.*
- Thiopentone can induce bronchoconstriction therefore, should be avoided.

The most important consideration is to prevent reflex stimulation of airways by laryngoscopy and intubation.

Maintenance: *Sevoflurane is the inhalational agent of choice for asthma patients.* Halothane, in spite of producing little more bronchodilatation than sevoflurane in asthma patients is not preferred because of the increase possibility of arrhythmias. As desflurane and isoflurane have irritating effects on airways therefore should be avoided.

Muscle relaxant: Steroidal class of muscle relaxant is preferred. Benzylisoquinolines by release histamine can precipitate bronchospasm.

To avoid immediate postoperative broncho-spasm extubation should be done when patient is deep (deep extubation).

Management of Intraoperative Bronchospasm

Diagnosis

Intraoperative bronchospasm is diagnosed by
- Wheezing
- Increase in peak airway pressure
- Decrease exhaled tidal volume
- Prolonged phase II (slowly rising CO_2) on capnography
- Decrease oxygen saturation in extreme cases.

Treatment

Step 1: Before starting therapy for asthma it is must to rule out other causes of increased airway pressure/bronchospasm like obstruction of endotracheal tube by secretions or kinking, inadequate depth of anesthesia, pulmonary edema, aspiration or embolus, pneumothorax.

Step 2: Once it is confirmed that bronchospasm is due to asthmatic attack it should *first be treated by increasing the depth of anesthesia with inhalational agent (preferably sevoflurane).*

Step 3: If not relieved by increasing the depth, inhaled β_2 agonist (with or without inhaled steroid) therapy should be instituted immediately.

Step 4: Still not relieved by inhaled β_2 agonist consider giving IV steroids, however, it should be kept in mind that the effect of steroids can take few hours.

Step 5: For refractory bronchospasm not responding to above said measures consider epinephrine, ketamine or aminophyline infusion.

CHRONIC OBSTRUCTIVE PULMONARY DISEASE (CHRONIC BRONCHITIS AND EMPHYSEMA)

Chronic obstructive pulmonary disease (COPD) is the most common pulmonary disease encountered in clinical practice.

The anesthetic management of COPD patients is similar to asthma patient with additional emphasis on the following points:
- Cor pulmonale must be ruled out and if there is any evidence of pulmonary hypertension then nitrous oxide should be avoided.

- Patients must be stabilized by stopping smoking, treating infection, correcting spasm (asthmatic bronchitis), improve pulmonary condition by physiotherapy before taking for elective surgery.
- *Nitrous oxide should not be used in emphysema.* It can cause expansion of bullae leading to rupture and pneumothorax.
- Ventilation principle of low tidal volumes and slow respiratory rate must be adhered.

RESTRICTIVE LUNG DISEASES

- These patients have low FRC therefore are more prone for hypoxemia during induction.
- As these patients are very vulnerable to barotrauma *avoiding large tidal volumes and inspiratory pressures* is the most important principle of ventilatory management during general anesthesia (GA).

TUBERCULOSIS

- *Elective surgery should be deferred in a patient of active (open) pulmonary tuberculosis.*
- Pulmonary damage caused by tuberculosis should be assessed in preoperative period.
- Antitubercular drugs should be continued however, assessment of liver functions is must.
- Emergency surgery of an active case should be performed in separate theater dedicated for infected cases. Equipment coming in direct contact with patient like mask, laryngeal mask airway (LMA), breathing circuits should be discarded after case while other equipment and theater should be sterilized properly.

RESPIRATORY TRACT INFECTION

Elective surgery is contraindicated in patients with lower respiratory tract infection (lung infections). The decision to go ahead with elective surgery in patient with upper respiratory tract infection (URTI) depends on the severity of the disease.

Patients with minimal URTI (viral infections), i.e. only running nose, occasional cough without expectoration and afebrile can go ahead with elective surgery however if the patient has significant URTI, i.e. significant cough or cough with expectoration, fever, signs of lower respiratory tract infection like crepitations, signs of upper airway obstruction like stridor then *elective surgery should ideally be deferred for 6 weeks.*

As airway remains hyperactive for 5–6 weeks after a significant URTI, deferring surgery for less than 6 weeks does not solve the purpose, therefore if surgery has to postponed then it should be deferred for 6 weeks otherwise take the patient with calculated risks; the incidence of respiratory complications in acute phase and recovery phase remains same.

Patients undergoing surgery with active URTI are prone to develop complications like laryngospasm (5 times), bronchospasm (10 times), hypoxia, increased bleeding from airways, post-intubation croup, lower respiratory tract infection (infection may spread to lower respiratory tract by intubation leading to pneumonitis, atelectasis or even septicemia).

To avoid these complications the following approach should be used in patients with active URTI undergoing surgery:

- *Anesthesia of choice is regional.*
- If GA is to be given then *prefer to get the surgery done under laryngeal mask airway* (LMA). *Avoid intubation* as far as possible, however, if intubation is necessary then *reflex stimulation of airways by laryngoscopy and intubation should be prevented.*
- Use of anticholinergic is strongly recommended.
- Humidification of gases is must.
- Be ready for cricothyroidotomy and/or tracheostomy should there occur significant upper airway obstruction.
- Keep the patients for longer periods in postoperative room for respiratory monitoring.

OPERATIVE CRITERIA FOR THORACOTOMY/PNEUMONECTOMY

The pulmonary pathology to the following extent usually requires surgical correction by thoracotomy/pneumonectomy.

- FEV1 < 2 liters
- FEV1/FVC ratio < 50% of predicted
- Maximum breathing capacity <50% of predicted
- PCO_2 > 45 and PO_2 < 50 mm Hg at room air
- Oxygen consumption < 10 mL/kg/min.

KEY POINTS

- Dyspnea at minimal activity and site of surgery are the two most important predictors of postoperative complications.
- Always rule out associated cor pulmonale in patients with pulmonary disease.
- Ideally smoking should be stopped 8 weeks before surgery however stopping smoking 12 hours before may be beneficial by reducing carboxyhemoglobin levels.
- The routine use of pulmonary function tests is not recommended.
- Regional anesthesia is always preferred over general anesthesia for respiratory compromised patients.
- Ventilation principle for COPD/asthma patients includes low tidal volume (6–8 mL/kg), low I: E ratio and slow respiratory rate of (6–10 breaths/min.) to allow adequate exhalation and prevent air trapping.
- Thoracic epidural is the most preferred approach to achieve analgesia for thoracic and upper abdominal surgeries while parenteral opioids should be avoided as much as possible.
- Ketamine in spite of its best bronchodilator property is generally avoided for asthma patients; its use is restricted to patients in active asthma (wheezing) undergoing life-threatening emergency surgeries.
- Propofol is preferred over ketamine for asthma patients in present day anesthesia practice.
- Thiopentone can induce bronchoconstriction therefore, should be avoided.
- Sevoflurane is the inhalational agent of choice for asthma patients.
- Intraoperative bronchospasm should first be treated by increasing the depth of anesthesia with inhalational agent (preferably sevoflurane).
- Nitrous oxide should not be used in emphysema.
- Elective surgery should be deferred in a patient of active (open) pulmonary tuberculosis.
- Elective surgery is contraindicated in patients with lower respiratory tract infection (lung infections). The decision to go ahead with elective surgery in patient with upper respiratory tract infection (URTI) depends on the severity of the disease.
- If surgery has to be deferred in a patient of URTI then it should ideally be deferred for 6 weeks.
- For patient of URTI general anesthesia (GA) with laryngeal mask airway (LMA) is always preferred over GA with intubation.

CHAPTER 20

Anesthesia for Central Nervous System Diseases

PARKINSON'S DISEASE

Parkinson occurs due to progressive loss of dopamine deficiency in brain.

- *All medications for Parkinson's disease (PD) including levodopa should be continued.* Discontinuing levodopa increases the chances of muscular rigidity in perioperative period.
- *Dopamine antagonists like droperidol and metoclopramide should not be used.*
- The PD patients are *prone for arrhythmias* [due to increased levels of dopamine in body (levodopa gets converted to dopamine)] and *hypotension* (due to depletion of catecholamines by chronically elevated dopamine levels). These patients are volume depleted (dopaminergic effect on kidneys) therefore, adequate fluid replacement is must.
- Anesthetic drugs which increase the muscle tone (ketamine, alfentanil) should be avoided.

ALZHEIMER'S DISEASE

The major concern of these patients is that they are geriatric, dementic, non-cooperative and more prone to develop postoperative psychosis. *The rising concern that general anesthesia worsens the dementia is not yet fully substantiated by studies.*

EPILEPSY

- As anticonvulsants affect the organ systems (especially liver function), evaluation of organ function is must in preoperative assessment.
- *All antiepileptic should be continued.*
- Anesthetic drugs with epileptogenic potential [Methohexitone, ketamine (due to its preservative), propofol (rare opisthotonous), etomidate (myoclonic activity), enflurane,

sevoflurane and atracurium (Laudonosine)] should not be used.
- Spinal/epidural can be given safely if there are no signs and symptoms of raised intracranial tension (ICT).
- Due to the anticonvulsant property *thiopentone in the induction agent of choice for epileptics.*
- Phenytoin and carbamazepine can potentiate the effect of non-depolarizing muscle relaxants.

STROKE

- *After cerebrovascular accident elective surgery should be deferred for 9 months.* The possibility of serious complications like another stroke, heart attack or even death is 14 times higher if elective surgery is performed within three months and 5 times higher if surgery is performed within 6 months after stroke. The odds are stabilized at 3 times after 9 months.
- Due to extrajunctional receptors suxamethonium is contraindicated for stroke patients.
- Patients with history of transient ischemic attacks must have at least carotid Doppler before considering for anesthesia.

HEADACHE

- Patients of chronic headache should be fully investigated to rule out any intracranial lesion and signs of raised ICT.
- As analgesics affect the organ systems (especially renal function) evaluation of organ function is must in preoperative assessment.
- These patients are prone to develop post-spinal headache therefore, spinal should be avoided.

MULTIPLE SCLEROSIS

Multiple sclerosis (MS) is an autoimmune disease characterized by demyelination of neurons.

- As immunosuppressant drugs affect the organ systems (especially hematologic) evaluation of organ function is must in preoperative assessment.
- Elective surgery should be avoided during the relapse of the disease.
- Patients with advanced disease having autonomic involvement are very liable for hypotension and bradycardia.

Choice of anesthesia: *Spinal anesthesia (but not epidural) and stress can precipitate multiple sclerosis*; spinal precipitates multiple sclerosis probably because of direct exposure of local anesthetic to sheath less spinal cord. As peripheral nerves are not involved in MS, peripheral blocks can be given safely.

General anesthesia:

- As stress can precipitate MS, blunting stress response to intubation and maintaining good depth of anesthesia is must.
- If there is spastic paresis/paralysis *suxamethonium becomes contraindicated.*
- Hyperthermia is one of a very important risk factor to precipitate MS therefore, must be avoided at any cost.

SYRINGOMYELIA

As there is lower motor neuron (LMN) paralysis suxamethonium must not be used and exaggerated response to non-depolarizer is expected. Neurological deficits and possibility of raised ICT warrants the avoidance of central neuraxial blocks however, associated scoliosis can cause ventilation perfusion mismatch during general anesthesia (GA).

AMYOTROPHIC LATERAL SCLEROSIS

It is a progressive disease involving upper and lower motor neurons therefore, succinylcholine is contraindicated. Central neuraxial can exacerbate the disease.

GUILLAIN-BARRÉ SYNDROME (GBS)

Central neuraxial blocks can worsen the already diseased nerve (double crush syndrome) therefore should be avoided. As there is lower motor neuron (LMN) paralysis suxamethonium must not be used.

AUTONOMIC DYSFUNCTION

The patients with autonomic dysfunction are very vulnerable for *severe hypotension*. Hypotension must be treated by directly acting vasopressors (phenylephrine), not by indirectly acting (ephedrine) vasopressors which act by releasing catecholamines.

SPINAL CORD TRANSECTION

Acute Transection

During first 1–3 weeks patients are in spinal shock due to sympathetic cut off therefore, are very vulnerable for hypotension and bradycardia.

Chronic Transection

Transection above T6 can precipitate autonomic hyper-reflexia manifested by severe hypertension and reflex bradycardia. Although these patients have no sensations below transection however, need anesthesia because surgery is a potent stimulus for developing *autonomic hyper-reflexia. Regional anesthesia and deep GA can prevent autonomic hyper-reflexia.* Due to extrajunctional receptors succinylcholine is contraindicated.

PSYCHIATRIC DISORDERS

Depression

- *All antidepressants including monoamine oxidase (MAO) inhibitors* (contrary to previous recommendation of stopping MAO inhibitors 2–3 weeks prior) *should be continued.*
- Antidepressants increase the level of brain neurotransmitters *increasing the anesthetic requirement.*
- Acute intake of tricyclic antidepressants (up to 3 weeks) by increasing the epinephrine and norepinephrine increases the chances of arrhythmias (particularly with halothane) and hypertensive crisis. Therefore drugs like pancuronium, ketamine and local anesthetics with adrenaline should not be used. However, chronic use causes catecholamine depletion increasing the risk of hypotension. *Patients on MAO inhibitors must not receive pethidine.*

Anesthesia for Electroconvulsive Therapy (ECT): *Methohexital*, being epileptogenic, is the induction agent of choice. If succinylcholine is used to prevent muscle contraction, tourniquet should be applied in one hand before giving succinylcholine to see the seizure activity.

Mania

- Patients are on lithium which can produce diabetes insipidus and electrolyte imbalance.
- Although lithium do enhances the block produced by muscle relaxants but this effect seems to be clinically insignificant therefore, in contrary to older guidelines of stopping lithium 48 before surgery current recommendation is to *continue lithium*. The other drug approved for bipolar disorder, i.e. Lamotrigine has to be continued.

Schizophrenia

- All antipsychotic drugs should be continued.
- Antipsychotic drugs by producing sedation decrease the anesthetic requirement. The patients on antipsychotic medications are more vulnerable for hypotension (α blocking property), arrhythmias (QTc prolongation and torsade de pointes).
- As these patients may not cooperate for regional blocks, general anesthesia is preferred.
- Ketamine is contraindicated because these patients can become very violent after ketamine in postoperative period.

Drug Abuse

- The drug abusers must have psychiatric consultation in preoperative period.
- *Patients must not be taken for elective surgeries in acute withdrawal.*
- *Acute intake decreases while chronic intake increases the anesthetic requirement.*
- Patients on cocaine are at high risk of arrhythmias and myocardial ischemia.
- These patients especially alcoholics must be evaluated for associated medical diseases like dilated cardiomyopathy, cirrhosis, pancreatitis, metabolic disorders (hypoglycemia), nutritional disorders (Wernicke-Korsakoff syndrome).

KEY POINTS

- Levodopa should not be stopped before surgery.
- Dopamine antagonists like droperidol and metoclopramide should not be used in patients with Parkinson's disease.
- The rising concern that general anesthesia worsens the dementia is not yet fully substantiated by studies.
- All antiepileptic should be continued.
- Thiopentone is the induction agent of choice for epileptics.
- After cerebrovascular accident elective surgery should be deferred for 9 months.
- Spinal anesthesia (but not epidural) and stress can precipitate multiple sclerosis; peripheral blocks can be given safely.
- Regional anesthesia and deep GA can prevent autonomic hyper-reflexia.
- All antidepressants including monoamine oxidase (MAO) inhibitors should be continued.
- Methohexital is the induction agent of choice for electroconvulsive therapy.
- Current recommendation is to continue lithium.
- Patients must not be taken for elective surgeries in acute drug withdrawal.
- Acute drug intake decreases while chronic intake increases the anesthetic requirement.

CHAPTER 21

Anesthesia for Hepatic Diseases

PREOPERATIVE EVALUATION

- Hepatic dysfunction can vary from mild impairment of hepatic functions to fulminant hepatic failure. *Child-Pugh classification is the gold standard scoring system to assess the severity of hepatic disease and hence the risk assessment* **(Table 21.1)**.
- The aim of preoperative evaluation is to not only to assess the severity of disease but also to assess the damage caused to other organs by hepatic dysfunction. Therefore, it is very important to rule out coagulopathy, renal damage (hepatorenal syndrome), pulmonary dysfunction (hepatopulmonary syndrome), portopulmonary hypertension, encephalopathy, ascites, gastroesophageal varices, cardiac functions, electrolyte and metabolic abnormalities.

- Always screen the hepatic patients for hepatitis B and C.
- Always rule out alcoholism and associated comorbidities in hepatic patient.

Timing of Surgery

There is no need to defer the surgery in asymptomatic patients with mild impairment of hepatic functions (mildly elevated liver enzymes). However, *elective surgery should be deferred in acute liver disease till the liver functions are stabilized*. Patients with moderate to severe chronic hepatic diseases should at least have *restoration of coagulation abnormalities* (by vitamin K, cryoprecipitate or fresh frozen plasma), correction of volume, electrolytes and metabolic disorder (especially *hypoglycemia*), correction of anemia, tapping of ascites (if significant enough to impair respiratory functions) and correction of encephalopathy (by lactulose and neomycin) before taking them for surgery.

Premedication

As hepatic patients may be oversensitive to the sedative effects of benzodiazepine premedication with benzodiazepines should not be given to these patients.

INTRAOPERATIVE

Universal precautions must be taken if the patient is positive for hepatitis B or C.

Monitoring: As there is fluid loss to 3rd space, the intravascular volume is depleted in these patients therefore, central venous pressure monitoring is highly recommended.

■ **Table 21.1:** Child-Pugh classification

	Group		
	A	B	C
S. bilirubin (mg %)	< 2	2–3	> 3
S. albumin (gm %)	> 3.5	3–3.5	< 3
Prothrombin time (Prolongation from control in seconds)	1–4	4–6	> 6
Ascites	None	Moderate	Marked
Encephalopathy	None	Moderate	Severe
Nutrition	Excellent	Good	Poor
Surgical risk	Minimal	Moderate	Marked
Mortality	2–5%	10%	> 50%

Choice of Anesthesia

Due to the possibility of existing coagulopathy and intravascular volume depletion *central neuraxial blocks should be avoided*. However, if there is no associated coagulopathy central neuraxial block can be considered if hypotension can be prevented.

General Anesthesia

Due to high volume of distribution the initial dose of intravenous agents is more while due to decreased metabolism the action of repeated/maintenance doses may be prolonged. Decreased albumin may increase the unbound fraction of the drug.

Induction: *Propofol,* due to its short half-life and extrahepatic metabolism is the induction agent of choice.

Maintenance: *Sevoflurane is the inhalational agent of choice* due to two reasons:
1. Maximum perseverance of hepatic blood flow. Maintaining hepatic blood flow should be the most important goal in these patients.
2. As sevoflurane does not produce Trifluoro-acetic acid on metabolism thereby avoiding any possibility of hepatitis.
   Desflurane because of its least metabolism and isoflurane because of perseverance of hepatic blood flow are good alternatives to sevoflurane. The amount of trifluoroacetic acid produced by desflurane and isoflurane is too minimal that hepatotoxicity appears to be just theoretical.
   Halothane must not be used due to two reasons—firstly, it may cause hepatitis and secondly it causes significant decrease in hepatic as well as portal blood flow.
   Nitrous oxide should be avoided for two reasons—firstly, it can increase the pulmonary artery pressure which may be already elevated in these patients (portopulmonary hypertension) and secondly it allows the anesthetist to use higher concentration of oxygen which is required due to significant right to left shunt (hepatopulmonary syndrome).

Muscle relaxants: *Succinylcholine can produce prolonged block due to decreased pseudocholine-sterase.* As *atracurium and Cis-atracurium are*

metabolized by Hoffman degradation they are the muscle relaxants of choice for hepatic patients.
- *Remifentanil* is the opioid of choice because it is metabolized by plasma esterases.
- As there is decreased metabolism of citrate (which can chelate calcium) these patients should receive calcium after blood transfusion.

Not Acceptable Intraoperatively

- *Hypotension*: Hypotension can severely impair hepatic blood flow. *Albumin is the preferred colloid.*
- *Alkalosis*: Alkalosis increases the conversion of ammonium to ammonia which crosses blood brain barrier to precipitate hepatic encephalopathy.
- *Hypoglycemia:* Hepatic disease patients have impaired gluconeogenesis and exhausted glucose stores therefore, they are prone for hypoglycemia.
- *Sepsis:* Sepsis can precipitate encephalopathy.
- *Decreased urinary output*: Can precipitate hepatorenal syndrome.

Postoperatively

- Renal functions and urine output should be monitored.
- Good antibiotic cover.
- *Oxygenation:* Cirrhotic patients have intra-pulmonary shunt therefore, are more prone for hypoxia.

ANESTHESIA FOR PATIENTS WITH BILIARY OBSTRUCTION

Whatever discussed above for the management of patients with hepatic disease, the same is applicable for patients with biliary obstruction with additional points to be taken care:
- These patients exhibit *bradycardia* because of direct effect of bile salts on Sinoatrial (SA) node.
- Just after the release of obstruction mannitol should be given to wash out the bile salts.
- Muscle relaxant, *vecuronium* which has 30–40% excretion through bile should not be used.
- Opioids cause constrictions of sphincter of Oddi increasing biliary duct pressure however, the studies have shown that incidence of

opioid-induced spasm of sphincter of Oddi is less than 3% therefore, strict guidelines of not using opioids for biliary colic has been questioned in current day practice.

KEY POINTS

- Child-Pugh classification is the gold standard scoring system to assess the severity of hepatic disease and hence the risk assessment.
- Elective surgery should be deferred in acute liver disease till the liver functions are stabilized.
- Due to the possibility of existing coagulopathy and intravascular volume depletion, central neuraxial blocks should be avoided in hepatic patients.
- Propofol, due to its short half-life and extrahepatic metabolism is the induction agent of choice for hepatic patients.
- Sevoflurane is the inhalational agent of choice for hepatic patients while halothane and nitrous oxide should be avoided.
- Atracurium and Cis-atracurium are the muscle relaxants of choice for hepatic patients.
- Albumin is the preferred colloid for a patient with compromised hepatic functions.
- As vecuronium has 30–40% excretion through bile, it should be avoided for patients with biliary obstruction.

CHAPTER 22

Anesthesia for Renal Diseases and Electrolyte Imbalances

ANESTHETIC MANAGEMENT OF PATIENTS WITH RENAL DYSFUNCTION

Preoperative Evaluation

The aim of preoperative evaluation is not only to assess the extent of renal impairment but also the damage caused to other organs by renal impairment and rule out associated comorbidities. The common manifestation/associated comorbidities seen in renal impairment which can increase the perioperative morbidity and mortality are:

- *Anemia*: The anemia is due to decrease erythropoietin or decrease intake due to anorexia seen in uremia.
- *Coagulopathies*: Uremic patients exhibit bleeding tendencies.
- Electrolyte and acid base abnormalities like *hyperkalemia*, hypocalcemia, hypermagnesemia and metabolic acidosis.
- *Endocrinal abnormalities*: Diabetes is the most common cause of chronic kidney disease.
- *Hypertension*: More than 80% patients with chronic renal disease exhibit hypertension.
- Cardiopulmonary abnormalities like pericardial or pleural effusion.
- *Associated liver disease*: Liver diseases are commonly associated with renal disease.
- Central nervous system (CNS) abnormalities like uremic encephalopathy, uremic polyneuropathy.

Timing and Preparation before Surgery

Patients with acute kidney injury (AKI) should not undergo elective surgery until the injury is fully resolved. Patients with chronic kidney diseases (CKDs) should at least have correction of electrolyte abnormalities (especially hyperkalemia), acidosis, coagulopathies, severe anemia, control of blood pressure (target should be < 130/80 mm Hg) and sugar and reversal of encephalopathy. Very often the patients of CKD are on dialysis. *Dialysis should be performed within 24 hours before surgery.*

Premedication

Premedication with benzodiazepines should be avoided as CNS of these patients is extremely sensitive to effect of sedatives and narcotics.

Intraoperative

Monitoring

- *Maintaining fluid balance is essential* in these patients; excess fluid can precipitate pulmonary edema and fluid deficiency can worsen kidney injury therefore, fluid should be given either by Goal directed therapy (stroke volume variation or pulse pressure variation) or at least by central venous pressure (CVP) if goal directed therapy is not possible.
- *Urine output:* Aim should be to maintain urine output > 0.5 mL/kg/hr. Urine output should be maintained by giving adequate fluids. The traditional use of dopamine in renal doses to maintain urine output is not recommended in current practice. If required (like for very major surgeries in renal patients) then fenoldopam (selective dopamine-1 agonist) is chosen over dopamine.
- If invasive blood pressure monitoring is required then *radial and ulnar artery should be spared as they may be required for hemodialysis*

in future. Dorsalis pedis is most often chosen in these patients.
- BP cuff should not be applied in the limb having AV fistula.

Choice of Anesthesia

Central neuraxial blocks should be avoided due to associated uremic coagulopathy, uremic polyneuropathy and intolerance of renal patients to extra fluids to treat hypotension. Peripheral nerve blocks should also be avoided if there is coagulopathy or neuropathy.

General Anesthesia

Induction: Due to shorter half-life and all inactive metabolites, *propofol is the induction agent of choice* however it may be required in small doses because of exaggerated response of CNS due to disrupted blood brain barrier in uremia.

Maintenance: *Desflurane is the inhalational agent of choice because it does not produce fluoride.* In case of non-availability of desflurane, isoflurane and halothane can be used safely. *Sevoflurane should be not be used in renal patients* as it produces high levels of fluoride approaching renal threshold of 50 µmol/L.

As these patients are anemic oxygen is required in high concentrations. Ensure normocapnia as respiratory acidosis can cause hyperkalemia and alkalosis can shift oxygen dissociation curve to left.

Muscle relaxants: As these patients exhibit hyperkalemia, *succinylcholine should not be used.*

Due to Hoffman degradation non-depolarizing muscle relaxant of choice are *Atracurium and Cis-atracurium.*

Opioids: *Remifentanil is the opioid of choice* because it is rapidly metabolized in plasma by esterases. Short acting like fentanyl, alfentanil and sufentanil can also be used safely while long acting like morphine and pethidine are not recommended.

Selection of Fluids

- The traditional concept of avoiding ringer lactate (as it contains potassium) and preferring normal saline (as it does not contain potassium) is no more valid in current day practice because recent studies have shown that normal saline by causing hyperchloremic metabolic acidosis produces more hyperkalemia. Therefore, *ringer lactate is preferred over normal saline however with close monitoring of potassium levels.* If ringer lactate cannot be used then 0.45% saline or 0.18% saline with dextrose is preferred over normal saline (0.9%).
- *Colloids (hydroxyethyl starch) have been found to exacerbate renal injury.* If it is mandatory to use a colloid then Gelatins (Gelofusine) is preferred. High molecular weight colloids (>MW 200 kDa) must not be used for renal patients.

Postoperative

Maintain fluid balance and urine output and avoid non-steroidal anti-inflammatory drugs (NSAIDs) for pain management.

ANESTHESIA FOR TRANSURETHRAL RESECTION OF PROSTATE

Spinal anesthesia is preferred over general anesthesia due to the following reasons:
- Old patients have decreased pulmonary reserve.
- Awake patient can tell central signs of transurethral resection of prostate (TURP) *syndrome* and bladder perforation.

TURP Syndrome

A large amount of irrigating fluid (most commonly-glycine) is used to distend the bladder and wash away blood and prostatic tissue. This fluid enters the systemic circulation through open prostatic sinuses and can produce *fluid overloading, dilutional hyponatremia and hypo-osmolality.* It is estimated that 10–30 mL of fluid is absorbed every minute. Glycine can also produce hyperglycinemia and hyperammonemia.

Signs and Symptoms

Hypo-osmolality (and hyponatremia) by producing cerebral edema produces restlessness, confusion or even seizures. Hyperglycinemia can produce visual disturbances including transient blindness. Fluid overload can cause hypertension and pulmonary edema.

Treatment

- Furosemide to treat fluid overload
- Hypertonic saline may be required to treat symptomatic hyponatremia and hypo-osmolality.

ANESTHESIA FOR PATIENTS WITH ELECTROLYTE IMBALANCES

In preoperative period, it is important to find the cause of electrolyte disturbances.

Hyperkalemia

Hyperkalemia must be corrected (serum potassium should be < 5.5 mEq/L) before taking the patient for surgery.

Anesthetic Considerations

- Potassium rich fluids should be avoided.
- As these patients are prone for cardiac arrhythmias, vigilant electrocardiographic (ECG) monitoring is must.
- *Succinylcholine is contraindicated.* Requirement of non-depolarizing muscle relaxants decreases due to muscle weakness.
- Mild hyperventilation is beneficial during general anesthesia because hyperventilation by causing alkalosis pushes the potassium intracellularly.

Hypokalemia

Correction of hypokalemia before surgery is one of the most debatable topic. The general consensus is not to treat mild (serum potassium >3 mEq/L) chronic hypokalemia if there are no ECG changes or any organ dysfunction because of hypokalemia. The exception is patients on digoxin where serum potassium should be >4 mEq/L before taking them for surgery.

Anesthetic Considerations

- As these patients are prone for cardiac arrhythmias, vigilant ECG monitoring is must.
- Dose of non-depolarizing muscle relaxant is decreased as prolonged block is expected due to muscle weakness.
- As hyperventilation and hyperglycemia can cause hypokalemia, they must be avoided.

Hyponatremia and Hypernatremia

- Hyponatremia and hypernatremia should be normalized before subjecting the patients for elective surgery. However, rapid correction must never be done; rapid correction can cause pontine myelinolysis.
- In case of emergency surgeries, considerations should be given to coexisting volume disturbances seen with hyponatremia (hypervolemia) and hypernatremia (hypovolemia). Accordingly the volume of distribution increases or decreases the doses of intravenous (IV) drugs.

Hypercalcemia

Anesthetic Considerations

- The key principle is maintenance of hydration and urine output.
- Increase requirement of non-depolarizing muscle relaxants may be expected.

Hypocalcemia

Anesthetic Considerations

- Symptomatic hypocalcemia should be corrected before surgery.
- Hypocalcemia can produce laryngospasm and hypotension.
- Hyperventilation and alkalosis can cause hypocalcemia therefore, should be avoided.
- Blood transfusion should be supplemented with calcium.

Hypermagnesemia

Anesthetic Considerations

- Acidosis and dehydration can lead to hypermagnesemia therefore, must be avoided.
- *Hypermagnesemia potentiates the action of both depolarizing and non-depolarizing muscle relaxants.*

Hypomagnesemia

Anesthetic Considerations

- Hypomagnesemia may be associated with refractory hypokalemia and hypocalcemia.
- Ventricular arrhythmias may be expected.
- Hypomagnesemia can prolong the block by non-depolarizing muscle relaxants.

KEY POINTS

- Patients with acute kidney injury (AKI) should not undergo elective surgery until the injury is fully resolved.
- Dialysis should be performed within 24 hours before surgery.
- Correction of hyperkalemia is of utmost importance in chronic kidney disease patients.
- Maintaining fluid balance is essential in renal patients; excess fluid can precipitate pulmonary edema and fluid deficiency can worsen kidney injury.
- If invasive blood pressure monitoring is required then radial and ulnar artery should be spared as they may be required for hemodialysis in future.
- Central neuraxial blocks should be avoided due to associated uremic coagulopathy, uremic polyneuropathy and intolerance of renal patients to extra fluids to treat hypotension.
- Desflurane is the inhalational agent of choice because it does not produce fluoride.
- Sevoflurane should not be used in renal patients as it produces high levels of fluoride approaching renal threshold of 50 µmol/L.
- Non-depolarizing relaxant of choice is atracurium/Cis-atracurium while suxamethonium is contraindicated due to associated hyperkalemia.
- Ringer lactate is preferred over normal saline with close monitoring of potassium levels. Colloids (hydroxyethyl starch) have been found to exacerbate renal injury.
- TURP syndrome is exhibited as fluid overloading, dilutional hyponatremia and hypo-osmolality.
- Hyperkalemia must be corrected before taking the patient for surgery while there is no need to correct mild chronic hypokalemia.
- Hypermagnesemia potentiates the action of both depolarizing and non-depolarizing muscle relaxants.

CHAPTER 23

Anesthesia for Endocrinal Disorders

DIABETES MELLITUS

Preoperative Evaluation

The basic goals of preoperative evaluation are:
- To assess the severity of disease by checking blood sugar and HbA_{1c} levels.
- To *rule out autonomic neuropathy.* Patients with autonomic neuropathy are hemodynamically unstable and can even suffer cardiac arrest.
- To rule out peripheral neuropathy as it can affect the choice of anesthesia.
- To rule out the organ damage caused by diabetes especially nephropathy.

Premedication

As diabetic patients have delayed gastric emptying, premedication against aspiration should be given.

Intraoperative

Management of Sugar

Patient on oral hypoglycemics: Oral hypoglycemics are continued omitting the morning dose on the day of surgery. However due to long half lives sulfonyl urea and metformin should be stopped 24–48 hours prior to surgery.

Patients on insulin: Majority of the patients are either on intermediate acting or mixed insulin. There are different protocols followed by different institutions:
- The most widespread traditionally employed regime is to give 1/2 of the AM dose of insulin on the morning of surgery after starting infusion of 5% dextrose at a rate of 125 mL/hour

(to avoid the possibility of hypoglycemia). Blood sugar is monitored every 2 hours and hyperglycemia is treated by intravenous regular insulin (1 unit of insulin decreases blood sugar levels by 25–30 mg/dL).
- As there is better control of sugar levels the *current guidelines are more in favor of regular insulin by continuous infusion.* Insulin is prepared in normal saline as 1 unit/mL and given by the following formula: Units/hour = plasma glucose (mg/dL)/150.

  For example, if plasma sugar is 300 then rate of infusion will be 2 units/hour.

  5% dextrose at a rate of 125 mL/hour and potassium chloride (KCL) 20 mEq/liter should also be given along with insulin infusion.
- The third regime is no insulin-no glucose, i.e. omit the morning dose of insulin and no need to start dextrose.
- If the patient is on insulin pump and posted for minor surgery there is no need to change the basal rate of infusion, however if the patient is posted for major surgery then pump should be stopped in the morning and patient is managed by continuous infusion of regular insulin.

Whatever may be the regime followed the *target should be to keep plasma sugar level between 150 and 180 mg/dL.*

Monitoring: ECG monitoring is more than mandatory because *myocardial ischemia is most common cause of death in perioperative period in diabetic patients.* The myocardial infarction (MI) may go silent in postoperative period if the patient is having autonomic neuropathy.

Choice of anesthesia: Patients not having peripheral and/or autonomic neuropathy can safely receive regional anesthesia. Maintaining asepsis during blocks is pivotal.

General Anesthesia

- Difficult intubation may be anticipated due to involvement of atlanto-occipital and temporomandibular joint (stiff joint syndrome).
- Hypotension and bradycardia in patients suffering from autonomic neuropathy may not respond to atropine and ephedrine; intravenous adrenaline may act as savior.
- Sympathetic stimulation can cause hyperglycemia therefore, drugs causing sympathetic stimulation like ketamine, pancuronium, atropine, desflurane >6% should be avoided. Sympathetic stimulation caused by intubation must be blunted by deep anesthesia, lignocaine, β blockers or calcium channel blockers.

Postoperative

Cardiac and regular blood sugar monitoring should be continued in postoperative period.

THYROID DYSFUNCTIONS

Hyperthyroidism

Elective surgery should be deferred till the patient is euthyroid.

Preoperative Evaluation

- *All antithyroid drugs should be continued as such including the morning dose.*
- Other than thyroid functions sleeping pulse rate should be brought down to normal with beta blockers before taking the patient for surgery.
- As large thyroid can produce tracheal compression therefore, airway assessment by indirect laryngoscopy, X-ray neck or CT scan is must.

Intraoperative

Monitoring: Other than routine monitoring, ECG to detect arrhythmias and temperature to detect hyperthermia is must in hyperthyroid patients.

Choice of anesthesia: Regional anesthesia can be safely given however, local anesthetics with adrenaline must not be used. In fact, central neuraxial blocks are preferred because of their capacity to block the sympathetic response.

General Anesthesia

- Sympathetic stimulation can precipitate thyroid storm therefore, drugs causing sympathetic stimulation like ketamine, pancuronium, atropine, desflurane >6% should be avoided. Sympathetic stimulation caused by intubation must be blunted by deep anesthesia, lignocaine, β blockers or calcium channel blockers.
- Exophthalmos increases the risk of corneal abrasion therefore eye protection is must.
- If there is airway compression due to large thyroid then awake intubation with fiberoptic bronchoscopy should be done.

Induction: As *Thiopentone* possess antithyroid property, it is the induction agent of choice.

Maintenance: As hyperthyroid patients are more prone for arrhythmias therefore, most cardiac stable, i.e. Isoflurane should be the preferred agent. The concern of increased toxicity of inhalational agents due to increased metabolism in hyperthyroid patient has not been substantiated in human studies. Minimum alveolar concentration (MAC) of inhalational agents remains same in hyperthyroidism.

Muscle relaxant: Vecuronium being most cardiac stable is most preferred.

Postoperative

Postoperative period in hyperthyroid patient can be risky due to the following complications:

- *Thyroid storm:* Thyroid storm is a life-threatening condition most often occurring in postoperative period however, can occur intraoperatively also. The management includes control of hyperthermia, arrhythmias, dehydration, antithyroid drugs (propylthiouracil) and dexamethasone (block conversion of T4 to T3).
- *Upper airway obstruction:* It is most often due to tracheal compression caused by expanding hematoma. It should be treated immediately by opening the sutures.

- *Recurrent laryngeal nerve palsy:* Unilateral palsy will just cause the hoarseness while bilateral can cause aphonia and stridor. Immediate ENT reference should be sought.
- *Hypoparathyroidism:* Hypocalcemia caused by hypoparathyroidism can precipitate laryngospasm.

Emergency Surgery in Hyperthyroid Patient

At least tachycardia should be settled with intravenous infusion of esmolol or intravenous propranolol (propranolol has added advantage of inhibiting the conversion of T4 to T3). However, if it is an urgent surgery (not life-threatening emergency surgery) then ipodate, propylthiouracil and dexamethasone should be given in addition.

The anesthetist should be prepared to handle thyroid storm in hyperthyroid patients undergoing emergency surgery.

HYPOTHYROIDISM

Ideally elective surgery should be deferred till the patient is euthyroid however mild hypothyroidism should not be a deterrent to postpone the surgery.

Preoperative Evaluation

- Associated conditions with hypothyroidism like congestive cardiac failure, anemia, hypothermia, hyponatremia and hypoglycemia should be ruled out.
- *Thyroxin preparations should be continued in preoperative period.*
- Hypothyroid patients can have very large glands therefore, indirect laryngoscopy or if required CT neck should be done to assess tracheal compression.
- These patients are extremely sensitive to depressant drugs therefore, premedication with benzodiazepines should be avoided.
- Due to delayed gastric emptying hypothyroid patients are more vulnerable for aspiration therefore, aspiration prophylaxis should be given.

Intraoperative

Choice of Anesthesia

Regional anesthesia is an appropriate selection provided that the intravascular fluid volume is well-maintained however, coagulation abnormality and platelet dysfunction should be ruled out.

General Anesthesia

- These patients are vulnerable to go into congestive cardiac failure therefore, for major surgeries fluid should be given by goal directed therapy or at least by central venous pressure (CVP).
- *As the metabolism of drugs is reduced in hypothyroidism they should be used in minimal possible doses.*

Induction: Normally done with propofol however, if there is evidence of low cardiac output then ketamine is preferred.

Maintenance: Isoflurane because of its cardiac stability is most preferred.

Muscle relaxant: As mivacurium, atracurium/Cis-atracurium do not have the possibility of accumulation therefore, are preferred muscle relaxants.

Postoperative

- These patients can go into hypoxia in postoperative period due to hypoventilation.
- Patients must be watched carefully for the postoperative complications of thyroidectomy like upper airway obstruction, recurrent laryngeal nerve palsy and hypoparathyroidism.

Emergency Surgery in Hypothyroid Patient

Intravenous T3 and T4 should be given in severely hypothyroid patients. As adrenal function is often decreased steroid cover also becomes must.

ADRENAL DYSFUNCTIONS

Pheochromocytoma

- Preoperatively patient's hypertension must be stabilized by α blocker; most often used is phenoxybenzamine. Tachycardia must be controlled by β blockers. β blockers must not be started before initiating the therapy with α blocker otherwise unopposed action can cause malignant hypertension.
- Agents causing sympathetic stimulation (ketamine, pancuronium, desflurane >6%)

are contraindicated. Sympathetic response to intubation must be blunted. *Halothane is absolutely contraindicated* because it sensitizes myocardium to catecholamines.
- Increase in catecholamines during tumor handing can cause profound hypertension and life-threatening arrhythmias.
- During adrenalectomy glucocorticoids infusion should be started at the beginning of the resection of tumor and then continued in postoperative period (100 mg/day of hydrocortisone) for 1–2 days for unilateral and 3–6 days for bilateral adrenalectomy.
- After the ligation of tumor vein, abrupt withdrawal of catecholamines can cause profound hypotension and hypoglycemia. In fact, *hypotension is the most common cause of death in immediate postoperative period in pheochromocytoma patient.* Dextrose normal saline should be started immediately after vein ligation.

Glucocorticoid Excess (Cushing Syndrome)

Glucocorticoid excess may be due to exogenous administration or increased endogenous production. The effects of cortisol, i.e. hypertension, hyperglycemia, volume overload and hypokalemia (mineralocorticoid effect of glucocorticoid) must be corrected before taking the patient for elective surgery. Due to osteoporosis there is possibility of fractures during positioning. Delayed wound healing and infections should be expected in these patients.

Glucocorticoid Deficiency

- Glucocorticoid deficiency may be due to primary adrenal insufficiency (Addison's disease) or secondary adrenal insufficiency due to inadequate adrenocorticotropic hormone (ACTH) secretion by pituitary. Exogenous steroids are the most common cause of secondary adrenal insufficiency.
- As exogenous steroids causes inhibition of hypothalamic pituitary axis (HPA) and

recovery of HPA takes 1 year, any patient who has taken steroid (prednisone in doses >5 mg/day or equivalent) for more than 3 weeks (by any route, even topical or inhalational) in last 1 year must receive intraoperative supplementation with hydrocortisone. 100 mg of hydrocortisone 8 hourly beginning on the day of surgery and continued for 24–48 hours is the conventional approach however continuous infusion at a rate of 10 mg/hour is considered better.
- *Etomidate is contraindicated* as it causes adrenocortical suppression.

Mineralocorticoid Excess

- Hypokalemia and hypertension should be corrected before taking the patients for surgery.
- Avoid hyperventilation as alkalosis can cause hypokalemia.
- Sevoflurane should be avoided if there is hypokalemic nephropathy.
- Hypokalemia may prolong the block of non-depolarizing muscle relaxants.

Mineralocorticoid Deficiency

Hyperkalemia should be corrected before taking the patients for surgery.

PITUITARY DYSFUNCTION

Acromegaly

- The most important concern for acromegaly patients is *difficult airway management* due to multiple reasons like prognathism, macroglossia, overgrowth of epiglottis, narrowed glottis due to overgrowth of vocal cords.
- Central neuraxial blocks may become difficult due to osteoarthritis of spine.
- As collateral circulation gets compromised radial artery cannulation should be done only after adequately performing Allen test.

KEY POINTS

- Ruling out autonomic neuropathy is one of the most important part of preoperative assessment in diabetic patient.
- Regular insulin by continuous infusion is the most recommended method to control intraoperative plasma glucose.
- The target plasma sugar level should be between 150–180 mg/dL in perioperative period.
- Myocardial ischemia is the most common cause of death in perioperative period in diabetic patients.
- Elective surgery should be deferred in hyper- or hypothyroid patient till the patient is euthyroid however, mild hypothyroidism should not be a deterrent to postpone the surgery.
- Thiopentone is the induction agent of choice in hyperthyroid patients.
- At least tachycardia should be settled in hyperthyroid patients undergoing emergency surgery.
- As the metabolism of drugs is reduced in hypothyroidism, all drugs should be used in minimal possible doses.
- Halothane is absolutely contraindicated in pheochromocytoma because it sensitizes myocardium to catecholamines.
- Increase in catecholamines during tumor handing can cause profound hypertension and life-threatening arrhythmias during pheochromocytoma surgery.
- Etomidate is contraindicated in adrenal insufficiency because it causes adrenocortical suppression.

CHAPTER 24

Anesthesia for Neuromuscular Diseases

MYASTHENIA GRAVIS

It is an autoimmune disease characterized by destruction of acetylcholine receptors by the antibodies against these receptors leading to weakness of the muscles.

Anesthetic Management

The myasthenic patient most often come for thymectomy as a part of their treatment.

Timing of Surgery

Elective surgery should be avoided in acute relapse. Patient's medical condition must be stabilized before considering them for anesthesia. Patients with significant respiratory or oropharyngeal weakness may even require intravenous (IV) immunoglobulin or plasmapheresis.

Preoperative Evaluation

- Other associated autoimmune diseases should be ruled out.
- Myasthenic patients may have weakness of respiratory muscles therefore, evaluation of pulmonary functions must be done in detail.
- Anticholinesterases (most commonly used is pyridostigmine) are the mainstay of treatment. Stopping these drugs can precipitate the myasthenic crisis while continuing can antagonize the effect of muscle relaxants therefore, *anticholinesterases should be continued in reduced doses.*

  Patients with advance disease may be on steroids and immunosuppressants which should also be continued

- Weakness of respiratory muscles makes these patients very vulnerable for respiratory depression therefore, premedication with benzodiazepines should be avoided.
- As these patients are vulnerable for aspiration prophylaxis for aspiration should be taken.

Intraoperative

Choice of Anesthesia

The basic problem of myasthenic patients is that they exhibit extreme sensitivity to respiratory depression by anesthetic agents and abnormal response to muscle relaxants therefore, *aim of anesthesia should be to avoid general anesthesia making local/regional anesthesia as the anesthetic technique of choice* however, all surgeries are not possible under regional anesthesia.

General Anesthesia

Monitoring: Other than routine monitoring *neuromuscular monitoring is mandatory.*

Induction: As Etomidate does not causes respiratory depression it is the preferred induction agent however, thiopentone and propofol can be used safely.

Maintenance: The aim should be to *avoid muscle relaxants.* Since myasthenia patients have weakness of muscles and inhalational agents have got muscle relaxation property therefore, in significant number of patients it is possible to intubate and maintain the surgical relaxation with inhalational agents alone.

Desflurane is the most preferred inhalational agent for maintenance because it produces maximum muscle relaxation among the currently used inhalational agents. In the absence of desflurane, sevoflurane or isoflurane can be used.

Muscle relaxants: Muscle relaxants should be used only if inhalational agents are not able to produce sufficient muscle relaxation. *Myasthenic patients are resistant to depolarizers* therefore suxamethonium is required in high doses (2 mg/kg instead of 1–1.5 mg/kg) and *hypersensitive to non-depolarizers* therefore, *only short acting with no risk of accumulation like mivacurium, atracurium, and Cis-atracurium* must be used. Long acting like pancuronium must not be used. The initial dose should be 1/3rd to ½ and further doses titrated as per neuromuscular monitoring.

A prolonged block by suxamethonium and mivacurium is expected in the patient on cholinesterase inhibitor because they inhibit pseudocholinesterase however, this prolongation is not very significant clinically.

As these patients are very prone for respiratory depression only short acting opioids (Remifentanil) should be used.

Postoperative

Many of these patients especially who have significantly compromised pulmonary functions (vital capacity <4 mL/kg) or on high doses of pyridostigmine (>750 mg/day) may require ventilation in postoperative period.

MYASTHENIC SYNDROME (EATON-LAMBERT SYNDROME)

It is an autoimmune disease in which antibodies to presynaptic calcium channel are produced leading to decreased production of acetylcholine.

These patients are sensitive to both depolarizing and non-depolarizing muscle relaxants.

Reversal requires a combination of anticholinesterase and 4-aminopyridine.

FAMILIAL PERIODIC PARALYSIS

Hyperkalemic Type

- Preoperatively normalize potassium levels.
- Avoid potassium containing solutions.
- Succinylcholine is contraindicated.

Hypokalemic Type

- Hypokalemic type is more common.
- Avoid anything which causes hypokalemia like hyperventilation and *glucose containing solutions.*
- Non-depolarizers will have prolonged effect.

MUSCULAR DYSTROPHIES

Muscular dystrophies patients are considered as high risk patients to develop malignant hyperthermia.

Duchenne's Dystrophy (Pseudohypertrophic Muscular Dystrophy)

This is the most common type of dystrophy of childhood. The involved muscles become hypertrophied due to fatty infiltration (pseudo-hypertrophy). It not only involves skeletal but cardiac muscles also get involved. Death usually occurs by 15–25 years of age due to congestive heart failure (CHF) or pneumonia.

Anesthetic Management

- Due to increased sensitivity to muscle relaxants general anesthesia (GA) should be avoided; if possible surgery should be performed under *regional anesthesia.*
- Due to respiratory muscle weakness opioids and benzodiazepines should be avoided.
- Due to weakness of laryngeal and pharyngeal reflexes these patients are prone for aspiration therefore, should be premedicated with metoclopramide and ranitidine.
- *Succinylcholine is absolutely contraindicated.* It may produce cardiac arrest due to hyperkalemia and rhabdomyolysis and can precipitate malignant hyperthermia.

Due to muscular weakness, non-depolarizing agent may exhibit increased sensitivity therefore, *short acting agents with no possibility of accumulation like mivacurium, atracurium, cis-atracurium (Mivacurium most preferred)* should be given with initial dose as 1/3 to 1/2 and further doses titrated as per neuromuscular monitoring.

- As there is involvement of cardiac muscle, most cardiac safe, i.e. isoflurane should be the most preferred inhalational agent. *Halothane is contraindicated as it can precipitate malignant hyperthermia.*

Myotonia Dystrophica

It is the most common and most serious dystrophy in adults characterized by persistent contracture after a stimulus. Contracture may not be relieved by general and regional anesthesia while local infiltration in effected muscle may induce relaxation.

The anesthetic management principles are same as for Duchene muscular dystrophy with an emphasis that *Succinylcholine is absolutely contraindicated* not only because it can produce hyperkalemia and precipitate malignant hyperthermia but can also induce severe muscle contractures.

Mivacurium, atracurium and cis-atracurium are not only preferred because of their short duration and no risk of accumulation but also they permit the avoidance of reversal agents. Reversal agents can precipitate contractures by causing muscle contraction.

As shivering can also precipitate muscle contractures it must be avoided at any cost.

KEY POINTS

- For myasthenic patients anticholinesterases should be continued in reduced doses.
- Local/regional anesthesia is the anesthetic technique of choice for myasthenia gravis patients.
- Desflurane is the most preferred inhalational agent for maintenance in myasthenia gravis patients because it produces maximum muscle relaxation among the currently used inhalational agents.
- Myasthenic patients are resistant to depolarizers and hypersensitive to non-depolarizers.
- Mivacurium, atracurium, and Cis-atracurium are safe non-deploarizers for myasthenia gravis patients.
- Myasthenic syndrome patients are sensitive to both depolarizing and non-depolarizing muscle relaxants.
- Succinylcholine is absolutely contraindicated for muscular dystrophies; it may produce cardiac arrest due to hyperkalemia and rhabdomyolysis and can precipitate malignant hyperthermia in these patients.
- Non-depolarizers exhibit increased sensitivity in muscular dystrophies making mivacurium, atracurium, cis-atracurium to be safer choices.
- Halothane is contraindicated in muscular dystrophies as it can precipitate malignant hyperthermia.

CHAPTER 25

Anesthesia for Immune Mediated and Infectious Diseases

RHEUMATOID ARTHRITIS

It is a disease characterized by immune-mediated synovitis.

Preoperative Evaluation

- Associated comorbidities like cardiac valvular lesions, pericarditis, and pulmonary fibrosis should be ruled out.
- As difficult airway is the most important concern, airway evaluation should be done very meticulously.
- Side effects of disease modifying anti-rheumatic drugs (DMARDs), nonsteroidal anti-inflammatory drugs (NSAIDs) and corticosteroids should be taken into consideration.

Anesthetic Management

Choice of anesthesia: *Regional anesthesia.* Lumbar spine is usually not involved in rheumatoid arthritis therefore spinal/epidural can be given easily.

General Anesthesia

General anesthesia is difficult and risky due to *difficult intubation* which in turn is due to:

- *Atlantoaxial instability: Patients of atlantoaxial subluxation cannot tolerate flexion.* Flexion of neck can cause odontoid process to compress spinal cord leading to quadriplegia. Therefore, intubation is best performed under topical anesthesia with awake patient. If intubation has to be done under general anesthesia then *intubation should be done with neck in extension.*

- Stiffness of cervical spine
- Temporomandibular and cricoarytenoid arthritis.
  - Arterial cannulation may be difficult due to calcified radial arteries and central venous cannulation may be difficult due to cervical spine fusion.

ANKYLOSING SPONDYLITIS

- From anesthesia point of view ankylosing spondylitis may turn out to be the most difficult case at times. *Fusion of lumbar spine may make central neuraxial blocks impossible and fusion of cervical spine may make intubation impossible.* Therefore, intubation in such patients should be performed in awake state under fiberoptic bronchoscopy.
- Aortic regurgitation and bundle branch block are common in ankylosing spondylitis.

SYSTEMIC LUPUS ERYTHEMATOSUS

The involvement of major organs functions determines the perioperative morbidity in systemic lupus erythematosus (SLE). Laryngeal involvement including cricoarytenoid arthritis and laryngeal nerve palsy can make intubation difficult.

SCLERODERMA

The multiorgan involvement, particularly pulmonary fibrosis and pulmonary hypertension can significant effect the perioperative morbidity. Small oral aperture can make intubation difficult. Dermal thickening can make intravenous (IV) cannulation difficult.

HUMAN IMMUNODEFICIENCY VIRUS AND ACQUIRED IMMUNODEFICIENCY SYNDROME

- Due to involvement of multiple organs all human immunodeficiency virus (HIV) positive patients are categorized as American Society of Anesthesiologists (ASA) grade II while patients with acquired immunodeficiency syndrome (AIDS) are categorized as ASAIII/IV
- Side effects of highly active antiretroviral therapy (HAART) including diabetes, coronary and cerebrovascular disease, deranged liver function must be ruled out in preoperative

period. The patients who have started HAART within 6 months of surgery suffer more from perioperative complications.
- *CD4 count and viral load* do affect the overall prognosis after surgery but *has not found to increase the perioperative anesthetic complications.*
- Regional anesthesia can be given safely if there are no associated neuropathies.
- Fat redistribution around the neck can make intubation difficult.
- *Maintaining universal precautions* and high degree of asepsis during any procedure is vital.

KEY POINTS

- Due to atlantoaxial instability intubation in patients with rheumatoid arthritis should be performed with neck in extension.
- In patients with ankylosing spondylitis fusion of lumbar spine may make central neuraxial blocks impossible and fusion of cervical spine may make intubation impossible.
- CD4 count and viral load do not determine the rate of perioperative anesthetic complications.

CHAPTER 26

Anesthesia for Disorders of Blood

ANEMIA

The most common anemia encountered in clinical practice in India is microcytic hypochromic due to iron deficiency.

Preoperative Evaluation

- One of a very important goal for preoperative evaluation is to find out the cause of anemia as it can affect the choice of anesthesia.
- Systemic effect of anemia particularly hyperdynamic circulation, which can lead to cardiac failure, must be ruled out.
- The most appropriate minimum hemoglobin at which patient can be safely taken for surgery is very difficult to define as there are number of compounding factors which effects the outcome in anemia patients like type of the surgery, chronicity of anemia, associated comorbidities however, for a normal patient without any comorbidity (especially ischemic heart disease) undergoing a surgery where major blood loss is not expected a *minimum hemoglobin of 8 g/dL is considered optimal to accept the patient for elective surgery.*
- Correction of anemia can be done by treating the cause, dietary modifications, medications (iron, folic acid, vitamin B_{12}) or blood transfusion depending on the severity of anemia and availability of time before surgery.

Intraoperative

- Blood loss should be minimized by adequate hemostasis or controlled hypotension.

- Maximum allowable blood loss is calculated by the following formula:

$$\frac{\text{Hematocrit of patient} - \text{desirable hematocrit (usually 30)}}{\text{Hematocrit of patient}} \times \frac{\text{Blood volume}}{(80\text{--}90 \text{ mL/kg})}$$

For example, allowable blood loss for a 70 kg patient with hemoglobin of 12 g% will be:

Patient hematocrit - $12 \times 3 = 36$

Desired hematocrit- 30

Blood volume - $70 \times 85 = 5950$ L

$$\text{Allowable blood loss} = \frac{36\text{--}30}{36} \times 5950 = 991 \text{ mL}$$

- Considering the complications associated with blood transfusion, the approach in present day practice is towards the minimum use of blood products (called as *restrictive approach to transfusion*). The general guidelines for transfusion are:

Blood loss greater than 20% of blood volume (however, the correct approach is calculate the allowable blood loss by above said formula) or hemoglobin level less than 8 g% in normal patient and less than 10 g% in a patient with major disease like ischemic heart disease.

Choice of Anesthesia

Regional anesthesia can be given safely however, due to possibility of neurological deficits regional anesthesia should be avoided for vitamin B_{12} deficiency anemia.

General Anesthesia

- The factors which can shift the oxygen dissociation curve to left (especially alkalosis caused by hyperventilation), which increases the oxygen requirement like shivering or which decreases the cardiac output should be avoided.
- As nitrous oxide can cause megaloblastic anemia therefore, should be avoided for vitamin B_{12} deficiency anemia.
- Increase uptake of inhalational agents is offset by increased cardiac output seen in anemia patients.

SICKLE CELL DISEASE

There is no increase in morbidity and mortality in patients having sickle cell trait while patients with sickle cell disease are at high risk of complications.

Preoperative Evaluation

The major goals of preoperative evaluation are:
- To assess the pulmonary (including acute chest syndrome), renal, splenic and cerebral damage caused by vasoocculsive episodes.
- Frequency of vasoocculsive episodes including the time lapse since last episode. *Patients in acute crisis phase must not be taken for elective surgery.*
- *Very commonly practiced policy of bringing HbS level to less than 50% by exchange transfusion does not hold valid now a days. The aim in current day practice is just to correct the anemia by giving red cell transfusion with the target hematocrit > 30 (Hemoglobin > 10 g%).*
- *The most important perioperative goal is to avoid the factors which can precipitate sickling, i.e. hypoxia, acidosis, dehydration, hypothermia, stress and pain.*
To avoid dehydration intravenous fluids should be started in preoperative period. To avoid stress and anxiety these patients must be premedicated with benzodiazepines.

Intraoperative

Choice of anesthesia: All regional blocks can be given safely. *The old recommendation of not giving intravenous regional anesthesia (Bier's block) to sickle cell patients does not hold true in current day practice.* Bier's block was not possible in sickle cell patients because use of tourniquet was contraindicated however as per current guidelines tourniquet can be used safely in sickle cell patients in spite of a little higher complications. To minimise the complication it is recommended to use tourniquet for minimal period with minimal possible pressure.

The factors which precipitate sickling must be avoided at any cost.

Postoperative

As pain can precipitate sickling, postoperative pain control becomes vital in these patients. Acute lung syndrome usually occurs after 48–72 hours in postoperative period.

THALASSEMIA

The patients with thalassemia minor are not high risk while with thalassemia major are high risk patients for perioperative morbidity and mortality.

Other than the severity of anemia it is important to assess the organ involvement like hepatosplenomegaly, skeletal involvement, congestive heart failure and consequences of iron overload like cirrhosis.

Skeletal abnormalities of maxilla (maxillary overgrowth) can make intubation difficult.

POLYCYTHEMIA

- Reduce hematocrit to <45 and platelet count (usually associated with polycythemia) to less than 4 lakhs before taking the patient for elective surgery.
- The patients with polycythemia are not only at high risk of thromboembolic complication but also at increased risk of bleeding due to decrease von Willebrand factor seen in polycythemia.

DISORDERS OF HEMOSTASIS

Disorders of Platelets

Thrombocytopenia

Platelet count of > 50,000/mm³ is recommended before considering for surgery. However, for minor surgeries where no blood loss is expected a count of 30,000 may suffice. Neurosurgical patients cannot be considered for surgery if their platelet count is <100000. Symptomatic patients (spontaneous bleeding) irrespective of their platelet count need platelet transfusion before surgery.

Choice of anesthesia: Patients with platelet count more than 80,000/cubic mm can be safely given central neuraxial blocks. Platelet count between 50,000 and 80,000/cubic mm is a relative contraindication while count less than 50000 is an absolute contraindication.

Disorders of Coagulation

Coagulation Deficiency Disorders

The deficit factor should be increased to at least 50% of the normal before considering the patient for surgery by administration of fresh frozen plasma, cryoprecipitate or recombinant factor.

Choice of anesthesia
- *Regional anesthesia is contraindicated.*
- Intramuscular route should be avoided.
- *Intubation should be performed by expert hand with minimum trauma,* otherwise there can be massive bleeding in oral cavity.

Hypercoagulable Disorders

Antithrombin levels should be > 80% at least for 5 days in postoperative period. Protein C and protein S deficiency should be corrected in preoperative period by fresh frozen plasma.

Central neuraxial blocks are preferred because they decrease the incidence of thromboembolic complications (due to increase blood in lower limb and pelvic veins).

All prophylaxis against deep venous thrombosis (DVT) should be started as early as possible.

G6PD DEFICIENCY

The anesthetic management of these patients includes assessing the severity of anemia and avoiding the drugs and conditions which can trigger hemolysis in G6PD deficient individuals. The drugs and conditions which can trigger hemolysis in perioperative period in these patients include:

- Diazepam; interestingly, midazolam is safe.
- Isoflurane and sevoflurane.
- Drugs which can cause methemoglobinemia can cause significant hemolysis in these patients. Therefore, prilocaine, benzocaine, lignocaine and nitroglycerine should be avoided.
- *Methylene blue:* Administrating methylene blue to these patients can be life threatening.
- Acidosis, hypothermia, hyperglycemia and infection can trigger hemolysis therefore, must be avoided throughout in these patients.

PORPHYRIA

Drugs which induce aminolevulinic acid synthetase can precipitate all kind of porphyrias except porphyria cutanea tarda and erythropoietic protoporphyrias. Drugs used in anesthesia which induce aminolevulinic acid synthetase and hence can precipitate all kind of porphyrias (except porphyria cutanea tarda and erythropoietic protoporphyrias) are:

- *Barbiturates* (Thiopentone/Methohexitone)— *Absolutely contraindicated.*
- Diazepam, etomidate, pentazocine—Should be avoided.
- Inhalational agents, ketamine, non-depolarizing muscle relaxants—although safety has not been established however, unlikely to precipitate porphyrias.
- *Fasting,* dehydration and infection can trigger acute crises.
- Regional anesthesia should be avoided in the porphyria patients with peripheral neuropathy.
- *Propofol,* opioids, suxamethonium are considered as safe agents.

KEY POINTS

- Minimum hemoglobin of 8 g/dL is considered optimal to accept the patient for elective surgery.
- Considering the complications associated with blood transfusion, the approach in present day practice is towards the minimum use of blood products called as restrictive approach to transfusion.

Contd...

Contd…

- Exchange transfusion is not practiced technique for sickle cell patient in current day. The approach is just to correct the anemia by giving red cell transfusion with the target hematocrit > 30 (Hemoglobin >10 g%).
- The most important perioperative goal in sickle cell patients is to avoid hypoxia, acidosis, dehydration, hypothermia, stress and pain.
- Intravenous regional anesthesia (Bier's block) can be utilized for sickle cell patients.
- Platelet count of > 50,000/mm^3 is recommended before considering the patients for surgery.
- The deficit coagulation factor should be increased to at least 50% of the normal before considering the patient for surgery.
- Regional anesthesia is contraindicated for patients with deficient coagulation factor disorders like hemophilia.
- Administrating methylene blue can be life-threatening in patients with G6PD deficiency.
- Barbiturates are absolutely contraindicated for all kind of porphyrias except porphyria cutanea tarda and erythropoietic protoporphyrias.
- Propofol, opioids and suxamethonium are considered safe for porphyrias patients.
- Fasting, dehydration and infection can trigger acute crisis of porphyria.

Subspecialty Anesthetic Management

CHAPTER 27

Neurosurgical Anesthesia

CEREBRAL PHYSIOLOGY AND PHARMACOLOGY

Cerebral Blood Flow (CBF)

Cerebral perfusion pressure (CPP) is the difference between mean arterial pressure and intracranial pressure. CBF is 50 mL/100 g of brain tissue. CBF is maintained at constant level by autoregulation when mean arterial pressure is between 60 mm Hg and 150 mm Hg.

Cerebral ischemia, head injury, hypercarbia, hypoxia, brain edema and *inhalational agents* can abolish this autoregulatory mechanism.

Cerebral blood flow is effected by:
- Cerebral metabolic rate
- Blood pressure (outside the limits of auto regulation)
- pCO_2 (pH): Each mm increase in pCO_2 above 40 mm Hg increases CBF by 15–30 mL/min
- pO_2: Increases CBF only if pO_2 is below 60 mm Hg
- *Anesthetics:* All inhalational agents, ketamine and opioids increase CBF while barbiturates, propofol, etomidate and benzodiazepines decreases the CBF.

Cerebral Metabolic Rate

Couples with cerebral blood flow. Hyperthermia, seizures increase the cerebral metabolic rate (CMR) while hypothermia and anesthetics decreases the cerebral metabolic rate.

Intracranial Tension

Intracranial tension (ICT) reflects relationship between volume of intracranial contents and cranial vault. *Normal* ICT is *10–15 mm Hg.* ICT > 20 mm Hg is significant and needs aggressive treatment.

Signs and Symptoms of Raised ICT

Headache, vomiting, altered sensorium, hypertension and bradycardia (Cushing reflex), papilledema, seizures, apnea, unconsciousness and death (at very high ICT) and midline shift > 0.5 cm on computed tomography (CT) scan.

Methods to Decrease Intracranial Tension

- *Hyperventilation:* It is the *most rapid method of reducing ICT.* Hyperventilation reduces the ICT by causing hypocapnia which in turn causes cerebral vasoconstriction to decrease the production of cerebrospinal fluid (CSF). Moderate hypocapnia is beneficial however excessive hypocapnia by causing excessive cerebral vasoconstriction can cause cerebral ischemia therefore *it is recommended to maintain pCO_2 between 25–30 mm Hg.*
- *Hyperosmotic drugs:*
  - *Mannitol, urea and hypertonic saline:* Among these agents most commonly used is mannitol. These drugs are retained in intravascular compartment increasing plasma osmolarity, drawing water from brain tissue decreasing brain edema however, if blood brain barrier is disrupted (head injuries, stroke) these agents can enter the brain tissue increasing the cerebral edema. Therefore, *the use of mannitol in head injury and stroke should be judicious.* Mannitol should be repeated only if there

is clear evidence for decrease in ICT or improvement in surgical conditions after 1st dose.

- *Diuretics:*
  - *Furosemide:* It is very effective method of reducing ICT particularly when blood brain barrier is disrupted.
- *Steroids:*
  - Dexamethasone
  - Methylprednisolone

  The exact mechanism by which steroids decrease the ICT is not clear; probably they act by membrane stabilization or reducing the production of CSF.
- *Barbiturates:* Thiopentone by causing cerebral vasoconstriction is effective in decreasing the production of CSF and hence ICT.
- *Posture:* Head up position by increasing venous drainage decreases ICT. Neck flexion by compressing jugular veins can increase ICT.
- *CSF drainage:* If ICT is not controlled by conservative measure it should be drained through ventricles (never through lumbar puncture, brain herniation can even cause death).

Pharmacology

Effect of anesthetic agents on cerebral blood flow (CBF), cerebral metabolic rate (CMR), cerebral oxygen consumption (CMO_2), CSF dynamics and intracranial tension (ICT):

Inhalational Agents

- *All inhalational agents (including nitrous oxide) increases the cerebral blood flow and hence ICT.* The order of vasodilating potency is- halothane >> Desflurane ≈ Isoflurane > Sevoflurane.
- All inhalational agents produce dose-dependent reduction in cerebral metabolic rate and cerebral oxygen consumption (CMO_2). Isoflurane and Sevoflurane can decrease CMR up to 50%.
- Halothane and desflurane have unfavorable effect on dynamics of CSF (increases production and decrease absorption). Sevoflurane has no effect while isoflurane has favorable effects on dynamics of CSF (increases absorption).

  Due to more favorable effects on cerebral hemodynamics (cerebral blood flow and ICT),

better preservation of autoregulation, equivalent reduction in cerebral metabolic rate and smoother *recovery sevoflurane is preferred over isoflurane as an inhalational agent of choice for neurosurgery in current day anesthetic practice.*

Intravenous Anesthetics

- Barbiturates, propofol, etomidate and benzodiazepines decrease CBF, CMR, CMO_2 and ICT. Barbiturates are most potent in this aspect.
- Opioids decrease CMR and CMO_2 but increases CBF (directly acting cerebral vasodilator) and hence ICT. This increase in CBF is significant when blood brain barrier is disrupted.
- Ketamine increases CBF and ICT very significantly (up to 60%). Ketamine also increases CMR and CMO_2.

Muscle Relaxants

- Succinylcholine increases the ICT.
- Non-depolarizing muscle relaxants do not cross the blood brain barrier.

Local Anesthetics

Lignocaine decreases CBF, CMR, CMO_2 (but at toxic doses it can induce seizure and can increase CMR).

Vasopressors
(Mephentermine, Ephedrine, Epinephrine)

Increase CBF indirectly by increasing cerebral perfusion pressure.

Vasodilators

Increase CBF and ICT by causing direct cerebral vasodilatation.

GENERAL CONSIDERATIONS IN NEUROSURGICAL PATIENTS

Fluids

It is difficult to determine the most ideal fluid for neurosurgery. As hyperglycemia can precipitate cerebral edema therefore, *Glucose containing solutions should be avoided.* Ringer lactate is hypoosmolar therefore, in large quantities can aggravate cerebral edema. Normal saline is large quantities can cause hyperchloremic metabolic acidosis. Therefore, *the best policy is to alternate ringer and normal saline liter by liter.*

The concern of colloids crossing disrupted blood brain barrier in head injuries or intracranial hemorrhages aggravating the cerebral edema is more theoretical, *therefore, if necessary colloids can be safely used for resuscitation,* however, their use should be limited because of their property to inhibit coagulation.

Hypothermia

The role of mild hypothermia is only restricted to the surgeries at high risk of ischemia. *Routine use of hypothermia is not recommended.*

Glycemic Control

Both hyperglycemia as well as hypoglycemia can be detrimental therefore, *blood sugar should be best maintained between 140 and 180 mg%.*

Monitoring

- Most important is *Capnography.* Hypercapnia is the most potent cerebral vasodilator therefore, can significantly increase the ICT. Moderate hypocapnia (pCO_2 between 25 and 30 mm Hg) is beneficial by decreasing ICT however excessive hypocapnia ($pCO_2 < 25$ mm Hg) can cause cerebral ischemia.
- *Pulse oximetry:* Hypoxia should be avoided as it increases ICT by causing cerebral vasodilatation.
- *Continuous (Invasive) blood pressure:* As autoregulation is often impaired in patients undergoing neurosurgery, cerebral perfusion pressure (CPP) becomes directly dependent on mean arterial pressure (MAP). Hypertension can increase ICT and hemorrhage while hypotension can cause cerebral ischemia. *The aim should be to maintain CPP (MAP-ICP) between 70 and 100 mm Hg* not only in intra-operative period but also in post-operative period for at least 2–3 days.

  To get CPP the *transducer should be zeroed at the level of external auditory meatus* not at right atrial level.
- *Central venous pressure (CVP):* CVP monitoring is needed only if large fluctuations in hemodynamics are expected. The concern of decreasing venous return and thereby increasing ICT with jugular venous calculation only appears to be theoretical.
- *Intracranial pressure (ICP):* ICP monitoring may be required if ICP is highly elevated and not getting controlled with conservative measures.

Emergence

Smooth emergence, i.e. emergence free of coughing, straining, and hypertension is must in neurosurgical patients. Coughing or hypertension during extubation not only significantly increase the ICT but can also cause massive bleeding. The best possible methods to achieve smooth emergence is to inject lignocaine before extubation, continue inhalational (at least N_2O) till dressing is over and use β blockers (Esmolol, Labetalol) if necessary.

ANESTHESIA FOR CONDITIONS WITH RAISED INTRACRANIAL TENSION

Usual conditions encountered with raised intracranial tension are:
- Intracranial space occupying lesions (ISOL).
- Head injuries.
- Cerebrovascular accidents.

Preoperative

If the patient is on steroids they must be continued and if not then *steroids must be started in preoperative period for ISOL but not for head injury;* preoperative steroids in head injury may prove to be detrimental. For edema due to ISOL 24–48-hour course of dexamethasone, 10 mg intravenously or orally every 6 hours, is optimal.

Intraoperative

Interventions to *decrease intracranial tension should be instituted at the earliest.* Hyperventilation should be started even from mask ventilation.

Choice of Anesthesia

Central neuraxial blocks are absolutely contra-indicated in raised ICT.

General anesthesia:
Premedication should to be avoided.

Induction: Although Thiopentone has more favorable effect on CMR and ICT than propofol but still due to shorter half-life *propofol is preferred over thiopentone for induction.*

Intubation: Intubation can significantly increase the ICT therefore, response to laryngoscopy and intubation must be blunted with lignocaine, adequate depth and β blockers.

Succinylcholine increases the ICT however, the increase is transient and can be revered with hyperventilation therefore *Suxamethonium is not absolutely contraindicated for neurosurgery* and can be safely used if there is clear indication like rapid sequence induction or possibility of difficult airway.

Maintenance: Oxygen, nitrous oxide and *sevoflurane.* However, if ICP is too high to be controlled or surgical field is too tight that inhalational agents should be avoided and anesthesia is maintained on IV agents.

Additional Considerations for Head Injury

Surgeries usually done are for drainage of extradural/subdural hematoma or for intracranial hemorrhage.

Management of head injury begins from emergency room. It includes:

- *Management of airway:* All patients of head injury should be assumed to be having cervical injury (incidence up to 15%) until proved otherwise and airway is to be managed accordingly (*for management of cervical injury see Chapter 5, page no. 56*).
- *Breathing:* Hyperventilation to be instituted at the earliest. *Nasal intubation should not be performed unless basal skull fracture has been ruled out.*
- *Circulation:* Hypotension associated with head injury is usually due to bleeding from other sites. Control of bleeding and management of hypotension takes priority.
- Rule out other major injuries like chest, abdominal or pelvic injuries and fracture of long bones.
- As *DIC* is commonly associated with head injury due to release of brain thromboplastin it must be ruled out in preoperative period.
- *Assessment of neurologic status:* The best method for assessing neurologic status is *modified Glasgow coma scale* which includes:

– Eye opening	*Score*
Nil	1
To pain	2
To speech	3
Spontaneously	4
– *Best motor response*	
None	1
Extension	2
Decorticate flexion	3
Withdrawal	4
Localizes pain	5
To verbal command	6
– *Best verbal response*	
Nil	1
Incomprehensible (garbled) sound	2
Inappropriate words	3
Confused	4
Oriented	5

Normal score is 15/15. Severe head injury is stated to be present if score is 7 or less and if persist for more than 6 hours is associated with more than 35% mortality.

- Number of times these patients may not be fasting requiring rapid sequence induction.
- Acute rise in ICT (>60 mm Hg) may cause irreversible brain damage or death in head injuries.

Additional Considerations for Posterior Fossa Surgery

Patients undergoing posterior fossa surgeries can have the following additional complications:

Venous Air Embolism

Posterior fossa surgeries are performed in sitting position. In sitting position dural sinuses are above the level of heart therefore, have subatmospheric pressure. Once the dura is opened, air from atmosphere can be sucked in causing venous air embolism.

The incidence of venous air embolism (VAE) can be as high as 20–40% in posterior fossa craniotomies however, fortunately the incidence of clinically significant VAE is very less. The major portion of the air gets absorbed through pulmonary circulation. *VAE can become clinically significant if the volume of entertained air > 100 mL* (however death has been reported with as low as 5 mL of air) or can be devastating if it becomes *paradoxical,* i.e. reaches left side of circulation (usually through patent foramen ovale). Paradoxical embolism can cause coronary block causing cardiac arrest or cerebral block causing massive infarcts.

Diagnosis:

- *The most sensitive tool to detect VAE is trans-esophageal echocardiography (TEE).* It can detect as low as 0.25 mL of air. Other advantage of TEE is that *it can measure the quantity of air, diagnose paradoxical embolism* and can assess cardiac function.
- *Precordial Doppler:* It is less sensitive than TEE.
- *End tidal carbon dioxide (ETCO$_2$):* Sudden drop in ETCO$_2$ values after the opening of dura strongly suggests venous air embolism.
- *End tidal nitrogen:* Sudden increase in end tidal nitrogen is more specific for VAE.
- Alveolar dead space, pulmonary artery pressure and CVP can increase due to blockage of pulmonary circulation.
- ECG may shows arrhythmias.
- *Clinical signs:*
  - Hypotension
  - Tachycardia
  - Cyanosis
  - *Mill wheel murmur*
  - Cardiovascular collapse

  Clinical signs appear late in venous air embolism.

  To conclude, the sensitivity of various tests for detection of air embolism in decreasing order is:

  TEE → Precordial Doppler → PAP, ETCO$_2$, ET nitrogen → CVP → ECG → clinical signs.

Treatment:

- Ask the surgeon to pack and flood the area with saline, apply wax to cut edges of bone to prevent further sucking of air.
- Stop *nitrous oxide* and start 100% oxygen. Nitrous oxide can expand the size of air embolus.
- Cardiopulmonary resuscitation, if cardiac arrest has occurred.
- Aspirate air through right atrial catheter (CVP catheter). That is why putting a CVP catheter makes sense in posterior fossa surgery.
- *Bilateral jugular venous compression and Trendelenburg position:* These maneuvers by increasing cerebral venous pressure will decrease air entrainment. Same way, positive end expiratory pressure (PEEP) will also reduce the air entrainment but avoided by most of the clinicians as it can increase the possibility of paradoxical embolism.

- Hypotension is to be managed with inotropic support like dopamine or dobutamine.
- Treat arrhythmias.
- Treat bronchospasm.
- Left lateral position (right chest up) to keep the air on right side of heart is now recommended only if right to left shunt is suspected.
- Hyperbaric oxygen to reduce size of air bubble. It is helpful if transfer to hyperbaric chamber is done within 8 hours.

Pneumocephalus

Like venous air embolism the incidence of pneumocephalus is high in sitting position. Once pneumocephalus develops air may remain in cranium up to 1 week. Using nitrous oxide during this period can be detrimental.

Injury to Brainstem

Injury to respiratory or cardiovascular centers during posterior fossa surgery may turn out to be fatal events.

Obstructive Hydrocephalus

Infratentorial masses can obstruct CSF flow leading to massive increase in ICT.

Additional Considerations for Stroke/Surgery for Cerebral Aneurysms

The patients after hemorrhagic stroke may come for emergency surgery for removal of clot or for control of bleeding or they may be posted for later date for aneurysmal clipping to prevent rebleeding or for carotid endarterectomy (CEA) to prevent another ischemic stroke.

Timing of Surgery

- *Emergency surgery* has to be conducted with the following considerations:
  - Blood should be available
  - Intracranial tension should not be reduced rapidly. Sudden shrinkage of brain may remove the tamponade effect causing re-bleeding.
  - *Avoid hypertension* (can cause re-bleeding) *as well as hypotension* (can cause ischemia)
  - Cardiac evaluation and ruling out syndrome of inappropriate antidiuretic hormone (SIADH) or salt wasting

syndrome is must in patients with subarachnoid hemorrhage

- If early intervention is not feasible due to any reason then *surgery should at least be delayed for 2 weeks to avoid the period of maximal vasospasm risk (4–14 days)*. Surgeries done in this period carries high morbidity and mortality. If it is mandatory to do surgery in this period than *"Triple H" therapy* (hypervolemia, hypertension and hemodilution) should be added to nimodipine for the treatment of vasospasm.
- Hypotensive anesthesia which used to be the cornerstone of aneurysm surgery is hardly used in current day anesthesia practice.
- Studies have shown that 6 weeks after a stroke there occurs reasonable recovery of autoregulation, blood brain barrier and CO_2 responsiveness therefore, *Carotid endarterectomy (CEA) can be undertaken after 6 weeks*. Delaying CEA surgeries beyond 6 weeks carries the risk of re-infarction. Other *elective surgeries should be deferred for 9 months after cerebrovascular accident*. The possibility of serious complications including another stroke, heart attack or even death remains significantly high up to 9 months. The odds of complications are stabilized at 3 times after 9 months.

ANESTHESIA FOR AWAKE CRANIOTOMIES (STEREOTACTIC SURGERY)

- Stereotactic surgeries are done for treating involuntary movements (Parkinsonism), intractable pain syndromes and epilepsy.

The surgeon need awake patient to locate the exact focus.

- Neuroleptanalgesia which used to be very popular technique in past is not used now a days due to QT prolongation (precipitating polymorphic ventricular tachycardia) seen with droperidol. The most commonly used technique used now a day is *"Asleep-awake-asleep"*. In this technique, patient is given anesthesia with short acting agents (Propofol, dexmedetomidine, remifentanil, etc.) for the painful part of craniotomy (reaching up to dura) then anesthetic agents are stopped so that patient becomes awake. Once the surgeon is done with the procedure patient is again given anesthesia for another painful part of surgery, i.e. closure.

ANESTHETIC MANAGEMENT OF SPINE SURGERIES

- Document all neurological deficits in preoperative sheet to avoid medicolegal litigations.
- Assess cervical movements in all planes if the disease involves cervical spine.
- The major concerns of spine surgery are related to prone position (*for complications related to prone position see Chapter 14, page no. 146*), excessive bleeding and possibility of neural damage. The assessment of neural functions should preferably be done by monitoring-evoked responses. However, if that facility is not available then keep the patient awake and avoid muscle relaxants during the crucial steps which can cause neurological damage.

KEY POINTS

- All inhalational agents inhibit autoregulation of cerebral blood flow while it remains largely preserved with most of the intravenous anesthetics.
- pCO_2 should be maintained between 25–30 mm Hg to achieve optimal hypocapnia.
- Hyperosmolar drugs like mannitol are not absolutely contraindicated in disrupted blood brain barrier like head injury or stroke however, should be used judiciously.
- All inhalational agents (including nitrous oxide) increase the cerebral blood flow and ICT. The order of vasodilating potency is- halothane >>Desflurane ≈ Isoflurane>Sevoflurane.
- Due to more favorable effects sevoflurane is preferred over isoflurane as an inhalational agent of choice in neurosurgery in current day anesthetic practice.

Contd...

Contd...

- All IV agents except ketamine decrease CBF, CMR and ICT.
- As hyperglycemia can cause cerebral edema, Glucose containing solutions should be avoided in neurosurgery.
- If necessary colloids can be safely used in neurosurgical patient however, there their use should be limited.
- Routine use of hypothermia is not recommended.
- Blood sugar should be best maintained between 140–180 mg%.
- Capnography is more than mandatory monitor for neurosurgical patients.
- The aim during neurosurgical procedures is to maintain cerebral perfusion pressure between 70 and 100 mm Hg.
- Not only induction, recovery should also be very smooth in neurosurgical patients.
- Steroids must be started in preoperative period in patients having brain edema due to brain tumor while preoperative steroids should be avoided if edema is due to head injury.
- Central neuraxial blocks are absolutely contraindicated in raised ICT.
- Suxamethonium is not absolutely contraindicated for neurosurgery.
- All head injury patients should be assumed to be having cervical injury and basal skull fracture until proved otherwise.
- Venous air embolism is the most bothersome complication of posterior fossa craniotomies.
- Venous air embolism can become clinically significant if the volume of entertained air > 100 mL.
- The most sensitive tool to detect venous air embolism is transesophageal echocardiography.
- After stroke surgery should avoided in period of maximal vasospasm risk (4–14 days) as far as possible.
- Carotid endarterectomy can be undertaken after 6 weeks while other elective surgeries should be deferred for 9 months after cerebrovascular accident.
- The major concerns of spine surgery are related to prone position.

CHAPTER 28

Anesthesia for Obstetrics

There are considerable physiological changes in parturient which can significantly increase the maternal morbidity and mortality.

PHYSIOLOGICAL CHANGES IN PREGNANCY

Cardiovascular System

- Intravascular fluid volume ↑ by 35%
- Cardiac output ↑ by 40%
- Systemic vascular resistance ↓ by 15%
- Heart rate ↑ by 15%
- Blood pressure ↓ by 5–20% (Diastolic decreases more than systolic)

↑: Increase; ↓: Decrease

The clinical implication of cardiovascular changes is that pregnant patients are more vulnerable for cardiac failure due to hyperdynamic circulation.

Respiratory System

Tidal volume	↑ by 40%
Respiratory rate	↑ by 10%
Minute ventilation	↑ by 50%
Functional residual capacity (FRC), Expiratory reserve volume (ERV) and residual volume (RV)	↓ by 20% (FRC, ERV and RV decreases due to gravid uterus causing diaphragmatic elevation and basal atelectasis)
Vital capacity	No change
Oxygen consumption	↑ by 20%

Blood gases	
pO_2	↑ by 10 mm Hg (Due to hyperventilation)
pCO_2	↓ by 10 mm Hg (due to hyperventilation)
pH	No change (due to compensation)

↑: Increase; ↓: Decrease

Anesthetic Implications of Respiratory Changes

- Due to increase minute ventilation the induction with inhalational agents may be faster.
- Due to decreased FRC, ERV and increased oxygen requirement pregnant patients are more vulnerable for hypoxia therefore, preoxygenation is must.
- Due to capillary engorgement in upper airways chances of trauma and bleeding during intubation are high.

Nervous System

- *Progesterone decreases the minimum alveolar concentration by 25–40% making pregnant patients more susceptible to anesthetic over dosage.*
- As the epidural veins are in direct communication with inferior vena cava, compression of inferior vena cava by gravid uterus causes engorgement of epidural veins decreasing the subarachnoid space leading the drugs to spread higher making *pregnant patients more vulnerable for high spinal. Therefore, to prevent high spinal the dose of local anesthetic for spinal has to be reduced by 30–40%.*

- Due to increased cerebrospinal fluid (CSF) pressure *pregnant patient are more vulnerable for post-spinal headache.*
- Due to decreased epidural space *chances for accidental dural puncture is high after epidural* in pregnant patients.

Gastrointestinal System

Parturients are very vulnerable for aspiration (sometimes they can even aspirate spontaneously called as *Mendelson syndrome*) due to the following reasons:

- Gastric emptying is delayed due to progesterone.
- Gravid uterus alters the normal gastroesophageal angle making lower esophageal sphincter (LES) to become incompetent.
- Progesterone relaxes the LES.
- Gastric contents are more acidic.

Anesthetic Implications

Pregnant patients are so vulnerable for aspiration that *all pregnant patients should be considered full stomach even if they are fasting for more than 8 hours and must be managed like a high risk case for aspiration.*

Hematological System

Pregnancy is a hypercoagulable state due to increase in factor I and factor VII. Increase in plasma volume causes dilutional thrombocytopenia and physiologic anemia of pregnancy.

Leukocytosis without infection is common in pregnancy.

Anesthetic Implications

Pregnant patients are more vulnerable for thromboembolism. Excessive thrombocytopenia (platelet count < 80,0000) may deter the anesthetist to give central neuraxial block.

Hepatic System

Plasma cholinesterase level is decreased by 25% theoretically prolonging the effect of succinylcholine however, clinically this effect is insignificant.

Kidneys

Because of increase in cardiac output there is increase in renal blood flow and glomerular filtration rate (GFR).

Uterus

In supine position gravid uterus can compress the inferior vena cava and aorta decreasing the cardiac output causing *supine hypotension syndrome* (SHS) which this *can cause severe hypotension or even cardiac arrest after spinal anesthesia.*

To prevent SHS the *pregnant patient should lie in left lateral position* which can be accomplished by putting a *15° wedge under right buttock* or by tilting the delivery table by 15° to left or by manually displacing the uterus to left.

EFFECT OF ANESTHETIC TECHNIQUE/DRUGS ON UTEROPLACENTAL CIRCULATION

Uterine blood flow is 500–700 mL/min (10% of cardiac output) and placental flow is directly dependent on maternal blood flow. Anything that causes hypotension like central neuraxial blocks, intermittent positive pressure ventilation (IPPV) during GA, inhalational agents, IV agents (Thiopentone and Propofol) or causes maternal vasoconstriction (vasopressors) or increases uterine tone (ketamine) can decreases the maternal flow and hence placental blood flow compromising the fetal wellbeing.

TRANSFER OF ANESTHETIC DRUGS TO FETAL CIRCULATION

All anesthetic drugs except muscle relaxants (only gallamine has significant transfer) and glycopyrrolate can be transferred to fetus from maternal circulation. Therefore, all drugs should be used in minimum concentration and dosage.

A large fraction of drug reaching the fetus is metabolized by fetal liver (75% of umbilical vein blood flows through liver) therefore less drug reaches to the vital structures like brain and heart. However, drugs like *local anesthetics and opioids can get accumulated in fetus.* Local anesthetics and opioids are bases; they crosses the placenta in unionized form, become ionized in fetal circulation (due to low pH) and cannot come back to maternal circulation leading to their trapping (called as ion trapping) and accumulation in fetus.

ANESTHESIA FOR CESAREAN SECTION

Regional anesthesia is preferred over general anesthesia.

Advantages of Regional (Spinal/Epidural) over General Anesthesia

- Risk of *pulmonary aspiration (which is 4 times more in obstetrics)* can be avoided.
- The possibility of *failed intubation (which is 8 times more in obstetrics)* can be avoided.

  Because of pulmonary aspiration and failed intubation *the mortality in obstetrics during general anesthesia (GA) is twice as compared to regional anesthesia.*

- Effect of anesthetic drugs on fetus can be avoided.
- Awake mother can interact with her newborn immediately after surgery.
- High inspired concentration of oxygen to mother can be delivered.

Disadvantages

- Increase procedure time makes spinal/epidural unsuitable for emergency situations like severe fetal distress.
- If hypotension is significant, it can compromise fetal circulation.
- *Pregnant patients are more vulnerable for high spinal and postspinal headache after spinal and accidental dural puncture after epidural.*

Anesthetic Considerations

- During cesarean there occurs handling of gut and mesentery therefore *level up to T4 is required.*
- As the pregnant patients are very vulnerable for high spinal *doses of local anesthetic should be reduced by 30–40%.*
- Left lateral tilt should be maintained to *prevent supine hypotension syndrome.*
- Hypotension can compromise fetal wellbeing therefore should be aggressively treated by fluids and vasopressors. However, disadvantage of vasopressors is that they not only produce vasoconstriction in maternal circulation but also in uteroplacental bed compromising fetal circulation except ephedrine which does not produces significant vasoconstriction in uteroplacental bed. Due to this reason Ephedrine had always been the vasopressor of choice in pregnancy however, recent human trials have shown phenylephrine to produce less fetal acidosis than ephedrine making *phenylephrine as a preferred vasopressor over ephedrine in pregnancy in current day anesthetic practice.*
- Onset of epidural takes a long time (15–20 minutes) therefore it is reserved for elective cases only or for specific conditions like pregnancy-induced hypertension (PIH).

General Anesthesia for Cesarean Section

GA is usually given for fetal distress when there is no time to given spinal or if there is contraindication for spinal anesthesia.

Premedication

All pregnant patients must be considered full stomach irrespective of their fasting status and must be managed like rapid sequence induction. Therefore, they must be premedicated with metoclopramide, sodium citrate (to neutralize pH) and ranitidine.

Induction

As induction is rapid sequence where bag and mask ventilation is contraindicated, preoxygenation becomes must. Due to dire emergency if it is not possible to preoxygenate for 3 minutes then patient must be asked to take 3–4 deep breaths with 100% oxygen as an alternative to preoxygenation.

Thiopentone had been the induction agent of choice in the past as propofol safety had not been proven in newborns however, now it is seen that at the doses used for induction *Propofol does not affect the APGAR therefore can be safely used in pregnancy.* Ketamine appears a good choice as it preserves upper airway reflexes however, generally avoided because of its hallucinogenic side effects and tendency to increase uterine tone at high doses.

Intubation is done with suxamethonium while assistant applies the cricoid pressure. *Anticipate difficult intubation* due to airway edema.

Maintenance

All inhalational agents in current use can relax the uterus in same magnitude and can cause postpartum hemorrhage (PPH) however it has been seen that at concentration less than half minimum alveolar concentration (MAC) they do not produces significant uterine relaxation therefore can be used safely in concentration <0.5 MAC. Traditionally isoflurane had been most preferred because of its cardiac stability however sevoflurane and desflurane are equally good alternatives.

Opioids can be given only after the delivery of baby. All muscle relaxant except gallamine can be used safely.

Anesthetic Considerations for Cesarean Section in Patients with Pregnancy-induced Hypertension/Preeclampsia

Before giving central neuraxial blocks it is important to rule out HELLP syndrome.

Anesthesia of Choice

Anesthetic technique of choice is epidural. Difficult intubation due to *laryngeal edema* can make GA to become risky. As PIH patients are hypertensive they are more prone for hypotension however, if necessary spinal can be given to PIH patients.

If the patient is having HELLP syndrome then epidural also becomes contraindicated and patient receives GA instead of laryngeal edema.

General Anesthesia

- As stated above intubation can be difficult due to laryngeal edema.
- Attenuation of cardiovascular response to intubation must be blunted, otherwise intracranial hemorrhage can occur.
- Many patients are on *magnesium which can potentiate the action of muscle relaxants* or can cause respiratory or cardiac arrest at toxic levels.
- If the patient presents with active seizures (eclampsia) induction should be done with thiopentone (anticonvulsant) and followed by general anesthesia in same way as for cesarean patient.

Anesthetic Considerations for Cesarean Section in Patients with Heart Diseases

The anesthetic considerations in patients with heart diseases depend on the existing lesions and the management is guided by the same principles applicable for cardiac patients. For example, in patients with severe fixed cardiac output lesion like mitral or aortic stenosis central neuraxial blocks should be avoided. Pregnant patients are more vulnerable for cardiac failure than nonpregnant patient.

LABOR ANALGESIA (PAINLESS LABOR)

Pain afferents from uterus and cervix travel up to *T10-L1*. Most commonly used technique is *continuous lumbar epidural.*

Lumbar Epidural

Timing to Start

Contrary to the previous recommendation that painless labor should be started once the labor is well established (i.e. cervix should be at least 3–4 cm dilated), the current recommendation is to start painless labor *when the patient demands* irrespective of the stage of labor.

Procedure

Epidural catheter is placed in lumbar space (usually L3-4) and 8–10 mL of bupivacaine (0.0625%–0.25%) or Ropivacaine (0.1-0.2%) (Ropivacaine preferred) + 2 µg/mL of fentanyl is given through catheter after confirming the position of catheter by test dose with 2-3 mL of lignocaine. Bolus dose is followed by the same concentration of bupivacaine/ropivacaine + fentanyl given as continuous infusion at a rate of 8–10 mL/hr. If the concentration of bupivacaine used is too low (0.0625%) it is called as *walking epidural* (means patient can move out of the bed and sit in recliner).

Lignocaine with adrenaline should be avoided for test dose in pregnant patient due to 2 reasons. Firstly, theoretically it can decrease uterine blood supply and secondly, as there is already so much variation in heart rate due to labor that it becomes impossible to differentiate whether the change in heart rate is due to intravascular injection or labor.

Complications

- *Accidental dural puncture* is a known complications. If there occur accidental dural puncture clinician is left with 2 options. First, to remove needle and try epidural in other space. Second, to pass a catheter in subarachnoid space and maintain analgesia with "continuous spinal" instead of "continuous epidural". The infusion rate used for continuous spinal is low, i.e. 1–3 mL/hr instead of 8–10 mL/hr used for epidural. The second option, i.e. continuous spinal should be preferred.

- *Low concentration epidurals neither increases the rate of cesarean section nor the rate of instrumental delivery* however, can delay the duration of labour by 30–60 minutes.

Combined Spinal Epidural

Some clinicians give spinal with a very small dose (2.5 mg, i.e. 0.5 mL) of hyperbaric bupivacaine + 10 μg of fentanyl before giving epidural. The advantage is immediate relief of pain due to rapid onset of spinal. Motor block does not occur with such a small dose of bupivacaine.

Other regional techniques like Double Catheter (first stage pain relief achieved by lumbar epidural and second stage by sacral epidural catheter), Pudendal Nerve Block (for second stage only) or Paracervical Block (can cause severe fetal bradycardia and cardiotoxicity) are hardly use in present day anesthetic practice.

Entonox Inhalation

The patients who cannot receive epidural are given entonox (combination of 50% oxygen and 50% nitrous oxide) through a self-inhaler mask.

Parenteral Narcotics

Intramuscular pethidine+ promethazine (phenergan) had been the very popular combination in past. Other short acting opioids like fentanyl, sufentanil and remifentanil can be used intravenously in small increments. As remifentanil is metabolized in maternal plasma, insignificant amount reaches the fetus making *remifentanil as a parenteral opioid of choice for pain relief in labor analgesia.* Parenteral narcotic should be used only as last resort as there is always a risk of fetal as well as maternal respiratory depression.

ANESTHESIA FOR MANUAL REMOVAL OF PLACENTA

Patients with retained placenta may bleed profusely. They need hemodynamic stability before considering for anesthesia. As all inhalational agents in current use are uterine relaxants therefore, anesthesia of choice is GA with inhalational agents. The choice of inhalational agents is guided by the hemodynamic parameters; for example, if the patient is in shock then inhalational agent preferred will be desflurane.

ANESTHESIA FOR NON-OBSTETRIC SURGERIES DURING PREGNANCY

The most common surgeries performed are appendectomies and cholecystectomies or patients may come for trauma surgeries.

- *Elective surgery should be deferred until postpartum period (6 weeks postdelivery) while urgent surgeries should be performed during the second trimester.*

In first trimester, there are increased chances of abortion and congenital abnormalities. During third trimester there are increased chances of preterm labor therefore only emergency operations should be performed in first and third trimester.

- *If any surgery has to be done from 14 weeks of gestation to 48 hours after delivery then aspiration prophylaxis should be taken.*

Choice of Anesthesia

The aim should be to *avoid general anesthesia therefore, anesthesia of choice is regional anesthesia.* Ensure that there does not occur hypotension after spinal as it can compromise fetal circulation.

General Anesthesia

The general principle is to use anesthetic drugs when absolutely necessary and in minimal possible doses. The concern of teratogenicity of nitrous oxide and benzodiazepines does not appear to be real in humans however, they should be avoided as far as possible. Similarly, propofol can also be used safely.

During laparoscopies ensure that surgeon uses minimum intra-abdominal pressure to prevent hypotension.

KEY POINTS

- Hyperdynamic circulation makes pregnant patients more vulnerable for cardiac failure.
- Decreased FRC, ERV and increased oxygen requirement makes pregnant patients more vulnerable for hypoxia.

Contd...

Contd…

- Minimum alveolar concentration decreases by 25 to 40% in pregnant patients making them more susceptible to anesthetic over dosage.
- Pregnant patients are very prone to develop high spinal.
- Supine hypotension syndrome (SHS) can cause severe hypotension or even cardiac arrest after spinal anesthesia. To prevent SHS the pregnant patient should lie in left lateral position.
- All anesthetic drugs except muscle relaxants (only Gallamine has significant transfer) and glycopyrolate can be transferred to fetus from maternal circulation.
- Due to alkaline pH local anesthetics and opioids can get accumulated in fetus.
- Regional anesthesia is preferred over general anesthesia for cesarean section because risk of pulmonary aspiration and possibility of failed intubation can be avoided.
- Because of pulmonary aspiration and failed intubation the mortality in obstetrics during GA is twice as compared to regional anesthesia.
- All pregnant patients must be considered full stomach irrespective of their fasting status and must be managed like rapid sequence induction.
- At concentration less than half minimum alveolar concentration (MAC) inhalational agents do not produces significant uterine relaxation.
- Contrary to old recommendations propofol can be safely used in pregnancy.
- Anesthetic technique of choice for PIH is epidural.
- Most commonly used technique for painless labor is continuous lumbar epidural.
- Maternal demand is sufficient indication to start painless labor.
- Low concentration epidurals neither increase the rate of cesarean section nor the rate of instrumental delivery.
- Nonobstetric elective surgery should be deferred until postpartum period (6 weeks postdelivery) while urgent surgeries should be performed during the second trimester.
- Anesthesia of choice for non-obstetric surgery is regional.

CHAPTER 29

Pediatric Anesthesia

Pediatric patients have number of physiologic and anatomic differences from adults which not only alter the anesthesia techniques but increase the anesthetic morbidity and mortality as compared to adults.

PHYSIOLOGICAL/ANATOMICAL CHANGES IN PEDIATRIC POPULATION

Respiratory System

Airway (Anatomical Differences)

As compared to adults, children (particularly infants) have large head size, large tongue, mobile, large and leafy epiglottis. The larynx is more anterior and high (at C4 compared to C6 in adults). *Subglottis* (at the level of *cricoid*) is the *narrowest* part. Vocal cords are more diagonal during infancy (not horizontal as in adults).

Physiologic Changes

See **Table 29.1**.

Anesthetic Implications of Respiratory Changes

- Due to large head and anteriorly placed larynx, intubation is easier in neutral or slightly flexed position of head.

■ **Table 29.1:** Respiratory physiologic changes

Parameter	Value		Comments
	Neonate	Adult	
Tidal volume	6–8 mL/kg	6–8 mL/kg	Oxygen consumption is twice that of adults and calorie requirement is three times. The tidal volume on body weight basis is same so important *determinant of high alveolar ventilation is respiratory rate*
Frequency (respiratory rate)	35/minute	14–16/minute	
Alveolar ventilation	120–140 mL/kg/minute	60–70 mL/kg/minute	
Oxygen consumption	6 mL/kg/minute	3 mL/kg/minute	
Calorie requirement	100 kcal/kg	30 kcal/kg	
Blood Gases			
pH	7.34–7.40	7.36–7.44	
pO_2	65–85 mm Hg (at birth) (intrauterine pO_2 is 25–40 mm Hg)	95–97 mm Hg	
pCO_2	30–36 mm Hg	35–45 mm Hg	Due to high respiratory rate

- Large tongue can obscure the view during laryngoscopy.
- Due to anatomical configuration of airway and large epiglottis intubation is preferred with *straight blade* (Magill) laryngoscope in neonates and infants.
- As subglottis (at the level of cricoid) is the narrowest part of larynx in children up to 6 years of age and tracheal diameter is narrow up to 10 years, the traditional approach had been not to use cuffed tube up to 6 years and avoiding cuffed tube up to 10 years. However, this *approach of not using cuffed tubes in children up to 10 years does not hold true in present day practice.* Many studies and development of better tube designs [especially microcuff tubes which have very soft and low lying cuff (placed below the cricoid)] has allowed the use of cuffed tubes even for infants. Nonetheless *a leak must be maintained around the cuff (inflated or not inflated) at a pressure of more than 15–20 cm H_2O. This* will not only prevent tracheal mucosal injury but also the barotrauma. However, excessive leak must not be allowed; excessive leak not only causes hypoventilation but can increase the risk of aspiration in high risk cases like full stomach child undergoing emergency surgery.
- Because of high alveolar ventilation induction with inhalational agents is faster.
- Due to high oxygen requirement and low reserve, children are very prone for developing *hypoxia.*
- The poor control of ventilation makes pediatric patients more vulnerable for hypoventilation in postoperative period.

Cardiovascular System
- Blood pressure in neonate is 60/40 mm Hg (50% of adult value) therefore, *cardiac output is mainly determined by heart rate* which is 120–140/minute at birth. *Bradycardia is the most common adverse cardiac event during perioperative period in pediatric patients.* Cardiac arrests are more common in pediatric age group as compared to adults.
- Vasoconstriction response is not so well developed therefore, pediatric patients may not tolerate shock.

Anesthetic Implications
- Bradycardia is not acceptable at any cost.
- Infants can develop severe hypotension and cardiac depression with inhalational agents.

Body Water
- Extracellular fluid (ECF) constitutes 40% of body weight (in adults ECF constitutes 20% of body weight). The high volume of distribution can dilute the initial intravenous drug therefore, the *initial dose requirement (on per kg weight basis) is higher than adults.*
- Fluid administration is very tricky in children. Less intake can make them easily dehydrated (because of high metabolic rate) and slightly excessive fluid can lead to *fluid overload* (heart is less compliant to tolerate volume loads). Therefore, fluid administration should be strictly on the recommended guidelines (See in fluid management section).

Metabolic
Due to inadequate glycogen stores and high metabolic rate children are comparatively more prone to hypoglycemia.

Thermoregulation
Children are very prone for *hypothermia* because of their decreased ability to produce and conserve heat and increased heat loss due to large body surface area. The only mechanism for heat production is metabolism of brown fat which is special fat present in posterior neck, interscapular and vertebral areas and around kidneys and adrenal glands.

To prevent hypothermia the operation theater temperature should be maintained at 28°C (usually maintained at 21°C for adults).

Blood
Hemoglobin at birth is 19 g% which falls to 10 g% at 2–3 months (physiologic anemia of infancy) thereafter it steadily increases to adult value by 12–13 years. Neonates have higher content of fetal hemoglobin which shifts the oxygen dissociation curve to left. Prolonged coagulation is expected in neonates due to vitamin K deficiency.

Central Nervous System

The neonates have immature brain and poorly developed blood brain barrier putting them at higher risk of over dosages.

Neonates have less minimum alveolar concentration (MAC) as compared to infants. Maximum MAC in human beings occurs in infancy peaking at the age of 6 months thereafter, decreasing steadily throughout the life (except a slight increase at puberty). So, the MAC requirement in decreasing order is *Infants > neonates > adults.*

The concern of apoptosis leading to long-term cognitive dysfunction after GA in young children has been shown only in animal models. Human studies still remains inconclusive.

Hepatic and Renal

Underdeveloped hepatic and renal functions may lead to prolonged effect of anesthetic agents. Moreover, decreased albumin increases the unbound fraction of the drugs.

Neonate is an obligate sodium loser and cannot conserve sodium, consequently may develop hyponatremia.

Neuromuscular Junction

Functional maturation of neuromuscular junction is not complete until 2 months of age therefore, newborns *are very sensitive to nondepolarizing muscle relaxants.*

ANESTHETIC MANAGEMENT

Fasting Recommendations

Fasting recommendations for children are:

Age	Milk and solid	Clear liquid (water)
< 6 months	4 hours (breast milk)	2 hours
6 months–3 years	6 hours	2 hours
> 3 years	8 hours	2 hours

Monitoring

Besides routine monitoring, temperature monitoring is very important in children.

Fluids

Considering the complexity of calculation of intraoperative fluid by traditional formula of 4-2-1 (calculate hourly maintenance then multiply by fasting hours and then add 3rd space losses) a simpler and probably more accurate method is to give *20–40 mL/kg of fluid during intraoperative period.* Thereafter, in postoperative period the fluid is given by the formula of 2-1-0.5, i.e. 0–10 kg @ 2 mL/kg, 10–20@1 mL/kg and > 20 kg @ 0.5 mL/kg. If the fluid has to be continued after 12 hours (child cannot be shifted to oral route) then 5% dextrose with 0.45% normal saline should be continued by the formula of 4-2-1.

However, if the clinician decides to give fluid by traditional 4-2-1 formula then to prevent fluid overload the child should *receive only two-thirds of the fluid requirement calculated by 4-2-1 formula.*

Choice of Fluid

As previously thought that children are very prone for hypoglycemia it is proven that they are not so prone therefore for *majority of the children ringer lactate may be the only fluid required.* Nevertheless if there is concern of hypoglycemia then 5% dextrose in 0.45% normal saline should be added as piggyback to balance salt solution and given at maintenance rates. It must not be used as replacement fluid for correcting deficit or third-space loss otherwise there can be significant hyperglycemia with it consequences.

Transfusion: Transfusion should be given only after exactly calculating the maximum allowable blood loss (*for details see Chapter 26, page no. 216*).

Choice of Anesthesia

Although regional nerve blocks are given frequently, often they are given only after giving GA.

General Anesthesia

Induction

Induction in children is a difficult task. Most commonly used techniques are:

- *Inhalational induction:* As the children will not allow putting IV lines *inhalational induction becomes the method of choice in majority of children.* Due to smooth and rapid induction, *sevoflurane (7–8%) is considered as the inhalational agent of choice* however, due to high cost, halothane is still very commonly used agent for induction in India. *Isoflurane and desflurane* have irritating induction and can produce severe laryngospasm therefore, *must not be used for induction.* If there is no IV access and the child develops laryngospasm then suxamethonium can be given intramuscular or sublingually.

A very important precaution is to put an intravenous line once the child falls asleep before proceeding to deeper plane.

- *Intravenous: Intravenous induction is always preferred over inhalational induction.* Older children may allow putting intravenous line. In smaller children if inhalational induction in contraindicated then IV line can be put by distracting the attention of child and by applying EMLA cream locally. Due to increase volume of distribution induction dose requirement will be higher.
- *Intramuscular:* Ketamine 5 mg/kg can be given IM when the child is in preoperative room with parents.
- *Rectal:* 10% Methohexital and midazolam can be used by this route however, not used in current day practice.

Intubation

As discussed above, intubation should preferably be done with neck in neutral position with straight blade in neonates and infants and with small Macintosh blade in children. Cuffed tubes can be used in pediatric age group.

Circuit: Jackson–Rees for children less than 6 years (or < 20 kg) and Bains for children more than 6 years (or >20 kg) are the semi-closed circuits used for children however, *preference should be pediatric circle system* (pediatric closed circuit).

Maintenance

Recent studies has shown a significant incidence of emergence agitation with sevoflurane (20%) and halothane (15%) making them unsuitable for maintenance. Therefore, *anesthesia is best maintained with desflurane* or isoflurane in case of nonavailability of desflurane.

To conclude—*sevoflurane and halothane are excellent agents for induction but not suitable for maintenance while desflurane and isoflurane are not suitable for induction but excellent for maintenance.*

Muscle relaxants

Atracurium and Cisatracurium are the relaxant of choice as they are not dependent on hepatic and renal functions.

Succinylcholine should be avoided in children due to presence of extrajunctional receptors and possibility of undiagnosed muscular dystrophy. The use of suxamethonium should be reserved for rapid sequence induction and for treating laryngospasm. Pediatric age group is very vulnerable for bradycardia after suxamethonium therefore, atropine must be given before injecting suxamethonium.

Postoperative Pain Management

In contrary to common misconception that children feel less pain, it has been very well proven that *pain perception in pediatric patients is same as adults*, rather due to underdevelopment of inhibitory control pathways it is more during infancy. Therefore, pain management considerations are equally important for children.

Regional nerve block is always a preferred option (Ropivacaine due to less toxicity is preferred over bupivacaine). If regional anesthesia is not possible then opioids can be used however, with closed monitoring. Short acting (fentanyl, remifentanil) should be preferred over long acting (morphine). Paracetamol or ketorolac/diclofenac suppositories or IV formulations should be used along with opioids to decrease their requirement.

REGIONAL ANESTHESIA IN PEDIATRIC PATIENTS

Age is no bar for regional anesthesia; any block can be given at any age. Regional anesthesia in pediatric population is given after GA to decrease the anesthetic requirement and achieve postoperative analgesia. Most commonly used blocks are caudal to be followed by ilioinguinal and penile.

Important differences from adults seen in pediatric population are:

- Onset of block is faster due to immature myelin sheath letting the drug to cross the sheath easily.
- Dose of local anesthetic required is less because drug can easily diffuse in the nerve due to lose sheath.

- Duration of block is less.
- Children are more vulnerable for toxicity due to increased systemic absorption (because of increased cardiac output) and decreased metabolism (due to underdeveloped hepatic functions).
- For differences in spinal anesthesia in pediatric patients *see Chapter 17, page no. 173.*

MANAGEMENT OF NEONATAL SURGICAL EMERGENCIES

Diaphragmatic Hernia

It results from incomplete closure of diaphragm leading to herniation of abdominal contents in thorax resulting in pulmonary hypoplasia, pulmonary hypertension and hypoplasia of left ventricle. Prognosis is very poor.

Anesthetic Management

- After preoxygenation *awake intubation* is done.
- *Bag and mask ventilation is contraindicated* (as it will increase the distension of bowels leading to more compression of lung).
- Positive pressure ventilation should be done with *airway pressure < 20 cm H_2O* otherwise pneumothorax can occur in hypoplastic lung. If available then ventilate with high frequency oscillatory ventilation.
- Anesthesia is maintained on oxygen and low dose volatile anesthetics or opioids like fentanyl. *Nitrous oxide is contraindicated* as it can diffuse into gut loop causing their distension and further compression of the lung.
- Postoperative elective ventilation is often required.

Tracheoesophageal Fistula

It is of five types, most common is upper end of esophagus is blind with fistula between lower esophagus and trachea.

Anesthetic Management

- Rule out associated abnormalities like atrial septal defect (ASD), ventricular septal defect (VSD), tetralogy of Fallot, coarctation of aorta.
- Nurse the baby in propped up position to minimize gastric regurgitation.

- Aspirate the upper blind pouch of esophagus to remove secretion from it.
- Ventilation with *bag and mask is contraindicated* as air can reach stomach through fistula causing gastric distension and aspiration.
- Intubation can be awake or after intravenous anesthetic. The position of *tube is most important; it should be below the fistula but above the carina.*
- These patients are very vulnerable for hypoxia as there occur significant V/Q mismatch in lateral position.

Pyloric Stenosis (Intestinal Obstruction)

- Due to repeated vomiting the patients with pyloric stenosis are dehydrated with hypokalemic, hypochloremic alkalosis therefore, *metabolic, fluid and electrolyte correction must be done* before taking the patient for surgery.
- Either awake intubation or rapid sequence intubation (crash intubation with Sellick's maneuver) is performed.
- *Ventilation with bag and mask is contraindicated* (can cause aspiration).

Anesthetic Considerations for Prematures

- Avoid elective surgeries till *50 weeks* of postconception.
- If the baby had developed hyaline membrane disease then defer elective surgery for 6 months.
- Premature are very vulnerable for postoperative apnea.

Anesthetic Considerations for Down Syndrome

- *Difficult airway* due to short neck, large tongue, irregular dentition, atlanto-occipital instability (avoid unnecessary flexion and extension of neck), small size trachea and subglottic stenosis.
- Associated congenital anomalies like congenital heart diseases (mainly endocardial cushion defects and VSD), tracheoesophageal fistula, mental retardation, seizures can increase morbidity and mortality.
- These patients may exhibit hypersensitivity to muscle relaxants due to hypotonia.

KEY POINTS

- The larynx is more anterior and high and subglottis (at the level of cricoid) is the narrowest part in children.
- Due to high oxygen requirement and low reserve, children are very prone for developing hypoxia.
- Contrary to previous recommendation cuffed tubes can be used in children but should allow a leak at a pressure of more than 15–20 cm H_2O.
- Bradycardia is the most common adverse cardiac event during perioperative period in pediatric patients.
- The high volume of distribution increases the initial dose requirement in children.
- MAC requirement in decreasing order is infants > neonates > adults.
- A simpler and probably more accurate formula than 4-2-1 is to give 20–40 mL/kg of fluid during intraoperative period. Thereafter, in postoperative period the fluid is given by the formula of 2-1-0.5.
- As children are not so prone for hypoglycemia ringer lactate may be the only fluid required.
- Inhalational induction is the most commonly utilized induction method in pediatric patients however, the method of choice for induction is always IV.
- Due to smooth and rapid induction, sevoflurane (7–8%) is considered as the inhalational agent of choice for induction.
- Isoflurane and desflurane has got irritating induction therefore, must not be used for induction.
- Sevoflurane and halothane are excellent agents for induction but not suitable for maintenance as they can cause postoperative agitation.
- Atracurium and Cisatracurium are the relaxant of choice as they do not depend on hepatic and renal functions.
- Succinylcholine should be avoided in children.
- Pain perception in pediatric patients is same as adults.
- Age is no bar for regional anesthesia; any block can be given at any age.
- Bag and mask ventilation is contraindicated for diaphragmatic hernia, tracheoesophageal fistula and pyloric stenosis.
- In diaphragmatic hernia positive pressure ventilation should be done with airway pressure < 20 cm H_2O.
- Nitrous oxide is contraindicated in diaphragmatic hernia surgery.
- The position of endotracheal in tracheoesophageal fistula should be below the fistula but above the carina.
- Metabolic, fluid and electrolyte correction must be done before taking the patient for pyloric stenosis surgery.
- Avoid elective surgeries in premature babies till 50 weeks of their postconception age.
- Airway management may be difficult in children suffering from Down syndrome.

CHAPTER 30

Geriatric Anesthesia

PHYSIOLOGICAL CHANGES IN OLD AGE

Cardiovascular System

Decreased ventricular compliance leading to *diastolic dysfunction* is the most common finding in old age. Hypertension, aortic stenosis and coronary artery disease are the often cause for diastolic dysfunction. Systolic function usually remains preserved. Blood pressure increases with age. Decrease heart rate, decreased adrenergic response and decreased cardiac reserve increase the incidence of cardiac complications.

Respiratory System

Decreased elasticity leads to alveolar distension and increase in residual volume and functional residual capacity. Increase in closing capacity increases the V/Q mismatch decreasing the pO_2. Kyphosis and scoliosis can cause difficulty in ventilation. Decreased respiratory muscle function decreases the cough reflex.

Central Nervous System

Loss of neurons decreases the brain reserve leading to dementia. There occurs increased sensitivity to anesthetic medications. The risk of perioperative delirium and postoperative cognitive dysfunction (POCD) is far more common in old age people.

Renal and Hepatic

There occurs age-related decrease in renal and hepatic functions.

Thermoregulation

Geriatric population is more prone for hypothermia.

ANESTHETIC MANAGEMENT

Age is not a contraindication for any surgery.

Preoperative

- Commonly coexisting diseases of the old age like hypertension, ischemic heart disease, diabetes mellitus, cerebrovascular diseases, chronic obstructive pulmonary disease (COPD), rheumatoid arthritis/osteoarthritis, Parkinson's disease, Alzheimer, malignancies must be ruled out by detailed preoperative assessment.
- Medical condition should be stabilized as far as possible.
- Many of the old age people are on polypharmacy. A detailed record of medication should be obtained and instructions are given accordingly.
- *Assessment of cognitive function is must.* Patients with preoperative dementia have higher incidence of postoperative delirium. Moreover, it can be used to compare if patient develops cognitive function in postoperative period.
- *Investigations: Age is not a criteria to do battery of routine investigations.* Investigations should be guided by associated comorbidity.

Intraoperative

Choice of Anesthesia

Regional anesthesia is preferred over general anesthesia due to the following reasons:
- Increased sensitivity of brain to anesthetic agents can prolong the recovery.
- Decreased metabolism and excretion due to decreased hepatic and renal function increases the chances of drug toxicity.

- Central neuraxial blocks decreases the risk of thromboembolism.
- Pulmonary complications associated with general anesthesia (GA) may be avoided.
- The incidence of postoperative delirium is less in regional anesthesia as compared to general anesthesia.

However, regional anesthesia, particularly central neuraxial blocks may be technically difficult due to degenerative changes in spine. Old age patients achieve higher level of spinal (and epidural) due to narrowing of spaces. Geriatric population is more sensitive to the effect of local anesthetics during nerve blocks.

General Anesthesia

Premedication: As the requirement of benzo-diazepines may be reduced by 50%, premedication with benzodiazepines should be done cautiously.

Induction: Increase sensitivity of brain, decrease volume of distribution, decreased unbound fraction of the drug (due to decreased albumin levels) and reduced metabolism and clearance not only decreases the dose of all IV agents but also increases the toxicity. *Propofol* because of shorter half-life is preferred. Decreased cardiac output may slow the onset with IV agents.

Intubation: Decrease pseudocholinesterase levels due to decrease hepatic functions may theoretically prolong the effect of suxamethonium however, clinically no prolongation has been seen.

Intubation and mask ventilation may become difficult due to edentulous jaw and decreased neck movements (due to rheumatoid arthritis and osteoarthritis).

Stress response to cope up with hemodynamic changes during surgery and anesthesia decreases.

Maintenance: *The minimum alveolar concentration (MAC) of inhalational agents decreases by 4–6% per decade. Desflurane* because of its rapid emergence and least metabolism is the preferred inhalational agent for geriatric patients.

Doses of opioids should be reduced by half. Remifentanil because of its ultra-short life is the most preferred opioid.

Muscle relaxant: Decrease cardiac output can delay the onset of muscle relaxants. Hoffman degradation makes *Atracurium and Cis-atracurium* to be the muscle relaxants of choice for old age patients.

Postoperative

Studies have shown that there occurs age related decrease in pain perception and moreover these patients are oversensitive to opioids, therefore opioids should be used very carefully.

Postoperative Complications

Geriatric population is more prone for hypoxia and urinary retention in postoperative period.

Postoperative Delirium

The overall prevalence of postoperative delirium in older patients is estimated to be 10%. This incidence of delirium can increase to more than 50% in patients shifted to ICU.

Important predisposing factors are age >65 years, male gender, major surgery, general anesthesia (compared to regional anesthesia), drugs like meperidine (pethidine), preoperative cognitive or functional impairment, dementia, associated comorbidities, polypharmacy, electrolyte imbalance, pain and sleep deprivation.

Postoperative Cognitive Dysfunction

Short-term (up to 3 months) changes in cognitive function have been very well-documented in 10–15% of geriatric population after surgery. Long-term (> 3 months) cognitive impairment can also occur in 1% of the patients.

The incidence of postoperative cognitive dysfunction (POCD) is independent of both surgery and anesthesia. Studies have shown no difference in the incidence of POCD in minor versus major surgery and regional versus general anesthesia.

At present there is no specific treatment available for POCD.

KEY POINTS

- Diastolic dysfunction, the most common cardiac finding in old age, is a significant determinant of morbidity.
- Chronological age is neither a contraindication for any surgery nor is a criterion to do battery of routine investigations.
- Assessment of cognitive function is must in geriatric patients.
- Regional anesthesia is preferred over general anesthesia.
- The requirement of benzodiazepines and opioids may be reduced by 50%.
- The minimum alveolar concentration (MAC) of inhalational agents decreases by 4–6% per decade.
- Desflurane because of its rapid emergence and least metabolism is the preferred inhalational agent for geriatric patients.
- Atracurium and Cis-atracurium are the muscle relaxant of choice for old age patients.
- The overall prevalence of postoperative delirium in older patients is estimated to be 10%.
- Short-term changes in cognitive function have been very well-documented in 10–15% of geriatric population after surgery.
- The incidence of POCD is independent of both surgery and anesthesia.

CHAPTER 31

Anesthesia for Obese Patients (Bariatric Anesthesia)

Obese patients may come to the operation theater for bariatric or nonbariatric surgery. As there has been a consistent rise in obesity, there is the parallel rise in bariatric surgeries.

Obese patients are one of the most challenging patients for anesthesiologist especially due to their associated comorbidities and difficult airway management.

Obesity is defined as body mass index (BMI) more than 30% and extreme/superobese as BMI more than 50%.

PREOPERATIVE ASSESSMENT

Preoperative assessment should be done in detail because of the associated comorbidities:

1. *Cardiovascular considerations:* Obese patients may have:
   i. Hypertension.
   ii. Coronary artery disease.
   iii. Left ventricular hypertrophy: Increase in cardiac output by 0.1 L/min to perfuse each kg of fat leads to increased stroke volume and hence left ventricular hypertrophy.
   iv. Right ventricular hypertrophy resulting from pulmonary hypertension which in turn is because of persistent hypoxia.
   v. Cor pulmonale because of right ventricular strain.
2. *Respiratory considerations:* Obese patients may have:
   i. Reduced expiratory reserve volume (ERV), functional residual capacity (FRC) and vital capacity.
   ii. Increased airway resistance.
   iii. Reduced oxygen saturation because of obesity and obstructive sleep apnea

hypopnea syndrome (OSAHS). *Patients with OSAHS are at increased risk of morbidity and mortality.*
3. *Gastrointestinal (GI) system considerations:* Obese patients may have associated hiatus hernia, gastroesophageal reflex, delayed gastric emptying and fatty infiltration of liver (may compromise liver functions).
4. *Blood:* There may be polycythemia because of chronic hypoxia.
5. Obese patients are very prone for thromboembolism in postoperative period.
6. *Evaluation of airways:* Obese patients often have *difficult airway* due to:
   i. Short neck (decreased thyromental distance).
   ii. Restricted mouth opening due to increased adipose tissue in neck and decreased mobility of temporomandibular joint.
   iii. Restricted neck movement because of decreased mobility of atlanto-occipital joint.

Investigations: *Obesity per se is not the criteria to order a battery of routine tests,* therefore investigation should be based on clinical assessment and associated comorbidities however, baseline oxygen saturation must be checked by pulse oximetry (if abnormal, then arterial blood gases should be done). *Polysomnography should be strongly considered in morbidly obese patients or in patients with a history of obstructive sleep apnea.*

Premedication: Premedication with respiratory depressant drugs like benzodiazepines should be avoided while premedication with metoclopramide and ranitidine should be considered.

INTRAOPERATIVE

Monitoring

Appropriate size BP cuff should be chosen.

Choice of Anesthesia

Due to difficult airway management, *anesthesia of choice is regional anesthesia* but unfortunately regional anesthesia is often difficult in obese patients. Due to reduced epidural and subarachnoid space obese patients are more vulnerable for high spinals.

General Anesthesia

Preoxygenation: Adding 10 cm H_2O of continuous positive airway pressure (CPAP) during preoxygenation has found to be beneficial in maintaining oxygenation in the perioperative period.

Induction: Lipid soluble drugs (IV induction agents, opioids) have increased volume of distribution, therefore given on actual body weight basis. Interestingly, this effect is not so marked on propofol as on thiopentone.

Achieving IV lines sometimes can become an arduous task.

Airway management: Airway management is the most challenging part in obese patients. The incidence of failed intubation is 3 times more in bariatric population, therefore be prepared for *difficult airway management. (For details see Chapter 5, page no. 54)*

As the *Ramped position* **(Fig. 31.1)** *provides a superior view of laryngoscopy it is preferred position for intubation for obese patients.* As the name suggests a ramp is created by commercially available device or by using sheets and blankets to elevate the upper back of the patient to the level when external auditory meatus lie in horizontal line with the sternal notch (that is why ramp position is also called as an *ear to sternum* position).

If intubation is anticipated to be difficult awake intubation with fiberoptic bronchoscopy should be considered.

Confirmation of intubation must be done by capnography as breath sounds may not be clearly audible on auscultation.

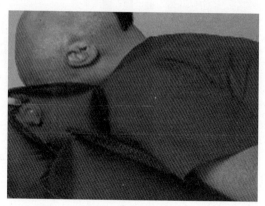

Fig. 31.1: Ramp position

Maintenance

- Inhalational agents are more extensively metabolized in obese patients therefore, the agent with least metabolism, i.e. *Desflurane is the inhalational agent of choice.* Increased metabolism of halothane makes obese patients more vulnerable for halothane hepatitis.
- Water soluble drugs (nondepolarizing muscle relaxants) have limited volume of distribution therefore should be given on *ideal body weight* basis.
- Application of 10 cm H_2O of positive end expiratory pressure (PEEP) during mechanical ventilation improves oxygenation by preventing alveolar collapse.
- 30° reverse Trendelenburg improves oxygenation particularly during laparoscopic surgeries.

POSTOPERATIVE

- Obese patients are very prone to *hypoxia* in postoperative period. Therefore, they should be nursed in 45° sitting (semi-reclined position) with supplemental oxygen. CPAP (continuous positive airway pressure) or BiPAP (bi level positive airway pressure) should be applied if the patient is not maintaining oxygen saturation on supplemental oxygen.
- Every precaution must be taken to prevent *thromboembolism.*
- Good antibiotic cover is must as these patients are prone for wound infection.

KEY POINTS

- To perfuse extra fat obese patients are in high cardiac output state.
- Obese patients may have extra parenchymal restrictive pattern in their pulmonary functions.
- Polysomnography should be strongly considered in morbidly obese patients or in patients with a history of obstructive sleep apnea.
- Due to difficult airway management, anesthesia of choice is regional anesthesia.
- Airway management is the most challenging part in obese patients.
- As the ramped position provides a superior view of laryngoscopy it is preferred position for intubation for obese patients.
- Lipid soluble drugs (IV induction agents, opioids) have increased volume of distribution, therefore given on actual body weight basis. Water soluble drugs (nondepolarizing muscle relaxants) have limited volume of distribution, therefore should be given on ideal body weight basis.
- Desflurane is the inhalational agent of choice for maintenance in obese patients.
- Obese patients are very prone to hypoxia in post- operative period.
- Application of CPAP and PEEP improves oxygenation in obese patients.

CHAPTER 32

Anesthesia for Laparoscopy

Laparoscopic surgeries have been on rise over a decade due to shorter hospital stay, avoidance of big surgical incision, less tissue trauma and less postoperative pain.

GASES FOR CREATING PNEUMOPERITONIUM

Carbon dioxide is most frequently used gas for laparoscopy because it is more soluble in blood leading to its rapid elimination from the body in cases of pneumothorax and accidental injection into vascular compartment. Other gases, which can used are air, helium, oxygen, nitrous oxide and argon. Since argon is an inert gas with no side effects *it is considered as most ideal gas for laparoscopy,* however because of its very high cost it is not used.

PATHOPHYSIOLOGICAL EFFECTS OF LAPAROSCOPY

Respiratory System

Increase intra-abdominal pressure due to pneumoperitoneum pushes the diaphragm upwards, leading to basal atelectasis producing ventilation perfusion (V/Q) mismatch and decrease in functional residual capacity (FRC). Thoracopulmonary compliance may be decreased by up to 50% during pneumoperitoneum.

Cardiovascular System

- *Decreased cardiac output:* Increase intra-abdominal pressure compresses the inferior vena cava leading to decreased venous return and cardiac output. Intra-abdominal pressure of 12–14 mm Hg can decrease the cardiac output by 30–35%.
- *Increased peripheral vascular resistance (PVR):* Increase in PVR occurs because of high pCO_2 and more importantly, because of increased catecholamines, vasopressin and prostaglandins.
- *Cardiac arrhythmias:* CO_2 by producing coronary vasoconstriction may produce any arrhythmia however, bradyarrhythmias occurring because of stretching of the peritoneum are more frequent.

Central Nervous System

CO_2 by producing cerebral vasodilatation can increase the intracranial tension.

Gastrointestinal System

Increased risk of aspiration: Increased Intra-abdominal pressure distorts the gastroesophageal junction making patient more vulnerable for aspiration.

COMPLICATIONS OF LAPAROSCOPY

Although laparoscopic surgeries have many advantages over open surgeries however, laparoscopic surgeries subjects the patients to certain complications attributed to laparoscopy.

1. *Pneumothorax (Capnothorax):* Carbon dioxide from peritoneal cavity can diffuse into the pleural cavity through embryonic remnants present between pleural and peritoneal cavity which gets open by increased intra-abdominal pressure or through pleural tears during surgery.

Diagnosis

i. Increased airway resistance on mechanical ventilation.
ii. Decreased oxygen saturation (SpO_2).
iii. Decreased air entry on auscultation.
iv. X-ray chest.
v. Abnormal movement of diaphragm as observed by surgeon.
vi. Associated subcutaneous emphysema of neck and chest.

Management

i. *Immediately stop nitrous oxide:* Nitrous oxide can expand the pneumothorax
ii. Start 100% oxygen.
iii. *Adjust ventilator setting:* Add positive-end expiratory pressure (PEEP) to correct hypoxia.
iv. Reduce intra-abdominal pressure as much as possible.
v. *Chest tube drainage should be reserved only for the cases not responding to conservative measures or the Pneumothorax is life-threatening* otherwise, usually capnothorax resolves by itself in 30–60 minutes (because of high diffusibilty of CO_2).

2. *Pneumomediastinum, pneumopericardium and subcutaneous emphysema:* The CO_2 can enter mediastinum and pericardium through esophageal, vena caval or aortic hiatus. Gas from mediastinum may diffuse cephalad to produce subcutaneous emphysema of face and neck.

   Management includes maintenance of vitals till CO_2 is absorbed from mediastinum or pericardial cavity.

3. *CO_2 embolism:* Gas embolism can be a fatal complication of laparoscopy; it carries a mortality of 30%. CO_2 embolism occurs because of accidental placement of a needle into the vessel during insufflation. Large volume of gas can cause 'gas lock' in the inferior vana cava leading to cardiovascular collapse.

Diagnosis

i. Most sensitive test to diagnose CO_2 embolism is transesophageal echocardiography.
ii. Doppler.
iii. Increased pulmonary artery pressure.

iv. *Capnography:* In CO_2 embolism, there is *biphasic response,* i.e. initial rise in end tidal CO_2 (due to direct injection of CO_2 in vessels) followed by fall.
v. Clinical signs like tachycardia, hypotension, right heart strain on ECG and Mill wheel murmur.
vi. *Aspiration of gas or foamy blood from central catheter is diagnostic.*
vii. Aspiration of blood from Veress needle (used for CO_2 insufflation) as needle is placed directly into vessel.
viii. Absence of abdominal distension in spite of CO_2 insufflation.

Management

Preventive:

i. The surgeon must ascertain the position of Veress needle before CO_2 insufflation.
ii. Rate of insufflation should not be more than 1 L/min.

Curative:

i. Immediately stop further insufflation.
ii. Start hyperventilation with 100% oxygen.
iii. Aspirate gas through central venous pressure (CVP) or pulmonary catheter.
iv. If possible place the patient in Durrant position (left lateral with Trendelenburg) so that gas get remains in right ventricle and can be aspirated.
v. Manage any co-existing arrhythmia.
vi. Hyperbaric oxygen therapy if there is cerebral embolism.
vii. For massive embolism cardiopulmonary bypass may be required.

4. *Complications related to patient's position:* Majority of the laparoscopic procedures are performed in either Trendelenburg or anti-Trendelenburg position.

5. *Abdominal organs trauma and hemorrhage:* Abdominal organs, especially intestines and stomach may be perforated by the needle or trocar. Moreover, bleeding and visceral trauma may go undetected.

6. *Consequences of increase pCO_2:* Increase in pCO_2 during laparoscopy can occur due to absorption from the peritoneal cavity and V/Q mismatch. Increase is pCO_2 is well-tolerated by young individuals, but can produce arrhythmias and ischemia in cardiac patients.

7. *Consequences of increased intra-abdominal pressure (IAP):* Intra-abdominal pressure of > 20 mm Hg can decrease the cardiac output by more than two-thirds producing even cardiac arrest.
   Intra-abdominal pressure of > 20 mm Hg can significantly impair renal, mesenteric and intestinal blood flow. Therefore, it is highly recommended that *intra-abdominal pressure should be kept between 12–14 mm Hg.*
8. *Nausea and vomiting:* Nausea and vomiting is the most common postoperative complication of laparoscopic surgeries; incidence can be as high as 40–75%.
9. *Shoulder pain:* Sub-diaphragmatic CO_2 irritating diaphragm causing shoulder pain in postoperative period is commonly complained by many patients.

ANESTHETIC MANAGEMENT

Laparoscopy can be performed under local, regional and general anesthesia.

Local Anesthesia

Laparoscopic surgeries of very short duration (<15 minutes) can only be considered under local anesthesia. Laparoscopic tubal ligation is the most common surgery performed under local anesthesia.

Regional Anesthesia

Patient discomfort (shoulder pain due to diaphragmatic irritation by CO_2) limits the use of central neuraxial blocks (spinal/epidural) for laparoscopy.

General Anesthesia

- *General anesthesia with endotracheal intubation and mild hyperventilation is most commonly used technique for most of the laparoscopic surgeries.* General anesthesia with second generation laryngeal mask airway (I-gel, proseal) can be considered if there is no risk of aspiration.

- $ETCO_2$ should be maintained at 35 mm Hg.
- Inhalational agents which depress cardiac function (like halothane) should be avoided.
- *Propofol because of its antiemetic properties is the induction agent of choice.*

CONTRAINDICATIONS FOR LAPAROSCOPY

Absolute

1. *Increased intracranial tension:* CO_2 can further increase the intracranial tension.
2. Congestive heart failure.
3. Severe hypovolemia and hypotension.
4. Right-to-left cardiac shunts or patent foramen ovale (risk of paradoxical embolism).
5. Generalized abdominal peritonitis.
6. Retinal detachment.

Relative

Ventriculoperitoneal (VP) or peritoneojugular (PJ) shunt: Insufflation in peritoneum can displace the shunt.

Contraindications of the Past

1. *Coronary insufficiencies:* A patient with the controlled *ischemic heart disease can be safely considered for laparoscopic surgeries* however, with enhanced perioperative cardiovascular monitoring.
2. *Pregnancy:* Although pneumoperitoneum may cause transient fetal acidosis, clinical studies suggest that additional risks to be very low for both mother and fetus. Therefore, *laparoscopy is considered safe during pregnancy.*
3. *Obesity:* Laparoscopy once used to be considered as contraindication in obese patients has now become the *preferred method over open surgeries.*
4. *Respiratory compromised:* Respiratory complications after laparoscopic surgery are significantly lower than open surgery.

KEY POINTS

- Carbon dioxide is the most frequently used gas for laparoscopy because it is more soluble.
- Argon is considered as most ideal gas for laparoscopy.

Contd...

Contd...

- Intra-abdominal pressure of 12–14 mm Hg can decrease the cardiac output by 30–35%.
- Capnothorax usually resolves by itself in 30–60 minutes; chest tube drainage should be reserved only for the cases not responding to conservative measures or which are life threatening.
- CO_2 embolism can be fatal complication of laparoscopy; it carries a mortality of 30%.
- In CO_2 embolism, there is a biphasic response on capnography.
- Intra-abdominal pressure of > 20 mm Hg can significantly impair renal, mesenteric and intestinal blood flow. Therefore, intra-abdominal pressure should be kept between 12 and 14 mm Hg.
- Nausea and vomiting is the most common postoperative complication of laparoscopic surgeries; incidence can be as high as 40–75%.
- General anesthesia with endotracheal intubation and mild hyperventilation is the most commonly used technique for most of the laparoscopic surgeries.
- A patient with the controlled ischemic heart disease can be safely considered for laparoscopic surgeries.
- Laparoscopy is considered safe during pregnancy.
- Laparoscopy once used to be considered as contraindication in obese patients has now become the preferred method over open surgeries.

CHAPTER 33

Anesthesia for Ophthalmic Surgery

PREOPERATIVE EVALUATION

- The patients usually posted for ocular surgeries are either pediatric or geriatric. Therefore, proper preoperative evaluation should be done in geriatric population to rule out coexisting medical diseases.
- History of ophthalmic medications must be recorded. Topical eye medications can have systemic effects. For example, echothiophate by inhibiting pseudocholinesterase can prolong the effect of suxamethonium, phenylephrine can cause hypertension, timololcan can cause bradycardia and bronchospasm and acetazolamide can cause hypokalemia.
- Cataract surgery can be performed safely in patients receiving warfarin. For other ocular surgeries warfarin should be stopped 4 days before.

INTRAOPERATIVE

- *Maintenance of intraocular pressure (IOP):* One of the most important goal during eye surgery is to reduce or at least maintain the intraocular pressure within normal range of 10–20 mm Hg. The factors which increase the IOP like hypertension, increased central venous pressure (coughing, straining), hypercapnia, hypoxia, anesthetic agents (ketamine, suxamethonium) and light anesthesia must be avoided.
- *Prevention of oculocardiac reflex:* It is triggered by pressure on globe or by *traction on extraocular muscle (especially the medial rectus)* during squint surgery. The afferents are carried by trigeminal and efferent by vagus.

It is manifested as bradycardia, atrioventricular (AV) block or even asystole. Treatment includes immediate cessation of manipulation and intravenous (IV) atropine if not reversed by cessation of manipulation. Pretreatment with atropine may be indicated in patients with a history of conduction blocks and β-blocker therapy.

ANESTHESIA

Most of the ocular surgeries are performed under *regional anesthesia* (topical, peribulbar, retrobulbar and sub-tenon blocks). Eye blocks are most often given by ophthalmologist themselves.

Peribulbar Block

Peribulbar block has now almost completely replaced retrobulbar block because of its less serious complications and avoidance of separate facial block to provide ocular akinesia.

Technique

Ask the patient to look straight ahead (neutral gaze). A dull short beveled needle is entered through the inferior fornix of conjunctiva at the junction of lateral 1/3rd and medial 2/3rd and 6–10 mL of drug is injected. The needle is never inserted beyond 25 mm because large vessels and optic nerve are encountered with deeper penetration. Orbital compression with Hanon ball or compression balloon (30–40 mm Hg) facilitates the block and decreases the IOP.

Advantages

- Serious complications seen with retrobulbar block like globe puncture, injury to optic artery or nerve are less with peribulbar block.
- Facial nerve need not be blocked separately.
- Less painful.

Disadvantages

- Slower onset.
- More chances of ecchymosis.

Retrobulbar Block

In retrobulbar block, the local anesthetic is injected at orbital apex, i.e. behind the eye into muscle cone.

Complications

- Oculocardiac reflex.
- Retrobulbar hemorrhage.
- Puncture of globe which can lead to retinal detachment.
- Optic nerve injury.
- Intraocular injection.
- Brain stem anesthesia [drug traveling along optic nerve sheath can enter central nervous system (CNS)].
- Retinal artery occlusion and blindness.
- Death.

Sub-tenon (Episcleral) Block

In sub-tenon block, the drug is injected beneath the Tenons's fascia. Complications are reported to be less than retrobulbar and peribulbar block.

Topical Anesthesia

The majority of the cataract surgeries (phacoemulsification) is possible under topical anaesthesia of the eye.

Local Anesthetics used for Blocks

A solution consisting of:
- 2% xylocaine for rapid onset.
- 0.5% bupivacaine for prolonged effect.
- 1 in 200000 adrenaline for vasoconstriction.
- Hyaluronidase for better spread.

GENERAL ANESTHESIA

Usual indications for general anesthesia are-pediatric patients, uncooperative patients not allowing regional anesthesia, retinal detachment surgeries and keratoplasties.

Premedication

Although benzodiazepines reduce the intraocular pressure, however they should be used cautiously in old age patients.

Induction

- All IV agents, except ketamine reduces the IOP. Propofol is most often used for induction. Ketamine increases the IOP, therefore should be avoided in ocular surgeries.
- Intubation and laryngoscopy can increase the IOP, therefore the response should be blunted by IV lignocaine and fentanyl.

Maintenance

- *All newer inhalational agents reduce the IOP therefore can be safely used for maintenance.*
- *Nitrous oxide should be avoided in retinal detachment surgery if air, sulfur hexafluoride or perfluoropropane bubble is used for correction.* Nitrous oxide can expand the bubble size and thus can raise the IOP significantly. As the bubble can persist for many days, nitrous oxide should not be used for 5 days after air, 10 days after sulfur hexafluoride and 30 days after perfluoropropane.

Muscle Relaxants

Succinylcholine increases the IOP, however the rise is transient (5–10 minutes), therefore if the patient is not fasting and risk of pulmonary aspiration is high, it is safer to use succinylcholine.

Non-depolarizing agents decrease the IOP.

Reversal

- Anticholinergics (atropine/Glycopyrrolate) when given IV or IM does not raise IOP significantly, therefore can be used safely with anticholinesterases.
- Recovery should be very smooth. Coughing and straining during extubation can be disastrous.

Position of patient: Head up by 10–15° decreases the IOP by reducing the venous pressure.

Postoperative: The incidence of postoperative nausea and vomiting is very high after strabismus surgery.

KEY POINTS

- Topical eye medications can have systemic effects.
- One of the most important goals during eye surgery is to reduce or at least maintain the intraocular pressure within normal range.
- Traction on extraocular muscle (especially the medial rectus) can precipitate oculocardiac reflex.
- Most of the ocular surgeries are performed under regional anesthesia.
- Peribulbar block has now almost completely replaced retrobulbar block.
- All IV agents (except ketamine) and inhalational agents reduce the IOP.
- Nitrous oxide should be avoided in retinal detachment surgery if air, sulfur hexafluoride or perfluoropropane bubble is used for correction.
- Succinylcholine increases the IOP, however the rise is transient (5–10 minutes), therefore if the risk of pulmonary aspiration is high, it is safer to use succinylcholine.

CHAPTER 34

Anesthesia for ENT Surgery

ENT anesthesia is one of the most difficult anesthesia because quite often airway is difficult, surgeon and anesthetist share the common field and complications are related to airway.

PANENDOSCOPY (PREVIOUSLY CALLED AS MICROLARYNGEAL SURGERIES)

As panendoscopy involves laryngoscopy, bronchoscopy, and esophagoscopy it is also called as triple endoscopy. It may be a diagnostic or therapeutic. The common procedures are laryngeal biopsies and removal of vocal cord polyp.

Anesthesia poses specific problems due to the following reasons:

- Due to the growth, the glottic opening may be reduced and sometimes to an extent that even insertion of the small size tube becomes impossible.
- Anesthetist and surgeon share the common field.
- Laryngeal manipulation causes sympathetic stimulation. Incidence of myocardial ischemia and arrhythmias is significant (2–4%).
- Laryngeal stimulation can induce laryngospasm.
- Chances of blood aspiration are very high.
- There may be additional complications related to laser.

Anesthesia for Panendoscopy

- During preoperative evaluation, assessment of airway by preoperative endoscopy or indirect laryngoscopy is must.
- Preoxygenation is very important.
- Intravenous (IV) lignocaine, IV fentanyl and topical anesthesia of the larynx are very important to prevent laryngeal reflexes.

Ventilation Techniques

The existing pathology and requirement of the working space for surgeons leaves the minimal space for ventilation.

1. *Microlaryngeal surgery (MLS) tubes*: MLS tubes are pediatric size tubes with cuff. They are available in 5, 5.5 and 6 mm size. *In the majority (>95%) of the patients it is possible to get the surgery done with MLS tube*. The disadvantage is that high ventilatory pressures are required to overcome the narrow size of tube.
2. *High frequency positive pressure ventilation (HFPPV):* In this technique small tidal volumes are delivered at high frequency (60–100 breaths/min) at a high pressure (60 psi) through a stiff 3.5–4.0 mm catheter passed through the vocal cord.
3. *Jet ventilation:* The tip of the jet is kept within the laryngoscope to avoid direct barotrauma to the trachea and gas is delivered at high pressure (50–60 psi).
4. *Insufflation:* Achieved by placing a catheter and gases flow at high pressure.
5. *Apnea technique:* In this technique intubation is done and after adequate ventilation tube is removed for short period (1–2 minutes or till oxygen saturation starts falling). In this period surgeon performs the procedure. If the procedure is not completed in this period, the patient is again intubated (or ventilated through the bag and mask) and the tube removed and so on.

Maintenance

Anesthesia is maintained with inhalational agent and repeated doses of succinylcholine for small procedures or nondepolarizing agent for prolonged surgery. *Nitrous oxide should be avoided* because it can increase the postsurgical edema by causing expansion of the cuff of endotracheal tube. Administration of Heliox is strongly considered in patients with stridor.

Concerns Related to Laser

Many of the panendoscopy surgeries uses laser. *The most important complication of laser surgery is fires,* therefore the most important aim should be to prevent fire by taking the following prophylaxis:

i. Use low FiO_2 (<30%)
ii. Avoid N_2O (N_2O can support fire)
iii. Use special kind of *laser resistant endotracheal tube*
iv. Fill the tube cuff with saline (instead of air)

In case there occurs fire, the following protocol should be followed:

i. Immediately remove tube and submerge in water
ii. Immediately stop oxygen (and nitrous oxide) and start ventilation of the patient with air by mask
iii. Flush pharynx with 50–60 mL of cold saline
iv. Do bronchoscopy to assess the damage and accordingly ventilate the patient with mask, laryngeal mask airway or by reintubation. Tracheostomy may be required if damage is severe enough not to allow intubation.
v. Steroids, antibiotics.

ANESTHESIA FOR BRONCHOSCOPY

- Flexible bronchoscopy, usually done for diagnostic biopsies, can be performed under topical anesthesia.
- Rigid bronchoscopy, usually done for foreign body removal is performed under general anesthesia. Ventilation is achieved with:
  i. High frequency jet ventilation through the oxygen port provided in bronchoscope.
  ii. Insufflation.
  iii. Apnea technique.

ANESTHESIA FOR ADENOTONSILLECTOMY/ TONSILLECTOMY

- Majority of the patients are pediatric.

- If there are no adenoids nasal intubation can be done, however due to increased chances of bleeding nasal intubation should preferably be avoided. Oral Ring-Adair-Elwyn (RAE) *preformed tubes* are most frequently used.
- Throat should be packed to prevent aspiration.
- In postoperative period to prevent aspiration and laryngospasm (by the blood tricking down the throat) *these patients are nursed in tonsillar position, i.e. on one side (preferably left lateral) with head low.*
- Sometimes post-tonsillectomy bleeding may require re-exploration of wound to control bleeding. Such patient should be resuscitated to stabilize hemodynamically and should be managed like full stomach patient considering that patient has swallowed enough blood which can cause significant aspiration.

ANESTHESIA FOR PERITONSILLAR ABSCESS AND LUDWIG ANGINA

General anesthesia (GA) should be avoided as intubation at times may be impossible due to trismus and patient can aspirate the pus. Therefore, the *abscesses should be drained under local anesthesia.* If GA is required than awake nasal intubation with fibreoptic bronchoscopy should be achieved before induction of anesthesia.

ANESTHESIA FOR EAR SURGERY

Nitrous oxide is 35 times more soluble than nitrogen. If the Eustachian tube is blocked, nitrous oxide can increase the middle ear pressure to 375 mm H_2O within half an hour. *Therefore, nitrous oxide should not be used in patients with blocked Eustachian tubes* (upper respiratory tract infection, adenoids, sinusitis and otitis media).

Increase middle ear pressure by nitrous oxide can displace the graft making nitrous oxide to be contraindicated for *Tympanoplasties.* However, if the surgeon is using "inlay graft" then increase in middle ear pressure is beneficial in holding the graft.

The incidence of postoperative nausea and vomiting is very high in ear surgeries; therefore prophylaxis with antiemetics is must.

ANESTHESIA FOR NASAL SURGERY

Most commonly performed nasal surgeries are correction of deviated septum, rhinoplasties, removal of nasal polyp or endoscopic sinus surgeries.

- In the preoperative evaluation always rule out the Samter triad (nasal polyps, asthma, and sensitivity to aspirin/NSAIDs).
- Throat pack is must to prevent aspiration of blood.
- The patients must be counseled and trained in the preoperative period to take breathing from mouth otherwise they can become very restless in the postoperative period after nasal packing.

ANESTHESIA FOR PAROTID SURGERY

Continuous monitoring of facial nerve function may deter the anesthetist to use muscle relaxants.

ANESTHESIA FOR OBSTRUCTIVE SLEEP APNEA SURGERY

All concerns related to obese patients (*for details see Chapter 31, page no. 245*) especially difficult airway management makes obstruction sleep apnea (OSA) surgeries (uvulopalatoplasties) to be very challenging to anesthetist.

ANESTHESIA FOR TEMPOROMANDIBULAR JOINT (TMJ) SURGERIES

Due to the limited mouth opening intubation mandates awake nasal intubation.

KEY POINTS

- In preoperative evaluation of patients posted for panendoscopy, assessment of airway by preoperative endoscopy or indirect laryngoscopy is must.
- In the majority (>95%) of the patients it is possible to get the panendoscopy surgery done with MLS tube.
- Nitrous oxide should be avoided in laryngeal surgeries because it can increase the post-surgical edema by causing expansion of the cuff of the endotracheal tube.
- The most important complication of laser surgery is fires.
- Laser resistant endotracheal tubes are not 100% protective against laser fires.
- Tonsillar patients should be nursed in tonsillar position in the postoperative period to prevent aspiration and laryngospasm.
- Post tonsillectomy bleeding re-exploration patients should be managed like full stomach patient.
- Nitrous oxide should not be used in patients with blocked Eustachian tubes and tympanoplasties.

CHAPTER 35

Anesthesia for Trauma and Burns

ANESTHESIA FOR TRAUMA

Management of trauma patients poses unique challenges due to the following reasons:

- *Inadequate medical history:* Attendant may not be present and patient may not be fit enough to give his/her medical history.
- Most often patients undergoing emergency surgery are not fasting.
- Patients may be intoxicated.
- Multiple injuries, especially lung, cardiac, brain, pelvic and abdominal injuries can make anesthesia complex and increases the morbidity and mortality.
- Airway may be very difficult due to facial and neck injuries.
- Presence of shock can significantly alter the outcome.
- Sometimes emergency may be so acute that there is not enough time to prepare the operation theater.

Preoperative Period

Unlike other patients the preoperative period of trauma patients is often turbulent. The involvement of anesthetist may begin from emergency room as a part of resuscitation team.

- If there is need, then airway must be secured and patient resuscitated before shifting to operation theater (OT). It is not uncommon to see intubated patients coming to OT. Although a *systolic blood pressure of at least 80–90 mm Hg is recommended before induction,* however sometimes the situation like damage control surgery (surgery is the only method to stop bleeding) warrants the induction at very

low or even nonrecordable blood pressure. The prognosis of such patients is very bleak.

- It is very important to rule out major injuries especially:
  - Chest injury like pneumo/hemothorax or lung contusion.
  - Head injury—presence of head injury can alter the anesthesia technique. For example, central neuraxial blocks may be absolutely contraindicated with elevated intracranial tension (ICT)
  - *Spine injuries:* Improper movements can produce devastating complications, including quadriplegia, paraplegia or even death.
  - Abdominal, pelvic injuries and major bone fractures, can produce massive hemorrhage
- As airway may be compromised detailed assessment of airway is must.
- Try to obtain medical history as maximum as possible.
- Obtain adequate blood and blood products.
- Correct acute traumatic coagulopathy (*for details see Chapter 40, page no. 286*)
- If fasting status cannot be obtained, premedicate the patient with metoclopramide and ranitidine/sodium citrate.

Intraoperative Period

- *Secure IV lines* with large bore cannulas. If peripheral access is not possible, then obtain central access (most often subclavian) or intraosseous access (if central access is also not possible).

- *Monitoring:* Although it may be difficult to cannulate artery in low output state but still every effort should be made to measure *continuous blood pressure by invasive monitoring.* As trauma patients are very prone for hypothermia, *temperature monitoring* becomes must.

Choice of Anesthesia

Except for limb saving surgeries which may be performed in regional anesthesia, majority of the trauma surgeries are done in general anesthesia.

General anesthesia: A trauma patient should always be considered full stomach until proved otherwise and should be managed like rapid sequence induction.

Induction: Selection of the induction agent is difficult in trauma patients. IV induction agents may produce profound hypotension (or even cardiac arrest) in shock patients. Requirement of doses is drastically reduced in hypotensive patients.

Etomidate (because of its cardiovascular stability) and *ketamine* (because of its sympathetic system stimulating property) *are the agents often selected for induction.* However, etomidate and ketamine can produce hypotension in shock patients who are already catecholamine depleted; etomidate by causing adrenocortical suppression and ketamine by causing direct myocardial depression in the absence of catecholamine.

Intubation

- All trauma patients should be assumed to be having cervical spine injury until proved otherwise and, therefore if cervical spine injury is not cleared they should be intubated with in-line manual stabilization. Similarly nasal route should not be acquired for intubation until basal skull fracture is ruled out.
- All equipment for difficult airway (including emergency cricothyrotomy) must be ready hand available because intubating a patient with face and neck trauma can become a big challenge. Mask ventilation in facial fractures at times becomes impossible.
  - Patients with maxillary fractures should not be intubated nasally; however most often can be easily intubated through oral route.
  - Patients with mandibular fracture are often intubated nasally due to two reasons. Firstly, the presence of trismus prevents oral intubation (however trismus can be relieved with anesthesia and muscle relaxants) secondly, most often maxillofacial surgeons do the dental wiring to close the mouth after mandibular surgery.
  - Patients with both mandibular and maxillary fracture may require tracheostomy. Intubation in pharyngeal and laryngeal trauma can worsen the injury or even lead to complete loss of the airway; the endotracheal tube can slip into the mediastinum through the defect. A low tracheostomy is the best solution in most of the cases. Application of cricoid pressure is also contraindicated in laryngeal trauma. Intubation guided by fiberoptic broncho-scopy appears to be a very promising method in patients with face and neck trauma, however becomes very difficult due to distorted anatomy and presence of blood and secretions in the airway.
- Chest tube must be inserted before intubation if there is pneumothorax because positive pressure ventilation can convert a small pneumothorax into tension pneumothorax.

Maintenance: Like IV agents patients in shock may exhibit extreme sensitivity to inhalational agents. *Desflurane is often the most preferred inhalational agent* because of its ability to maintain blood pressure by causing sympathetic stimulation and least metabolism.

Muscle relaxants: In spite of succinylcholine causing hyperkalemia in crush injury and increasing intraocular and intracranial pressure, it remains the muscle relaxant of choice for intubation in trauma patients with difficult airway and high risk of aspiration. The consequences of failed intubation and aspiration can be devastating.

Atracurium and Cis-atracurium are preferred non depolarizers because of their independency on hepatic and renal functions.

- As trauma patients are very prone for hypothermia OT temperature should be maintained and fluids/blood should be warmed to room temperature before infusion.
- Patients with spine injuries should be shifted with utmost care.

Postoperative Period

Extubation in trauma patients is a tricky exercise. Deep extubation can cause aspiration while extubation under light anesthesia can increase intraocular, intracranial pressure and restart the hemorrhage by increasing blood pressure.

It is not uncommon to see trauma patients getting electively ventilated in postoperative period.

ANESTHESIA FOR BURNS

Emergency Management of Burn Patient

- Burn patient may present with acute respiratory obstruction due to smoke inhalation in whom gentle intubation with expert hand should be tried to prevent further exaggeration of edema. If edema is severe tracheostomy may be required.
- Carbon monoxide poisoning is the most common immediate cause of death if burns occur in closed space. Therefore, immediate treatment with oxygen or hyperbaric oxygen (in severe cases) may be required.
- Hypovolemia is another important cause of death. Fluid should be given by the standard Parkland formula which recommends fluid replacement at a rate of 4 mL/kg/% burn. (50% of this fluid is given in first 8 hours and next 50% in next 16 hours). However studies have shown fluid overload by this method therefore current recommendation is to start fluid by Parkland formula but immediately start

tapering once urine output becomes >0.5–1 mL/kg/hr. *Ringer lactate is the fluid of choice. Colloids if necessary can be given in acute phase* (contrary to previous recommendation of not giving colloid for first 48 hours).

- Patients with electrical burns can present with cardiac arrhythmias or even cardiac arrest.

Anesthetic Management

Usual surgeries done in burn patients are release of post-burn contractures and split skin grafts.

- Venous access may be very difficult and may require central line.
- Intraoperative monitoring of ECG is mandatory in electric burns as there are high chances of arrhythmias.

Choice of Anesthesia

Lower limb surgeries can be performed under central neuraxial blocks. Patients with electrical burn can have neurological injuries. They should be evaluated for neurological deficits before giving regional anesthesia.

General anesthesia

Induction

Dose of intravenous induction agent may be slightly higher because of the large volume of distribution (hyperdynamic circulation) and increased metabolism. Increased protein loss can lead to an increased unbound fraction of benzodiazepines and thiopentone.

Intubation: Airway may be difficult due to contracture of face and neck. Awake intubation under fiberoptic bronchoscopy may be required. If that is not possible then contracture is released under intravenous ketamine and then intubation is done.

Muscle relaxants: Presence of extrajunctional receptors *contraindicates the use of succinylcholine for one year and decreases the sensitivity (increase dose requirement) of nondepolarizers.*

KEY POINTS

- Management of trauma patients poses unique challenges due to difficulty in obtaining a medical history, inadequate fasting, intoxication, multiple injuries and shock.
- Systolic blood pressure of at least 80–90 mm Hg is recommended before induction.

Contd...

Contd...

- Invasive blood pressure and temperature monitoring is highly recommended for trauma patients.
- Requirement of IV induction doses is drastically reduced in hypotensive patients.
- Etomidate and ketamine are the agents often selected for induction.
- All trauma patients should be assumed to be having cervical spine injury and basal skull fracture until proved otherwise.
- Patients with maxillary fractures can be easily intubated through oral route; patients with mandibular fracture are often intubated nasally. Patients with both mandibular and maxillary fracture may require tracheostomy.
- Desflurane is often the most preferred inhalational agent in trauma patients.
- Succinylcholine remains the muscle relaxant of choice for intubation if there is risk of aspiration or difficult airway while atracurium and Cis- atracurium are preferred non depolarizers in trauma.
- Airway may be difficult in burn patients due to contracture of face and neck.
- In burns succinylcholine is contraindicated for one year while dose of nondepolarizers is increased.

CHAPTER 36

Anesthesia for Orthopedics

Orthopedic anesthesia poses special problems due to lengthy procedures, increase blood loss, positioning, tourniquet-related problems, complications like fat embolism and deep vein thrombosis, increased age and associated diseases like rheumatoid arthritis and ankylosing spondylitis.

COMPLICATIONS OF ORTHOPEDIC SURGERY

Excessive Hemorrhage

In orthopedic procedures not done under tourniquet, there may be excessive blood loss.

Tourniquet-related Problems

Tourniquet is used to decrease the intraoperative bleeding. Complications associated with tourniquet are:

During inflation: Hypertension, increased cardiac output and increased pulmonary artery pressure. This is due to increased blood volume associated with exsanguination.

During tourniquet:
   i. *Metabolic changes:* Local tissue ischemia leads to acidosis (mitochondrial pO_2 becomes zero within 6 minutes of tourniquet inflation).
   ii. Pain is due to cellular acidosis, therefore may not be relieved by intravenous analgesics. It is relieved only by deflation.

During deflation:
   i. *Hypotension* because of sudden release of accumulated metabolites like thromboxane and substance P.

   ii. Hypothermia due to heat loss as acid metabolites are vasodilators.
   iii. Transient metabolic acidosis.
   iv. Increase in end tidal CO_2 (which is accumulated in limb).
   v. Transient decrease in central venous oxygen tension (because of acidosis).
   Deflation is the most crucial period. Cardiac arrest may occur at the time of deflation due to hypotension and release of acid metabolites.

Post-tourniquet: Neuropraxia may occur if tourniquet pressure is high or time is prolonged. *Pressure in tourniquet should not exceed more than 2 hours for both upper and lower limbs.* If re-inflation is needed, then it should be should be deflated for at least 30 minutes before re-inflating. Pressure in tourniquet should not exceed more than 100 mm Hg above systolic (maximum–250 mm Hg).

Fat Embolism Syndrome

Usually seen after fracture of long bones and pelvis. Incidence of significant embolism after long bone and pelvic fractures may be as high as 15%. Fat embolism classically presents within 24–72 hours of fracture. Due to rimming the incidence of fat embolism syndrome (FES), is higher in nailing as compared to plating.

Pathophysiology

Fat emboli released from long bone causes endothelial injury in the lungs and brain, which can precipitate acute respiratory distress syndrome (ARDS) and cerebral edema respectively. In some cases fat emboli may cause renal failure.

Signs and Symptoms

Dyspnea, chest discomfort, tachycardia, hypotension, mental clouding, restlessness, seizures, delirium, petechial hemorrhage on upper chest, axilla and conjunctiva, hypoxia and finally coma and death. *The triad of fat embolism syndrome is dyspnea, confusion and petechial hemorrhages. Petechial rash is pathognomonic of FES.*

Investigations

- The fat globules in urine are helpful in diagnosis, but may not necessarily indicate the progression to fat embolism syndrome.
- X-ray chest shows diffuse interstitial infiltrates.
- ECG shows the right ventricular strain.
- *Capnography shows fall in end tidal CO_2* (ETCO$_2$ may become zero if embolus is large enough to block the main pulmonary artery).
- Coagulation abnormalities like increased clotting time and decreased platelets.
- Serum lipase is increased (but has no relation to the severity of disease).

Treatment

Stabilization of fracture: Early stabilization of fracture may prevent fat embolism.

Treatment includes:
  i. Oxygen therapy
 ii. If hypoxia persists on oxygen therapy consider intermittent positive pressure ventilation (IPPV) with positive end expiratory pressure (PEEP).
iii. Reduction in raised intracranial tension (if there are CNS symptoms).
 iv. Corticosteroids, heparin (which stimulates circulating lipase that breaks neutral fat), ethanol (act as a lipase inhibitor in suppressing rise in fatty acids) and hypertonic saline (acts as alternative metabolic fuel thereby blocking mobilization of fatty acid) are now considered as outdated treatment modalities.

Cement Implantation Syndrome

Cement implantation syndrome (CIS) occurs more commonly in total hip replacement where cemented prosthesis is used. There occurs hypoxia, profound hypotension or even cardiac arrest. It may occur because of embolization of bone marrow debris, microemboli or fat due to increased intramedullary pressure created by cement or due to reaction to cement (methyl methacrylate).

The treatment includes Oxygenation, adequate hydration and adrenaline for severe reactions.

Deep Vein Thrombosis and Pulmonary Embolism

The incidence of deep vein thrombosis (DVT) and pulmonary embolism (PE) is highest in orthopedic patients particularly after hip surgery due to prolonged immobilization. *The incidence of fatal PE after hip surgery can be as high as 1–3%.* Many centers start low molecular weight heparin before 12 hours or more in preoperative period and restart 12 hours after surgery. *For diagnosis and treatment of pulmonary embolism see Chapter 14, page no. 139.*

Complications of Different Positions

Spine surgeries are done in the prone position while majority of hip surgeries in lateral position (*for complications of different positions see Chapter 14, page no. 146*). There have been case reports of stroke or even brain death in shoulder surgeries done in beach chair position due to ischemia. Therefore, invasive blood pressure is highly recommended for shoulder surgeries done in the beach chair position with transducer zeroed at the level of external auditory meatus to denote cerebral perfusion pressure.

CHOICE OF ANESTHESIA

Most of the orthopedic surgeries are performed under regional anesthesia. *Regional anesthesia is always preferred over general anesthesia due to decrease incidence of thromboembolism,* decrease blood loss, respiratory complications and better control of pain.

Upper limb surgeries can be performed under brachial plexus block. Small procedures lasting less than 30–45 minutes can be performed under Bier's block. Lower limb surgeries are performed under spinal/epidural or combined spinal epidural (most preferred technique).

General anesthesia is required either for very prolonged surgeries of upper limb, shoulder or spine surgeries or when regional is not possible.

Pain management: Postoperative pain management is one of the standards to define the quality of care in orthopedics. Other than continuous epidural various nerve blocks like continuous adductor canal block for knee replacement, fascia iliaca/femoral nerve block for hip surgeries, brachial plexus block for upper limb surgeries are frequently utilized for postoperative analgesia.

ANESTHESIA FOR SPINE SURGERY

Spine surgery is performed under general anesthesia in prone position. Therefore, complications related to prone position like endotracheal tube dislodgement, airway edema, injury to brachial plexus and peroneal nerve, injury to genitalia and breast, ocular injury (postoperative vision loss), hypotension do occur.

Monitoring

Other than routine monitoring, monitoring of spinal cord function is required for major spine surgeries like scoliosis. Wake up test done in the past is not performed in current day practice. The function of the spinal cord is monitored by evoked responses like somatosensory evoked potential (SSEP), motor evoked potential (MEP) and electromyogram (EMG).

As inhalational agents can depress these evoked responses their concentration should be kept at half minimum alveolar concentration (MAC). IV agents preserve evoked responses except a little inhibition seen with Propofol. Muscle relaxants cannot be used during MEP monitoring.

KEY POINTS

- Cardiac arrest can occur at the time of tourniquet deflation.
- Pressure in tourniquet should not exceed more than 100 mmHg above systolic pressure and duration should not exceed more than 2 hours for both upper and lower limbs.
- The triad of fat embolism syndrome is dyspnea, confusion and petechial hemorrhages. Petechial rash is pathognomonic of FES.
- Cement implantation syndrome may be characterized by hypoxia, profound hypotension or even cardiac arrest.
- The incidence of fatal PE after hip surgery can be as high as 1–3%.
- There have been case reports of stroke or even brain death in shoulder surgeries done in the beach chair position.
- Regional anesthesia is always preferred over general anesthesia due to less incidence of thromboembolism, less blood loss, fewer respiratory complications and better control of pain.
- The function of the spinal cord is monitored by evoked responses like somatosensory evoked potential (SSEP), motor evoked potential (MEP) and electromyogram (EMG).

CHAPTER 37

Anesthesia at Remote Locations

ANESTHESIA AT LOW BAROMETRIC PRESSURE (HIGH ALTITUDE)

The patients at high altitudes (low barometric pressure) have chronic hypoxia which can lead to polycythemia, pulmonary hypertension, decreased pCO_2 (due to hyperventilation) and lower bicarbonate concentration (as a compensatory mechanism to low pCO_2).

General Anesthesia

- Potency of anesthetic gases is proportional to their partial pressure. Therefore, at high altitudes where the barometric pressure is decreased, the potency also decreases. The potency of nitrous oxide is reduced to 50% at altitudes >3,300 meters. Therefore, it is recommended that nitrous oxide should not be used at altitudes more than 2,000 meters.
- Density of gases decreases at high altitudes, therefore, *rotameter under reads the actual flow rate* and this error may be up to 4 liters/minute.
- At altered barometric pressure, all vaporizers (except desflurane) deliver fixed partial pressure of vapor. Therefore, *vaporizer settings need not be changed at low or high barometric pressure except for desflurane,* which needs an upward adjustment at high altitude.
- Venturi type devices deliver higher oxygen (because of decreased density and resistance).
- Blood loss during surgery is more due to high venous pressure and blood volume.
- In the postoperative period, chances of hypoxemia are high due to low ambient partial pressure of oxygen.

Regional Anesthesia

The incidence of postspinal headache is high due to increased CSF pressure.

ANESTHESIA AT HIGH PRESSURE (IN HYPERBARIC CHAMBER)

General Anesthesia

- Tissues can become supersaturated with nitrous oxide causing significant diffusion hypoxia. The effect of supersaturation is more evident in helium atmosphere, therefore *nitrous oxide should not be used in helium atmosphere.*
- Rotameter will falsely give high values due to increased gas density.
- Endotracheal tube cuff should be filled with water or saline.
- The vaporizer output becomes less.
- Regional anesthesia is safe.

ANESTHESIA OUTSIDE OPERATING THEATER

Nonoperating room anesthesia means all procedures done outside the operation theater. For example, anesthesia services utilized in radiology (MRI, CT scan), gastroscopy suites, intervention cardiology and neurology, etc. Anesthesia outside Operation Theater possesses following challenges to an anesthetist:

- Procedure rooms are often small and crowded making placement of anesthesia machine, drug trolley, emergency cart and patient access difficult.
- Nonavailability of adequate equipment, monitors, technical support and help in case of emergency.

- Many times, like MRI suites, anesthetist stands far away from the patient.
- Unlike surgeons, many of the medical proceduralists do not understand the intricacies and importance of anesthesia. Any demand by anesthetist is often considered as obstructive by medical specialist. Majority of the patients undergoing medical procedures are even sicker than surgical patients. In spite of that, they are seldom evaluated and medically optimized in preoperative period.
- Risk of exposure to radiation.
- Contrast-related anaphylaxis can occur in radiology procedures.
- Majority of the times, cases come as unbooked and so, disturbing the schedule.
- Patients may not be adequately fasting.
- In spite of the high risk and adverse working circumstances, anesthetists are almost always undercompensated financially as compared to surgical cases.

Fasting

Inadequate sedation leading to conversion to general anesthesia is very common, therefore, *full fasting recommendation,* i.e. 6 hours for light food, 8 hours for a full meal, and 2 hours for water *is mandatory.*

Monitoring

- Other than pulse oximetery, ECG and BP, *capnography* (nasal capnography for spontaneously breathing patients) *is highly desirable;* capnography can pick up life-threatening complications very early.

Anesthesia

- Most often either sedation with midazolam or total intravenous anesthesia (TIVA) with Propofol + Remifentanil (in India fentanyl, due to nonavailability of remifentanil) is utilized for nonoperating room procedures.
- For MRI suites, everything including anesthesia machine, monitors, oxygen cylinders must be MRI compatible, i.e. nonferrous. *The equipments used in MRI suites are made up of aluminum.*

KEY POINTS

- At high altitude, rotameter under reads the actual flow rate.
- Vaporizer settings need not be changed at low or high barometric pressure, except for desflurane.
- The incidence of postspinal headache is high at high altitude.
- Nitrous oxide should not be used in helium atmosphere.
- Small and crowded space, nonavailability of adequate equipment, monitors, technical support and help in case of emergency, inadequate preoperative evaluation of patients and inadequate knowledge of anesthesia intricacies by medical proceduralists make nonoperating room anesthesia very challenging and least preferred by majority of anesthetists.
- Full fasting recommendations are required for non-operating room anesthesia.
- Capnography is highly desirable for nonoperating room anesthesia.
- Most often, either sedation with midazolam or total intravenous anesthesia (TIVA) with Propofol + Remifentanil is utilized for nonoperating room procedures.
- For MRI suites, anesthesia machine, monitors and oxygen cylinders should be made up of aluminum.

CHAPTER 38

Anesthesia for Day-care Surgery (Outpatient/Ambulatory Surgery)

In day-care surgeries/procedures the patient is admitted, procedure done and is discharged on the same calendar day. If the patient stays for one night, it is called as "short-stay surgery/procedure". Over the years, there has been tremendous increase in day-care surgeries/procedures due to the following reasons:

- Decreased hospitalization and hence the cost.
- Early ambulation (that's why called as ambulatory anesthesia) decreases the complications like pulmonary embolism.
- Less incidence of hospital-acquired infections.
- Hospital beds can be utilized for other needy patients.

SELECTION OF SURGERY/PROCEDURES AND PATIENTS

- Surgeries associated with major hemodynamic alterations, postoperative complications, requiring prolonged immobilization and parenteral/epidural analgesics, are not considered for day-care surgeries. *Duration of surgery is no longer a parameter to exclusion.*
- Although the American Society of Anesthesiologists (ASA) grading is not an absolute parameter, however, usually ASA grade I, II and III (with their disease well controlled) patients are considered for day-care procedures. Obesity (not even the morbid obesity with obstructive sleep apnea) is a barrier to daycare procedures.
- Age is no bar for day-care surgery; even a newborn or 100-year-old patient can be considered. The *only exclusion is prematures up to 50th postconception week* because

prematures are at high risk of apnea up to 50th postconception week.

- Patients not accompanied by responsible attendant cannot be considered for day-care surgery.

PREOPERATIVE ASSESSMENT AND PREMEDICATION

Prior assessment of a patient for day-care surgery should be done to avoid on-the-spot cancellation, which is very uncomfortable to the patient.

Investigations: As for other patients, there are *no routine investigations* for day-care patients too; investigations should be guided by the existing comorbidity and the nature of surgery.

Premedication: Like indoor patients, the most important goal for premedication for day-care patients is to relieve the anxiety. As Benzodiazepines can delay the recovery, the preferred method of relieving anxiety should be nonpharmacological (taking to the patient in detail to clear his/her doubts). If deemed necessary, then only benzodiazepines should be used. Because of the shorter half-life, *midazolam is the benzodiazepine of choice for day-care patients.* Patients who are at high risk of aspiration should be given prophylaxis with ranitidine and metoclopramide.

Premedication with oral NSAIDs has been found to be very useful in reducing the requirement of opioid analgesics.

Nil orally guidelines are same, i.e. 6 hours for light meal, 8 hours for full meal and 2 hours for clear fluids (water).

ANESTHESIA FOR DAY-CARE PATIENTS

Monitoring

Other than routine monitoring, bispectral index (BIS) monitor to measure the depth of anesthesia is suggested for day-care surgery, however, still considered optional because of its high cost and insignificant difference in awake time in patients whom BIS was used vs. in whom BIS was not used.

GENERAL ANESTHESIA

To avoid the complications of intubation (especially postoperative sore throat), *general anesthesia (GA) with laryngeal mask airway (LMA) is always preferred over intubation.* It is now considered safe to do even laparoscopic surgeries in LMA in patients who are adequately fasting and do not have a risk factor for aspiration.

Induction: *Propofol is the agent of choice for induction* because of its rapid, smooth recovery and antiemetic property. Propofol autoco-induction, the technique in which 30 mg of propofol is given as an initial dose, has been found to reduce the requirement of propofol, hastening the recovery.

Maintenance: Due to lowest blood gas coefficient, *Desflurane has earliest induction and recovery, therefore, is the inhalational agent of choice for day-care patients.* In case of nonavailability of desflurane, sevoflurane serves as an excellent alternative.

Use of nitrous oxide decreases the requirement of other anesthetic agents hence fastening the recovery (nitrous oxide itself is eliminated from body in 3–5 minutes).

Intravenous analgesics: Nonopioids like NSAIDs, can be used safely. Opioids should be avoided if possible. *Remifentanil* because of its ultra-short half-life (10 minutes), is the most preferred opioid.

Muscle relaxants: Short duration of action (10 minutes) makes *mivacurium as preferred muscle relaxant for day-care surgery.* Succinylcholine, in spite of having short duration, is usually not preferred due to high incidence of postoperative myalgia.

TOTAL INTRAVENOUS ANESTHESIA

This is the technique where only intravenous anesthetics are used (no inhalational, no muscle relaxant). The combination of choice for total intravenous anesthesia (TIVA) is *Propofol + Remifentanil.*

REGIONAL ANESTHESIA

Regional nerve blocks are simple and safe techniques for day-care surgery. In current-day practice, *spinal anesthesia is frequently used for day-care patients,* however, with small gauge pencil tip-needles and short/intermediate-acting agents like prilocaine or chloroprocaine. Lignocaine in spite of intermediate duration is not preferred due to the possibility of transient neurologic symptoms (TNS). If a long-acting agent like bupivacaine has to be used, then the spinal should be "selective spinal anesthesia (SSA)" which entails giving minimal doses to block only the required segments. Epidural is hardly used for day-care patients.

MONITORED ANESTHESIA CARE

Many times, the services of anesthetist are utilized for monitoring with or without sedation while surgery/procedure is performed under local anesthesia. *Most preferred drug for sedation is midazolam.* Sometimes, propofol may be required in low (sedative) doses.

POSTOPERATIVE PERIOD

The common problems seen in postoperative period are *pain (most common),* nausea and vomiting (2nd most common), sedation, myalgia, weakness and bleeding.

Discharge

The decision for discharge should be with common consensus between the surgeon and anesthetist. The aim should be *fast-track discharge,* which means shifting the patient directly from operation theater to phase II (step down) postanesthesia care unit (PACU). This will decrease the cost and facilitate early discharge.

The incidence of unexpected admission (unable to discharge) varies from 1% to 6%. The two *most common causes of unexpected admission are uncontrolled pain and nausea and vomiting.*

Criteria for *home readiness* are:
  i. Vital signs are stable for more than 60 minutes.
 ii. There is no nausea (or minimal nausea) for at least 30 minutes.
iii. Patient should be well oriented in time, place and person.
 iv. Able to walk without dizziness.
  v. Should be pain-free (or minimal pain) on oral analgesics.
 vi. There should not be any active bleeding.
vii. Must be accompanied by a responsible attendant.
viii. Should be able to stay in the vicinity of the hospital for first 24 hrs.
   • Able to accept liquids orally without vomiting is not a mandatory criterion in current-day practice. Similarly, able to pass urine is also not considered as mandatory criteria even after spinal, except for high-risk patients like urology/urogynecology, inguinal or perianal surgery, age >70, history of urinary dysfunction or dose of bupivacaine used for spinal is > 7 mg.
   • Patients with obstructive sleep apnea should be monitored for more than 3 hours and more than 7 hours, if there is even a single episode of desaturation on room air.

Postoperative Instructions for Day-care Patients

The patients should be instructed not to do important and skillful work like driving, operating a machine for at least 24 hours. Patients coming from outstation should be advised to stay for one day near the hospital so that if any problem arises, they can be brought back to the hospital.

Although > 50% of the patients complains of little drowsiness after discharge, the incidence of re-admission (or emergency visit) is 2–3%. *Most often the re-admission is due to surgical complications, such as surgical site infection.*

KEY POINTS

- Duration of surgery, the American Society of Anesthesiologist (ASA) grading and age (except prematures) are not considered as absoulte parameters to deny a surgery on day-care basis.
- Midazolam is the benzodiazepine of choice for day-care patients.
- Nil orally guidelines for day-care patients are same as for indoor patients.
- GA with laryngeal mask airway (LMA) is always preferred over intubation.
- For day-care patients, propofol is the most preferred agent for induction, desflurane for maintenance and mivacurium for muscle relaxation.
- The combination of choice for TIVA is Propofol + Remifentanil.
- Spinal anesthesia is frequently used for day-care patients, however, with small gauge pencil tip needles and short/intermediate acting agents.
- The aim of discharge should be fast-track discharge.
- The two most common causes of unexpected admission are uncontrolled pain and nausea and vomiting.
- Able to accept liquids and pass urine is not considered as mandatory criteria for discharging a patient after day care surgery.
- Most often the re-admission is due to surgical complications such as surgical site infection.

CHAPTER 39

Pain Management

Pain has been designated as the fifth vital sign.

ASSESSMENT OF PAIN

Pain is a subjective feeling; there may be up to 10-fold variation in pain perception among individuals. Various scales and questionnaires are available to assess the pain. The most commonly used scales are:

- *Visual analog scale*: It is a horizontal line divided into 10 equal points (0–10). At one end, (0 end), the label is no pain while at the other end (10 end) the label is worst pain imaginable. The patient is asked to mark the point where the pain lies.
- *McGill pain questionnaire (MPQ)*: It contains 20 sets of descriptive words. It not only determines pain intensity but also effective and cognitive components of pain.
- Pediatric scales such as *smiley scale* with different faces (at one end the crying face and other end the most smiling face); the child has to choose the face as per his/her pain.
- For younger children (usually less than 3–4 years), who even cannot identify the faces, pain has to be assessed objectively. The most commonly used scale to objectively assess the pain in these children is Children's Hospital of Eastern Ontario Pain Scale (CHEOPS). It includes cry, facial expression, verbal response, torso (body position), touch (touching wound) and Legs position.

Pain management may be acute pain management or chronic pain management.

ACUTE PAIN MANAGEMENT

Acute pain management is usually synonym with postoperative management; however, acute pain management is sometimes utilized for trauma patients too. Inadequate pain control in postoperative period can elicit the stress responses which can manifest as immunosuppression, poor wound healing, increased myocardial oxygen demand, decreased gastrointestinal motility and chronic postsurgical pain.

METHOD OF RELIEF

Postoperative pain management should have multimodal approach, which means combination of different modalities to control postoperative pain.

- *Nonsteroidal anti-inflammatory drugs (NSAIDs)*: Whatever the method of analgesia used, NSAIDs or cyclo-oxygenase-2 (COX-2) inhibitors should always be the part of multimodal analgesia because of their anti-inflammatory property. They can reduce the dose requirement of opioids by almost one third.
- *Acetaminophen (paracetamol)*: Acetaminophen along with the NSAIDs or regional nerve blocks may omit the need for opioids. It may serve as an alternative to NSAIDs in the patients where NSAIDs are contraindicated.
- *Opioids*: *Opioids still remain the mainstay of treatment for postoperative analgesia.* Although opioids can be given by almost all routes, however, *epidural route is the most preferred route for postoperative analgesia.* Bupivacaine (0.125–0.25%) or ropivacaine (0.2%) with/without fentanyl is the most frequently used combination for controlling postoperative pain.

In case of non-feasibility of epidural, IV route is most often utilized for postoperative analgesia. Excellent patient satisfaction seen with *patient-controlled analgesia (PCA) has made it a method of choice for postoperative analgesia if opioids have to be given by parenteral route.* PCA is an automatic system which is connected to an IV line. As the name suggests, the patient himself/herself presses a button which delivers a prefixed amount of opioid (usually morphine). A lockout interval (during which drug will not be delivered) is set to avoid over dosage.

The rationale for the success of PCA is that pain is best controlled when the analgesic is delivered either before or just at the beginning of pain. The delays in the delivery of analgesics by nurses leading to escalation of pain (making analgesic to become less effective) can be avoided with PCA devices.

- *Regional nerve blocks*: Regional nerve blocks with local anesthetics as a single shot or continuous infusion provide excellent postoperative analgesia. In fact, the nerve block given before skin incision (called as *pre-emptive analgesia*) not only decreases the stress response and requirement of anesthetics (if surgery is done in general anesthesia) but also decreases (or abolishes) the requirement of opioids (and hence their side effects) and incidence of acute pain getting converted into chronic pain. Commonly used nerve blocks for achieving postoperative analgesia are:
  - *Thoracic paravertebral block*: Thoracic paravertebral block is used to provide analgesia for thoracic, breast and upper abdominal surgeries.
  - *Transversus abdominis plane (TAP) block*: TAP block is very effective to produce analgesia for abdominal surgeries such as cesarean section, hernia repair, etc. TAP block is given in the fascial sheath deep to the internal oblique muscle and superficial to the transversus abdominis muscle.
  - Lumbar plexus block (also k/a psoas compartment block) is given to provide analgesia for hip and knee surgery.
  - *Femoral nerve block and fascia iliaca (modified femoral) block*: These blocks are utilized for hip fractures and hip surgeries.
  - *Brachial plexus blocks*: Brachial plexus blocks are utilized to provide analgesia for upper limb surgeries.

- *Other techniques*: Other techniques which are occasionally utilized to achieve postoperative analgesia, are:
  - Transcutaneous electrical nerve stimulation (TENS)
  - Acupuncture
  - *Cryoanalgesia*: It is produced by cryoprobes which use compressed carbon dioxide (CO_2) or nitrous oxide (N_2O). They cool the peripheral nerves to –5 to –20°C to produce analgesia.
  - *Ketamine infusion* in analgesic doses.

CHRONIC PAIN MANAGEMENT

Incidence of chronic pain can be as high as 25–30%. Chronic pain has most tangled and complicated pathophysiology. Chronic pain not only causes physical pain but damages the patient psychologically and emotionally also.

The main role of anesthetist in chronic pain management is to give neurolytic (damaging nerve) or diagnostic blocks (temporary blocks with local anesthetics). Neurolysis can be done with chemical agents (5% phenol in glycerin or absolute alcohol) or with radiofrequency probes, which ablate the nerve by burning at 60–90°C. As chemical Neurolysis can damage adjacent structures *radiofrequency ablation (RFA) is always preferred over chemical neurolysis*. Neurolytic blocks usually provide analgesia for 6 months to 2 years.

The most commonly encountered conditions in clinical practice are:

LOW BACKACHE

Low backache is one of the most commonly encountered conditions in clinical practice. Before treating low backache, neurosurgical and/or orthopedic consultation should always be sought to rule out any surgical problem.

The most common interventions done for low backache patients are:

- *Epidural steroids*: Usual indication for epidural steroid is chronic disc prolapse with nerve root compression. Studies have shown that only 40–50% of drug reaches the nerve roots if steroids are given through epidural route, therefore, now-a-day's *transforamina route (drug injected as the nerve exit through foramina) is always preferred over epidural route.*

- Facet joint injection with steroids and *radiofrequency (RF) ablation of medial branch of posterior ramus of spinal nerve* (supplying the facet joint) for facet arthropathy.
- Ozone/percutaneous discectomy for prolapsed discs.
- Sacroiliac joint injection for sacroiliitis.
- Vertebroplasty/kyphoplasty (injection of cement) for vertebral prolapse.

NEUROPATHIC PAIN

Most common neuropathy encountered in clinical practice is diabetic neuropathy. Drug of choice for neuropathic pain is pregabalin followed by gabapentin (except trigeminal neuralgia which still responds best to carbamazepine).

Trigeminal Neuralgia

Most often the pain is in maxillary division.

Treatment

- Drug of choice is carbamazepine.
- Patients not responding to carbamazepine are subjected to radiofrequency ablation of Gasserian ganglion or neurolytic block (radiofrequency/glycerol) of involved segment of trigeminal nerve (maxillary, mandibular or very rarely ophthalmic).

Postherpetic Neuralgia

Treatment

- Tricyclic antidepressants.
- Intercostal nerve blocks.
- Transdermal lignocaine patch/topical application of eutectic mixture of lignocaine and prilocaine (EMLA) cream.
- Topical application of capsaicin cream or patch.

Complex Regional Pain Syndrome (CRPS)

It is a group of diseases; most of them have sympathetically mediated pain. It is classified as Type I, which includes reflex sympathetic dystrophies such as Raynaud's phenomenon/disease, Berger's disease, phantom limb, Sudeck's dystrophy; and, Type II, which includes causalgia (neuralgic pain after direct nerve injury is called as causalgia).

The hallmark of CRPS is extremely painful limb. The limb becomes extremely sensitive to pain *(hyperalgesia)*; even a light touch can produce pain *(allodynia)*, pain may persist after the end of stimulus *(hyperpathia)* or patient may feel pain in anesthetized area *(anesthesia dolorosa)*.

Other clinical features of CRPS are of sympathetic overstimulation of limb like burning pain, increased sweating, edema, decreased blood flow, hair loss and limb weakness.

Treatment

- *Sympathetic blocks: The mainstay of treatment is sympathetic blocks. For upper limb CRPS, stellate ganglion block is performed; and, for lower limb dystrophies, lumbar sympathetic chain block is performed.* Usually 3–7 blocks are required to break the cycle of pain.
- Alpha blockers, pregabalin/Gabapentin
- Ketamine infusion
- TENS, spinal cord stimulation, surgical sympathectomy for refractory cases.

Intravenous regional sympathetic block (chemical sympathectomy) with guanethedine, which was popular in past, is not recommended in current-day practice; however, intravenous regional block with local anesthetic is still performed occasionally.

CANCER PAIN

Treatment of cancer pain requires multifaceted approach.

- *Pharmacologic therapy*:
  The WHO recommends *step ladder* for control of cancer pain.
  - Nonopioids like NSAIDs, paracetamol for mild pain.
  - Weak opioids like codeine for moderate pain.
  - Strong opioids like morphine for severe pain.

  Opioid remains the mainstay of treatment for cancer pain. Depending on the severity and feasibility, opioids are given through many routes.
  - *Oral*: Reserved for mild to moderate cancer pain.
  - *Transdermal fentanyl/butorphanol patch*: Patch is a very good alternative to oral route. Fentanyl patch provides analgesia for 48–72 hours while butorphanol patch provides analgesia for 6–7 days.
  - *Parenteral*: Parenteral route is utilized for severe pain.

– *Neuraxial*: Preservative-free morphine is used through epidural/spinal catheter. If this is effective in relieving pain, the spinal catheter may be surgically implanted for long-term use.

- *Regional blocks* like celiac plexus block for pancreatic and stomach malignancy, hypogastric block for pelvic malignancies.
- *Neurolytic blocks*: If block with local anesthetic is successful. then only neurolytic block should be considered.
- Adjuvant therapies like antidepressants, pregabalin/gabapentin and ziconotide (directly acting calcium channel blocker).
- For intractable pain, surgical intervention (cordotomy) should be considered.

MYOFASCIAL PAIN SYNDROME

It is a syndrome characterized by muscle pain and muscle spasm. Painful points (*trigger points*) are typical of myofascial pain syndromes.

Treatment includes physiotherapy, transcutaneous electrical nerve stimulation (TENS), acupuncture, topical cooling of muscle and *trigger point injection with local anesthetic*.

FIBROMYALGIA

Fibromyalgia is a very common pain disorder characterized by pain in different groups of muscles, easy fatigability and sleep deprivation. *The multiple trigger points are pathognomonic of fibromyalgia.*

Treatment includes trigger point injection with local anesthetics, pharmacotherapy (pregabalin, duloxetine, milnacipran and antidepressants), physiotherapy and cognitive–behavioral therapy.

COMMONLY USED PAIN BLOCKS

STELLATE GANGLION BLOCK

Stellate ganglion is formed by the fusion of lower cervical and first thoracic ganglion.

Indications

Usually employed for complex regional pain syndromes (CRPS) of upper limb. Other indications may be intra-arterial thiopentone injection and hand pallor (ischemia) following radial artery cannulation for invasive blood pressure monitoring.

Technique

It is blocked anterior to the tubercle of transverse process of C6 vertebra called as *Chassaignac tubercle.*

Signs of Successful Block

- *Horner syndrome,* which consists of:
  – Miosis.
  – Enophthalmos.
  – Ptosis.
  – Anhydrosis over the ipsilateral face and neck up to T3.
  – Absence of pupillary dilatation on shading the eye.
  – Absence of ciliospinal reflex (dilatation of pupils when skin over neck is pinched).
- Flushing of face.
- *Conjunctival congestion (most often the first sign).*
- Nasal stuffiness *(Guttmann's sign).*
- Congestion of tympanic membrane *(Mueller's syndrome).*
- Increased skin temperature.
- Lacrimation (due to involvement of superior cervical ganglion by cephalad movement of drug).

Complications

- Brachial plexus block causing unnecessary sensory and motor block.
- Recurrent laryngeal nerve block causing hoarseness of voice.
- Phrenic nerve block, however, unilateral phrenic nerve block is not bothersome; it just reduces the vital capacity by 20–25%.
- Epidural and intrathecal (subarachnoid) block.
- Pneumothorax
- Esophageal perforation and mediastinitis
- Hypotension due to sympathetic block and bradycardia due to blockade of cardioaccelerator fibers (T1-T4) by downward spillage of drug.
- Bleeding, hematoma and intravascular injection.

TRIGEMINAL NERVE BLOCK

Trigeminal nerve has three main branches—ophthalmic, maxillary and mandibular.

Indications

The principal indication of trigeminal nerve block is trigeminal neuralgia. Depending on the site of involvement block may be given at Gasserian ganglion level (*at foramen ovale*) or at one of the branches (usually maxillary or mandibular).

Technique for Maxillary and Mandibular Nerve Block

8 cm long 22 G needle is inserted at the inferior edge of coronoid notch till lateral pterygoid plate is encountered (usually at 5 cm). Needle is walked off anteriorly for 0.5 cm to block maxillary nerve and posteriorly to block mandibular nerve (and hence its branches viz., buccal, auriculotemporal, lingual and inferior alveolar).

Complications

Block of maxillary nerve can cause temporary blindness due to optic nerve involvement. While blocking mandibular nerve pharynx may be entered superior to superior constrictor.

INTERCOSTAL NERVE BLOCK

Indications

Intercostal nerve block is performed for post-operative analgesia, rib fractures and herpes zoster.

Technique

Usually performed in mid or posterior axillary line at the inferior border of rib.

Complications

- Pneumothorax
- After intercostal block, *highest blood level of local anesthetic is achieved per volume of drug injected.*

CELIAC PLEXUS BLOCK

Celiac plexus block is usually given for pain relief in gastric and pancreatic malignancy. *Most common complication is hypotension.*

LUMBAR SYMPATHETIC CHAIN BLOCK

Lumbar sympathetic chain block is usually utilized for CRPS of lower limb, especially Berger's disease. It is blocked anterior to lumbar vertebral bodies.

SUPERIOR HYPOGASTRIC BLOCK

Superior hypogastric block is performed for pain relief for pelvic malignancies.

GANGLION IMPAR BLOCK

Ganglion impar (ganglion of Walther) is used for pain relief of perineal area.

KEY POINTS

- Visual analog scale is the most commonly used scale for pain assessment.
- Postoperative pain management should have multimodal approach.
- Opioid remains the mainstay of treatment for post-operative analgesia.
- Epidural route is the most preferred route for postoperative analgesia.
- Patient-controlled analgesia (PCA) is the method of choice if opioids have to be given by parenteral route.
- Regional nerve blocks with local anesthetics as a single shot or continuous infusion provide excellent postoperative analgesia.
- Radiofrequency ablation (RFA) is always preferred over chemical neurolysis.
- Transforamina route for the delivery of steroids is preferred over epidural route.
- Radiofrequency (RF) ablation of medial branch of posterior ramus of spinal nerve is the most definitive modality of treatment for facet arthropathy.
- Most common neuropathy encountered in clinical practice is diabetic neuropathy.
- Drug of choice for neuropathic pain is pregabalin followed by gabapentin.
- Trigeminal neuralgia still responds best to carbamazepine.
- For upper limb CRPS, stellate ganglion block is performed; and, for lower limb dystrophies, lumbar sympathetic chain block is performed.
- Opioid remains the mainstay of treatment for cancer pain.
- The multiple trigger points are pathognomonic of fibromyalgia.
- Highest blood level of local anesthetic is achieved after intercostal nerve block.

Cardiorespiratory Care

CHAPTER 40

Intensive Care Management

INTENSIVE CARE UNIT

First intensive care unit (ICU) was started in 1953. Total number of beds in ICU should be 10% of hospital beds. Each bed should have 20 m² floor area. The patients usually coming to ICU are:

- Those who are in respiratory failure and need mechanical ventilatory support.
- Those who require very high level of monitoring.
- Those who are at high risk of going in cardio-respiratory failure.

ACUTE RESPIRATORY FAILURE

DEFINITION

Respiratory failure is the inability of lungs to maintain adequate oxygenation with or without acceptable elimination of carbon dioxide.

As a guideline, *acute respiratory failure* is considered to be present if partial pressure of oxygen (pO_2) is less than 60 mm Hg, pCO_2 over 50 mm Hg and pH less than 7.30 (however pCO_2 may be normal or even decreased in early phases of acute respiratory failure).

Elevated pCO_2 in presence of normal pH constitutes *chronic respiratory failure* (as pH is compensated by renal tubular reabsorption of bicarbonate).

CLASSIFICATION

Respiratory failure is classified in three types:

Type I or Oxygenation Failure

This is characterized by:
- Low pO_2 (<60 mm Hg).
- Increased pAO_2 (alveolar)—paO_2 (arterial) gradient.
- Increased dead space (increased VD/VT) and venous admixture.
- CO_2 is usually normal or even low (due to compensatory hyperventilation) but can be high in advance cases.

Causes

- Acute respiratory distress syndrome (ARDS).
- Chronic obstructive pulmonary disease (COPD).
- Pulmonary edema.
- Asthma.
- Pneumonitis.
- Pneumothorax.
- Pulmonary hypertension.
- Pulmonary embolism.
- Interstitial lung disease.

Type II or Hypercapnic Ventilatory Failure

This is characterized by increase in pCO_2 (> 50 mm Hg), pO_2 is usually normal (but may be low if pCO_2 rises to more than 75–80 mm Hg). pAO_2–paO_2 is normal.

Causes

- Overdosage of narcotics/barbiturates/benzodiazepines/anesthetics.
- Residual paralysis of muscle relaxants.
- Central causes, such as brainstem infarction/hemorrhage.
- Disorders affecting the signal transmission to respiratory muscles like Guillain-Barré syndrome, myasthenia gravis, multiple sclerosis, spinal cord injury.

- Disorders of respiratory muscles such as poliomyelitis, muscular dystrophies.
- Injury to chest wall like flail chest.

Type III or Combined Oxygenation and Ventilatory Failure

Theoretically any condition causing type I and type II failure can progress to type III failure, however, the usual causes of type III failure are:
- ARDS.
- COPD.
- Asthma.

MANAGEMENT OF RESPIRATORY FAILURE

- Supplemental oxygen with or without continuous positive airway pressure (CPAP).
- Mechanical ventilation, including addition of positive-end expiratory pressure (PEEP).
- Inotropic support to heart.
- Management of shock.
- Nutritional support.
- Control of infection/secretions.
- Maintenance of other organ functions.
- General nursing care.

SUPPLEMENTAL OXYGEN

For mild to moderate cases, supplemental oxygen therapy may be able to achieve pO_2 of 80 mm Hg. Supplemental oxygen can be delivered by various oxygen delivery devices like mask, nasal cannula, Venturi mask or by T piece attached to endotracheal or tracheostomy tube during the trial of weaning from ventilator.

Ideally, *inspired oxygen concentration (FiO_2) should not exceed more than 50%*, otherwise oxygen toxicity can occur. If the patient is not able to maintain oxygen saturation by oxygen delivery devices, noninvasive positive pressure ventilation (NIPPV) should be tried, if situation permits (see section of NIPPV) before proceeding to intubation and mechanical ventilation.

Oxygen therapy is helpful in improving oxygen saturation in all types of hypoxia except histotoxic hypoxia, maximum benefit is seen in hypoxic hypoxia. *Hypoxia produced by shunts* (whether intracardiac or intrapulmonary) *is not fully corrected even by inhalation of 100% oxygen.*

MECHANICAL VENTILATION OF LUNGS

Indications

Putting a patient on ventilator is more or less a clinical criterion however the general *guidelines are*:
- *On the basis of blood–gas analysis*:
  - pO_2 <50 mm Hg on room air or <60 mm Hg on FiO_2 (inspired oxygen) > 0.5 (50%).
  - pH <7.25 (acute respiratory failure).
  - pCO_2 >50 mm Hg.
  - pO_2/FiO_2 <250 mm Hg (normal >400)
  - p (A – a) O_2 gradient >350 mm Hg on 100% oxygen.
- *On the basis of pulmonary functions*:
  - Respiratory rate >35/minute.
  - Vital capacity <15 mL/kg.
  - Dead space volume (V_D/V_T) >0.6 (60%).
  - Peak negative pressure < –20 cm H_2O.
  - Tidal volume <5 mL/kg.
- *Other*:
  - Excessive fatigue of respiratory muscles.
  - Loss of protective airway reflexes which makes patient vulnerable for aspiration.
  - Inability to cough adequately.

Mechanical ventilation of lungs is carried out by intubating the patient by nasal or oral route or through tracheostomy and connecting endotracheal or tracheostomy tube to ventilator.

Ventilators

The breath by ventilator is governed by three factors (called as variables):
1. What initiates (triggers) breath? Patient spontaneous breath (therefore called as assist ventilation) or ventilator (therefore called as control breath).
2. What sustains breath? Preset volume (fix preset tidal volume is delivered therefore called as volume targeted or volume controlled ventilation) or preset pressure (ventilator will deliver till preset pressure is attained, therefore, called as pressure targeted or pressure controlled ventilation).
3. What terminates inspiration or other words what cycles ventilator to start expiration (therefore called as cycling)? The variable may be preset tidal volume (ventilator will start expiration once the preset tidal volume is delivered), preset pressure (ventilator will start

expiration once preset pressure is attained), set inspiratory time is lapsed (can be set by adjusting inspiratory to expiratory ratio, I:E ratio) or preset inspiratory flow is delivered.

So, broadly speaking, *ventilatory breath can be volume preset (volume targeted/controlled) or pressure preset (pressure targeted/controlled) breath.*

The chief advantage of volume preset breath is assurance of delivery of preset tidal volume and hence decreased chances of hypoventilation; however, the chief disadvantage is increased chances of barotrauma, if airway pressure increases or lung compliance decreases.

The chief advantage of pressure targeted ventilation is maintenance of preset airway pressure throughout the inspiration thereby decreasing the chances of barotrauma. Since tidal volume varies to maintain the preset pressure, the chief disadvantage of pressure controlled ventilation is the increased possibility of hypoventilation.

Depending upon the mode of ventilation selected ventilator will combine these three variables to deliver it breath.

1. *Time/patient initiated and volume cycled:* Triggering (initiation) factor for start of respiration is either time {determined by setting the respiratory rate (for example, if set frequency is 10 breaths/min, ventilator will initiate breath after every 6 second} or patient spontaneous breath.

   Inspiration is terminated (or other words ventilator cycles to expiration) when a preset tidal volume is delivered.

   As discussed above the main advantage of volume cycled ventilation is less chances of hypoventilation while the disadvantage is more chances of barotrauma.

2. *Time/patient initiated and pressure cycled:* The breath is initiated by time or patient spontaneous breath. Ventilator will cycle to expiration after attaining preset pressure for preset time (pressure preset time cycled) or till the delivery of preset flow (pressure preset flow cycled). As discussed above, that tidal volume can vary depending on the airway pressure and lung compliance the patient is more vulnerable for hypoventilation but at decreased risk of barotrauma.

3. *Dual control:* New ventilators can combine the benefits of both volume and pressure ventilation.

Initial Setting of Ventilator

The usual initial parameters set on ventilator are:

Tidal volume	: 6–8 mL/kg
Respiratory rate (frequency)	: 10–12 breaths/min.
Inspiratory (I) : Expiratory (E) ratio	: 1 : 2
Inspiratory flow rate	: 60–80 liters/min.
Trigger sensitivity (sensitivity of ventilator to detect patient spontaneous breath)	: –1 to –2 cm H_2O
FiO_2 (delivered concentration of oxygen)	: < 0.5 (50%). Initially, patient is started with 100% oxygen (FiO_2–1.0) but should be reduced to less than 0.5 at the earliest if patient maintains oxygen saturation >90%

Modes of Ventilation

- *Controlled-mode ventilation (CMV); also called as intermittent positive pressure ventilation (IPPV)* **(Fig. 40.1):**

  As the name suggests, in this mode the total breathing of the patient is controlled by ventilator at preset tidal volume (or preset pressure) and respiratory rate; there is no spontaneous effort by the patient.

  The major disadvantage of this mode is that the intrathoracic pressure always remains positive decreasing the venous return and cardiac output.

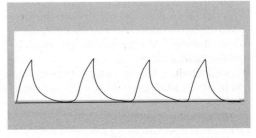

Fig. 40.1: Controlled-mode ventilation (CMV)

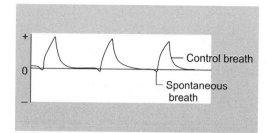

Fig. 40.2: Assist-control ventilation (AC)

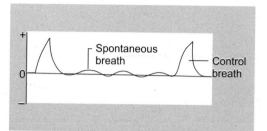

Fig. 40.3: Synchronized intermittent mandatory ventilation

- *Assist-controlled (A/C) ventilation* (also called as continuous mandatory ventilation) **(Fig. 40.2)**:
  As the name suggests, in this mode, ventilator assists the patient spontaneous breath to a preset tidal volume and can also deliver control breath, if required.
  For example, if the preset rate with ventilator is 10 breath/minute and patient's spontaneous breath are 5 then ventilator will assist those 5 breaths and remaining 5 breaths it will deliver in control mode (means ventilator need to work in assist as well as control mode). If the patient's spontaneous rate exceeds the set rate, say, it becomes 12 then ventilator will assist those 12 breaths (means ventilator is working in only assist mode). If patient becomes apneic then all 10 breaths will be delivered in controlled mode (means ventilator is working in controlled mode).
  In A/C mode, ventilator breath is initiated (triggered) by patient spontaneous breath. Ventilator detects patient's spontaneous effort by either detecting negative pressure in airway (trigger sensitivity) or by detecting inspiratory flow generated by patient's spontaneous breath.
- *Synchronized intermittent mandatory ventilation (SIMV)* **(Fig. 40.3)**:
  In this mode, the ventilator delivers the preset mandatory breaths; however, these breaths are synchronized with the patient's spontaneous breaths, meaning by that ventilator will deliver its breath either between patient's spontaneous efforts or will coincide with inspiration, never during expiration.
  The advantages of SIMV over CMV are:
  - *Less hypotension*: As there occurs good venous return during spontaneous breath,

the hypotension is less as compared to CMV.
  - As there is no synchronization with patient breath in CMV, the patient need to remain heavy sedated or to receive muscle relaxants in CMV.
  - As there is spontaneous breaths, patient do not feel the sense of breathlessness in between ventilatory breaths.
  Disadvantages of SIMV:
  - Increased hyperventilation (patient spontaneous breath + ventilator mandatory breaths) can cause hypocapnia and increases the work of breathing.
- *Inverse ratio ventilation (IRV)*: The normal I : E ratio of 1 : 2 is reversed to 2 : 1. Doubling the inspiratory time will double the gas exchange time. Like in CMV, the patients in IRV also need heavy sedation or muscle relaxants.
- *Pressure support ventilation (PSV)* **(Fig. 40.4)**:
  As the name suggests, a preset pressure is delivered to each breath of the patient to attain a desired tidal volume. The ventilator will cycle to expiration once the predetermined flow falls below 25% (flow cycled).
  To begin with usually a pressure of 8 cm H_2O is applied and then titrated to achieve the desired tidal volume. The aim of PSV is to decrease the work of breathing and to overcome the resistance offered by endotracheal tube and ventilator tubing. PSV can be used alone or in combination of SIMV.
- *Proportional-assisted ventilation (PAV)*: PAV is similar to PSV, the only difference is that in PAV, ventilator delivers the required pressure by calculating the lung compliance, not a fixed pressure as in PSV further decreasing the chances of barotrauma.

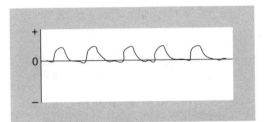

Fig. 40.4: Pressure support ventilation (PSV)

- *Pressure-controlled ventilation (PCV)*: In PCV, ventilator maintains a constant preset pressure for a preset time. Ventilator will cycle to expiration once preset time is lapsed (time cycled). Tidal volume is determined by set inspiratory flow and inspiratory time. As tidal volume is variable the patient is more prone for hypoventilation but less prone for barotrauma.
- *Neurally adjusted ventilatory assist (NAVA)*: The diaphragm activity is sensed by a sensor placed in distal esophagus to trigger ventilatory breath.
- *Dual mode ventilation:* New ventilators can combine the benefits of both pressure and volume ventilation to deliver mixed breaths. Although the different terminologies used by different manufactures have made these mode complicated but the most fundamental characteristic of these modes is that *the breath delivered is volume guaranteed (decreasing the chances of hypoventilation) and pressure regulated (decreasing the chances of barotrauma).*

  The most commonly used dual mode in India is *pressure-regulated volume control (PRVC)*. In this mode, upper level of pressure is set to prevent barotrauma and lower level of pressure is set to prevent alveolar collapse. The ventilator adjusts between these pressure limits to deliver the preset tidal volume at preset rate. As PRVC offers the combined benefits of volume and pressure *PRVC can be considered as mode of choice for ventilation in current day critical care practice.*
- *High-frequency ventilation*: This mode is applicable in conditions in which adequate tidal volume cannot be delivered; therefore, minute volume is compensated by high frequency. High frequency ventilation is delivered through special high-frequency devices. High-frequency ventilation may be:

- High-frequency positive-pressure ventilation where frequency is 60–120 cycles/min.
- High-frequency jet ventilation where frequency is 100–300 cycles/min with gases at high pressure of 60 psi. *This is the most commonly used mode for high frequency ventilation.*
- High frequency oscillations where frequency is 600–3,000 cycles/min.
Indications:
  - *Bronchopleural fistula*: Large tidal volumes can cause pneumothorax.
  - *Bronchoscopies*: Patient has to be ventilated through a very small port in bronchoscope which cannot deliver sufficient tidal volume.
  - *Microlaryngeal surgery*: At times glottic opening is so narrow to just allow a catheter through which it is not possible to deliver adequate tidal volume.
  - Emergency ventilation through cricothyroid membrane.

ADD ON MODES/POSITIVE PRESSURE AIRWAY THERAPY

These modes can be used alone or in conjugation with above mentioned modes.
- *Positive end-expiratory pressure (PEEP) (Fig. 40.5)*:
  During expiration the alveoli collapses and there is no gas exchange. In PEEP, as the name suggests positive pressure is given at the end of expiration to prevent alveolar collapse leading to gas exchange even during expiration. PEEP is very useful for situations like pulmonary edema or ARDS where gas exchange is impaired. PEEP can also be used in thoracic surgeries to minimize bleeding.
  Side effects of PEEP:
  - *Hypotension and decreased cardiac output*: Increase intrathoracic pressure produced by PEEP can significantly reduce the venous return and cardiac output.
  - *Increase pulmonary artery pressure (PAP)*: Compression of alveolar capillaries by PEEP can increase PAP producing right ventricular strain.

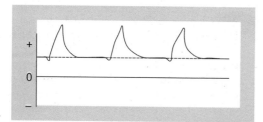

Fig. 40.5: Assist-control ventilation with PEEP

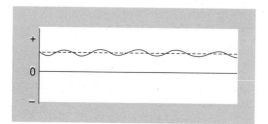

Fig. 40.6: Spontaneous ventilation with continuous-positive airway pressure

    – *Increase dead space*: Excess PEEP can lead to over distension of alveoli increasing the dead space.

    – Increase barotrauma

    Considering these side effects the *ideal PEEP is considered as the PEEP which maintains oxygen saturation > 90% without decreasing the cardiac output significantly. Usually it is 5–12 cm H_2O.*

- *Continuous-positive airway pressure (CPAP) (Fig. 40.6)*:
CPAP is a misnomer. It is just the PEEP given to a nonintubated patient or other words it is the noninvasive method of giving PEEP. It is given through a tight fitting mask.

- *Bilevel positive airway pressure (BIPAP)*: As the name suggests, BIPAP means positive pressure during inspiration (IPAP) as well as expiration (EPAP). Typical settings are 8–20 cm H_2O positive pressure during inspiration and 5 cm H_2O cm during expiration. *In very simple words it can be considered as combination of pressure support ventilation and PEEP or CPAP.*

    It is possible to deliver BIPAP to the non-intubated patient (NIPPV, see below) as well as intubated patients. The machine (ventilator or BIPAP machine) will maintain EPAP until a spontaneous breath is sensed and then it switches to IPAP. IPAP will be terminated either by preset time (time cycled) or if flow falls by certain level (flow cycled).

- *Airway pressure release ventilation (APRV)*: It is applied to patients on very high PEEP or CPAP where there is periodic release of PEEP or CPAP to decrease the incidence of barotrauma and hypotension.

NONINVASIVE POSITIVE PRESSURE VENTILATION: VENTILATION WITHOUT INTUBATION OR TRACHEOSTOMY

Since intubation and tracheostomy carries their multitude of complications; therefore, whenever possible, a trial of noninvasive positive pressure ventilation (NIPPV) should be given. Ideal candidates for trial of NIPPV are:

- The patients who are in respiratory failure but there is no urgent need of intubation
- Conscious and cooperative patients
- Patients in whom there is no risk of aspiration
- Face mask could be tightly fitted

NIPPV is contraindicated in:

- Cardiac or respiratory arrest
- Severe hypoxemia
- High risk of aspiration
- Facial trauma
- Inability to protect airways
- Upper GI bleed.

Common Indications

Although NIPPV can be used in respiratory failure due to any cause; however, most often in chronic setting it is very effectively used for sleep apnea syndrome while *in acute setting NIPPV is most frequently applied for acute exacerbation of COPD.* Other usual indications are immunocompromised patients who are very prone for respiratory infections following intubation or tracheostomy and cardiogenic pulmonary edema (because patients with cardiogenic pulmonary edema may recover early).

Recently it has been proven by studies that *prophylactic CPAP in preterm* babies can avoid intubation and allows the clinician to use low FiO_2 (<0.4) (this is very important consideration as preterm babies may develop retinopathy following the use of high oxygen concentration).

Equipment

NIPPV can be given through special CPAP/ BIPAP devices or through ventilators (most of the ventilators used now a day have option for delivering NIPPV).

Most commonly used for NIPPV is tight fitting face mask in acute setting and nasal mask in chronic setting (for sleep apnea syndrome). Other options are full face mask and helmet.

Modes of Ventilation

Modes of ventilation utilized for NIPPV are CPAP and BIPAP (already described above).

Protocol and Principles for NIPPV

- Explain the procedure to patient
- Mask should be tight fitting
- Preferably keep head end in propped up position
- Usual settings are:
    - *Inspiratory pressure (IPAP)*: 8–20 cm H_2O. Do not exceed above 20 cm H_2O (aspiration can occur).
    - *Expiratory pressure (EPAP)*: 5–10 cm H_2O
    - *FiO_2*: 1.0 to begin with
    - *Trigger sensitivity (ability of ventilator to detect spontaneous breath)*: Maximum
    - Titrate IPAP, EPAP and FiO_2 as per tidal volume and blood gases.
    - Give a trial for 1–2 hours, if there is no improvement or deteoration consider intubation. If there is improvement reassess after every 4 hours.

Complications

- *Leakage:* This is a major problem during NIPPV. Although most of the machines compensates for mild-to-moderate leaks; however, significant leaks can cause hypoventilation. It is best avoided by using tight fitting masks.
- Patients inconvenience and claustrophobia (particularly with full face mask and helmets).
- Increased chances of aspiration
- Skin breakdown, facial edema on prolonged use.
- Delay in intubation.

WEANING FROM VENTILATOR

Weaning means discontinuing the ventilatory support. Generally accepted parameters for

weaning are (these are simply the reversal of criteria for putting the patient on ventilator):

- pO_2 >60 mm Hg (and oxygen saturation >90%) on FiO_2 <50% and PEEP <5 mm Hg.
- pCO_2 <50 mm Hg.
- Respiratory rate <35/min.
- Vital capacity > 15 mL/kg.
- VD/VT <0.6.
- Tidal volume >5 mL/kg.
- Inspiratory pressure < –25 cm H_2O.
- Rapid shallow breathing index (RSBI)

$$= \frac{\text{Respiratory rate (breaths/min)}}{\text{Tidal volume (in liters)}}$$

RSBI should be <100.
- Normal arterial pH
- Normal hemoglobin.
- Normal cardiac status, i.e. at the attempt of weaning patient should not have tachycardia, hypertension.
- Normal electrolytes.
- Adequate nutritional status.

Method of Weaning

There are numerous methods of weaning and weaning varies from patient to patient. *It is possible to wean patient in any mode of ventilation except control mode ventilation.*

The most common process followed for weaning includes shifting from control mode ventilation to assist control and SIMV and then keep on decreasing the rate of breath delivered by ventilator gradually till it becomes 1–2 breath/min. If the tidal volume is not sufficient then pressure support ventilation may be instituted. The pressure support may be decreased gradually till the patient achieves adequate tidal volume. Once the patient's frequency and tidal volume is adequate then ventilator can be disconnected and T tube is attached to endotracheal tube.

If patient is able to maintain normal pulmonary and cardiac functions and shows normal blood gas analysis for more than two hours, extubation can be attempted.

COMPLICATIONS OF MECHANICAL VENTILATION (AND ASSOCIATED PROBLEMS)

- *Pulmonary barotrauma*:
  Incidence is 7–10%. Barotrauma may manifest as pneumothorax, pneumomediastinum,

pneumopericardium, pneumoperitoneum, bronchopleural fistula and air embolism (pulmonary/systemic).

- *Infections: The most common source of nosocomial infections in ICU are urinary tract infections* accounting for 35–40% of total ICU infections followed by pulmonary (25–30%) and bloodstream infections (20%) {occurring due to CVP, arterial or IV lines}. *Majority of nosocomial infections are caused by gram-negative organisms* except for IV related infections which are caused by staphylococcal epidermidis.

Ventilator-associated pneumonia (VAP): It is defined as pneumonia developing in patients on ventilators for >48 hours with no evidence of preintubation pneumonia. The incidence of VAP is around 20%. Most often it is due to gram-negative organisms. Pooling of secretions from oral cavity or due to gastric reflux is the main reason for VAP, therefore, preventive measures includes:

  - Positioning of the head of the bed at 30 degrees: By decreasing the gastroesophageal reflux *positing head at 30 degrees proves to be simplest and most cost effective method to decrease VAP.*
  - Use of endotracheal tubes with subglottic suctioning appears to be very effective method for the prevention of VAP.
  - Oral hygiene with chlorhexidine can significantly decreases the load of bacteria
  - *Early* (6–8 days after intubation) *vs. late* (13–15 days) *tracheostomy has no effect on the incidence of VAP* as well as mortality in ICU.

- *Complications due to prolonged intubation/tracheostomy* like airway edema, sore throat, laryngeal ulcer, granuloma or web, tracheal stenosis, fibrosis or tracheomalacia.
- *Complications due to inadequate ventilation like* hypoxia, hyperoxia, hypercarbia or hypocarbia, acidosis or alkalosis.
- *GIT:*
  - Stress ulcers.
  - Paralytic ileus.
- *Cardiovascular*: Positive pressure ventilation by increasing the intrathoracic pressure *decreases venous return and hence cardiac output.* Right ventricular strain or even right ventricular failure can occur due to increase in pulmonary artery pressure.

- *CNS:* IPPV and PEEP by decreasing venous return from brain increases the intracranial pressure.
- *Liver and kidney dysfunctions* may occur due to decreased cardiac output.
- *Intensive care acquired weakness:* It may be due to prolonged immobilization, use of muscle relaxants, electrolyte imbalances.
- *Ciliary activity* is impaired if nonhumidified oxygen is used for prolonged periods.
- *Deep vein thrombosis,* Thromboembolism and *bed sores* due to prolonged immobilization.
- *Psychological:* Depression and emotional trauma.
- *Financial burden* on patient and relatives.

MONITORING

Usually used monitors are:
- Pulse rate
- *Blood pressure:* Mostly invasive. Arterial cannulation is not only required for blood pressure monitoring but also to take frequent samples for blood gas analysis and other investigations.
- ECG
- Oxygen saturation
- Respiratory parameters like tidal volume, minute volume, frequency, airway pressure, FiO_2, etc.
- CVP
- Urine output
- Other special monitoring depends on specific indications.

INOTROPIC SUPPORT TO HEART

Maintenance of normal cardiac function is important in the patient of respiratory failure. Dopamine or dobutamine infusion may be required to maintain normal cardiac output.

SHOCK

Shock often accompanies respiratory failure or vice versa; therefore, often the management of shock goes parallel with respiratory management.

Definition

Shock is defined as the state in which ineffective tissue perfusion leads to first reversible and then irreversible cellular injury.

Classification

It is classified into four major types:
1. Hypovolemic
2. Cardiogenic
3. Distributive
4. Obstructive.

Causes of Shock

Hypovolemic

- Hemorrhage.
- Fluid loss in diarrhea, vomiting, excessive sweating, diabetic ketoacidosis, polyuria, etc.
- Third space loss in ascites, pancreatitis.
- Burns.

Cardiogenic

- Pump failure (left ventricular failure or right heart failure).
- Arrhythmias.
- Myocardial trauma/rupture.
- Severe valvular diseases (of regurgitant type).

Distributive

- Neurogenic.
- Septic.
- Anaphylactic.
- Acute adrenal insufficiency.
- Vasodilators.

Obstructive

- Cardiac tamponade/constrictive pericarditis.
- Tension pneumothorax.
- Pulmonary embolism or pulmonary hypertension
- Valvular disease (obstructive type especially Aortic stenosis).
- Aortic dissection.

Hypovolemic shock is characterized by decreased circulatory volume leading to low central venous pressure (CVP), low pulmonary artery occlusion pressure (PAOP, previously called as PCWP) and hence decreased cardiac output/index. There is reflex vasoconstriction leading to increased systemic vascular resistance (SVR) therefore BP may be normal initially.

In *cardiogenic shock* poor pump function leads to increased CVP, increased PCWP (in LVF PCWP is >25 mm Hg), BP is again normal initially due to sympathetic stimulation which also leads to increased SVR.

In distributive shock poor vascular tone (decreased SVR) is the hallmark. Decrease SVR decreases the afterload increasing the CO. PCWP may be normal or low.

Septicemic shock is usually hyperdynamic type (increased CO) but hypodynamic is also seen. In septicemic shock pulmonary hypertension is also prominent.

In *obstructive shock* CVP is raised, PCWP is usually low, cardiac output is decreased, SVR is elevated.

Hemodynamic parameters in shock

Type	CVP	PCWP	CO/CI	SVR	BP
Hypovolemic	↓	↓	↓	↑	↓ or normal (initially)
Cardiogenic	↑	↑	↓	↑	↓ or normal
Distributive	↓	↓	↑	↓↓	↓
Obstructive	↑	↓	↓	↑	↓ or normal

Abbreviations: CVP, central venous pressure; PCWP, pulmonary capillary wedge pressure; CO, cardiac output; CI, cardiac index; SVR, systemic vascular resistance; BP, blood pressure. ↑, increase; ↓, decrease

Compensatory Mechanism in Shock

Increased sympathetic activation (and also increased release of adrenaline, vasopressin, angiotensin), tries to maintain intravascular volume and increases cardiac contractility.

Clinical Features

- *Mild shock (loss <20% of blood volume)*: Tachycardia, cold skin, postural hypotension and concentrated urine (osmolarity >450 mosmol/L).
- *Moderate (loss 20–40% of blood volume)*: Tachycardia, supine hypotension, oliguria (output <0.5 mL/kg /hr), metabolic acidosis.
- *Severe (>40% of blood volume)*: Restlessness, agitation, confusion to coma, tachypnea (rapid shallow breathing), ARDS and finally respiratory arrest.

MANAGEMENT OF SHOCK

The goals for resuscitation can be classified as early goals and late goals.

Early Goals

- *Target blood pressure*: In hemorrhagic shock increasing the blood pressure to normal level can lead to increased bleeding due disruption of clots removing the tamponade effect and reversal of compensatory vasoconstriction. Therefore, the current guidelines for hemorrhagic shock are in favor of *hypotensive resuscitation*, which means maintaining systolic blood pressure (SBP) between 80–100 mm Hg and mean arterial pressure (MAP) between 60–65 mm Hg. Hypotensive resuscitation should be avoided in ischemic heart disease patients and patients with brain or spinal cord injury. *For other type of shock the target should be to achieve normal blood pressure or at least systolic blood pressure >100 mm Hg.*

- *Maintain coagulation and platelet:* Life-threatening coagulopathy is one of the serious complications seen in profound shock; therefore, the correction of coagulopathy from the very beginning is of utmost importance and is called as *hemostatic resuscitation*. In fact, some clinicians have even suggested a preemptive resuscitation with blood products in a ratio of 1:1:1 (RBC: FFP: Platelets); however, FFP and platelets should be transfused only after assessing the coagulation and platelet deficiency. PT, APTT and INR are the universally performed test to assess coagulation but not considered as reliable as thromboelastography. *Platelet count should be kept >50,000.* Antifibrolytic therapy with tranexamic acid have shown the survival benefit if given within 1 hour. *This newer concept of hypotensive and hemostatic resuscitation is called as balanced resuscitation.*

- *Maintain hematocrit of 25–30%:* Hyperviscosity as well as excessive hypoviscosity are detrimental therefore hematocrit should be maintained between 25% and 30%.

- Arterial O_2 saturation >90% and venous oxygen saturation (SVO_2)> 60%.

- *Other goals* are to avoid hypothermia (keep core temperature >35° C), prevent worsening of acidosis and increase in serum lactate levels.

Late Goals

Late resuscitation begins once bleeding is definitively controlled.

- Maintain systolic blood pressure >100 mm Hg
- Maintain *urine output > 0.5 mL/kg/hr.*
- Maintain hematocrit
- Correct coagulation, electrolyte imbalance and acidosis
- Normalize body temperature
- Decrease lactate to normal range
- Assess the tissue perfusion by measuring:
    - *Mixed venous oxygen tension (SVO_2): Mixed venous oxygen saturation is considered as best guide to assess tissue perfusion (i.e. cardiac output) however it is technically difficult.*
    - *Urine output: Urine output is considered as best clinical guide of tissue perfusion.*
    - Acid-base status
    - *Serum lactate levels:* Results are delayed; however, serum lactate levels not only provide excellent assessment of tissue perfusion but also assess the results of resuscitation.
    - Gastric tonometry
    - Skeletal muscle partial pressure of oxygen.

Treatment

Fluids

Titration of fluid therapy

The current concept is to give fluids by *Goal directed therapy (GDT)* which means giving fluids by measuring dynamic cardiac functions like cardiac output or stroke volume and pulse pressure variation (means variation in stroke volume and pulse pressure during inspiration and expiration). *Variation >10–15% confirms hypovolemia. Stroke volume variation is considered as most reliable to assess fluid status and titrate fluid therapy* however due to technical feasibility and cost the static parameter, i.e. CVP is still most commonly used.

Choice of fluids

Fluid remains the mainstay of treatment for shock.

For hemorrhagic shock if loss is >20% of blood volume it should be replaced by blood. A normal patient without any systemic disease like ischemic heart disease and normal hemoglobin well tolerates blood loss up to 20% of blood volume therefore should be managed by crystalloids/colloids.

Crystalloids are preferred over colloids due to the following reasons:

- They not only replace intravascular volume but they also replace extravascular volume (and cellular hydration depends on extravascular volume).
- They do not interfere with clotting while all colloids in high doses can interfere with clotting.
- Colloids are expensive.
- There is risk of anaphylactic reaction with colloids.

Due to the above said reasons *colloids are reserved only for severe shock* where maintenance of intravascular volume is vital.

Ringer is the most preferred crystalloid as it is more physiological except for hypochloremic alkalosis (seen in vomiting) and brain injury where normal saline is preferred solution (Ringer contains calcium which can worsen neurological injury in case of brain injury). Glucose containing solutions should not be used (they exacerbate ischemic brain damage).

Drugs

- *Vasopressors*: Vasopressors should be used for severe shock or if hypotension is not responding to fluid therapy. Vasopressors in common use are:
  - *Phenylephrine: Phenylephrine is considered as first-line drug in neurogenic shock*
  - *Ephedrine and mephentermine: Ephedrine is most preferred for spinal shock*
  - *Norepinephrine (noradrenaline): Noradrenaline is the vasopressor of choice for septicemic shock*
  - *Vasopressin*: It can be tried in hypotension refractory to norepinephrine.
- *Inotropes*: Inotropes in common use are dopamine, dobutamine, dopexamine and milrinone (phosphodiesterase III inhibitor). *Inotropes are very useful for cardiogenic shock.*
  Adrenaline is used for treatment of shock when inotropes and vasopressors fail.
- *Steroids*: Steroids are effective for septicemic shock refractory to fluids and vasopressors,

not useful in hyperdynamic and hypovolemic shock and contraindicated in cardiogenic shock (they can alter healing process of myocardium).

Acid Base Management

The patients of shock are in metabolic acidosis; however, *this metabolic acidosis should not be treated by sodium bicarbonate* (unless severe, pH<7.15), *rather treated by improving the tissue perfusions by fluids and drugs*. Sodium bicarbonate by producing CO_2 may worsen cellular acidosis.

Prediction of Outcome in Shock

Shock index (SI) which is heart rate (HR) divided by systolic blood pressure (SBP) is often used as predictor in calculating the outcome in severe shock however recently studies have shown the equal role of diastolic blood pressure in predicting the mortality bringing the concept of *modified shock index (MSI), which is a ratio of heart rate to mean arterial pressure (MAP)*.

NUTRITIONAL SUPPORT

The malnutrition in mechanically ventilated patient may be seen in more than half of the patients. Nutritional support can be accomplished by enteral or parenteral route.

Enteral Route

For short-term feeding large bore nasogastric (Ryle's) tubes may suffice but for long term feeding jejunostomy tubes should be used. Jejunostomy tubes may be inserted through nasal route or can be placed surgically through gastrotomy or percutaneously under endoscopic guidance.

Enteral route is always preferred over parenteral route due to the following reasons:

- It is the natural route of food intake
- *Atrophy of luminal brush border of GIT can be prevented.*
- Less expensive
- More nutrients can be provided.

Parenteral Route

Parenteral nutrition is used when the enteral route is not possible or is unable to provide sufficient caloric intake. Parenteral nutrition can be provided through peripheral vein if osmolarity of solution is < 750 mosm/L (making it useful only for short duration feeding) or through central vein if energy requirement are higher and total osmolarity of solution is > 750 mosm/L. Due to large diameter (and hence less chances of thrombophlebitis due to lipid emulsions) *subclavian is the vein of choice for parenteral nutrition.*

Calculation of Energy Requirement

Ideally exact energy calculation should be done by calorimetery and estimation should be based on resting energy expenditure (calculated by using Harris–Benedict equation and is approximately 10% greater than basal energy). However, a simple formula to calculate energy requirement is:

Energy expenditure = Basic metabolic requirement × activity factor (1 for resting and 1.5 for ambulatory) × Injury factor (1.2 for minor and 1.8 for major) × temperature (1 for 37°C and multiply by 1.07 for each degree).

For clinical purposes, calorie requirement for normal 70 kg man is 1,800 kcal/day. For major surgery, trauma and sepsis, it is increased by 40% (2,500 kcal/day) and for burn patients it becomes double (3,600 kcal/day).

Substrates for Providing Energy

Out of the total energy required *60–70% should be provided by carbohydrates (dextrose) and 30–40%* by fats. *Amino acids are given as supplement (never as a substrate for source of energy) at a rate of 1–2 g/kg/day.* Multivitamins and trace elements should be given along with. Parenteral glucose solution provides 3.5 kcal/g (compared to dry carbohydrate which provide 4 kcal per g).

Complication of Enteral and Parenteral Nutrition

See **Table 40.1**.

PULMONARY CARE

- Frequent suctioning to remove secretions. This is very important as endotracheal or tracheostomy tube can be blocked by secretions and can cause hypoxia and death. Close suctioning devices can decrease the incidence of infection. Patient on ventilator remains apenic during suctioning therefore suctioning duration should not exceed more than 20 seconds.
- Regular chest physiotherapy.
- Postural drainage of secretions.
- Steam inhalation.
- Bronchodilators.

GENERAL NURSING CARE

Care of bladder, bowel, intravascular fluid volume and other organ functions.

■ **Table 40.1:** Complications of enteral/parenteral nutrition

Complication	Cause	Comments
Dextrose-related		
1. Hyperglycemia	Due to excessive dextrose and decreased insulin and corticoids	Hyperglycemia can increase CO_2. Therefore glucose should not provide >60–70% of energy
2. Hypoglycemia	It is rebound due to excess insulin release which is because of prolonged stimulation of pancreas by high glucose	Leads to hyperventilation and muscle fatigue making weaning difficult
3. Ketoacidosis, nonketotic coma	Due to hyperglycemia	
4. Respiratory acidosis	Due to increased CO_2 production by excessive glucose	
Fat-related		
5. Hyperlipidemia	Due to excessive fat	Excess fat can produce cholestatic jaundice, lipoid pancreatitis and lipoid pneumonitis
6. Hypolipidemia	Due to deficient fat	

Contd...

Contd...

Amino acid-related		
7. Hyperammonemia and azotemia	Due to excess of amino acids	
8. Hypoproteinemia	Due to deficient amino acids	It is very difficult to wean off a patient with hypoprotenemia
9. Hyperchloremic metabolic acidosis	Due to excessive chloride content of amino acid solutions	
Others		
10. Hypophosphatemia	Inadequate phosphorus administration	Hypophosphatemia can cause respiratory failure
11. Hypokalemia	Inadequate potassium	Normal Potassium is needed for weaning
12. Hyperkalemia	Due to excessive administration	
13. Hypomagnesemia	Deficient administration	Normal magnesium is needed for weaning
14. Hypermagnesemia	Excessive administration	
15. Hypocalcemia	Deficient administration	Normal calcium is needed for weaning
16. Hypercalcemia	Excessive administration	
17. Anemia	Due to iron and vitamin B_{12} deficiency and anaemia of prolonged illness	
18. Hypernatremia and water loading	Stress is a sodium retaining condition	
Catheter-related		
19. Infection at site, endocarditis	Due to faulty septic insertion and low maintenance of asepsis	Central lines should be inserted with highest aseptic precautions
20. Catheter misplacement and catheter embolism		
During catheter insertion		Catheter should be placed with expert hands and always obtain a X-ray chest after catheter insertion
21. Pneumothorax		
22. Pneumomediastinum		
23. Hemothorax		
24. Cardiac tamponade		
25. Injury to major vessels (subclavian, carotid) and hematoma formation		
26. Air embolism		
27. Cardiac injury		
28. Arrhythmias		
29. Nerve injuries (phrenic, brachial plexus)		

SPECIFIC CONDITIONS

SEPSIS

Sepsis is the leading cause of death in ICU. ARDS and renal failure are the most common causes of death in septicemia. In hospitalized patients, septicemia most often results from gram-negative organisms. The most common sources of sepsis are urinary tract infections and pneumonitis.

The sepsis patient's coming to ICU are most often in *septicemic shock* which is defined as systolic blood pressure <90 mm Hg or mean arterial pressure (MAP) <60 mm Hg. The mainstay of management of septic shock is fluids given by goal-directed therapy. *Colloids especially hydroxyethyl starch (HES) should be avoided,* because it may increase kidney injury. If a colloid has to be used then it should be albumin.

Antibiotics should be instituted at the earliest. If MAP remains <65 mm Hg in spite of fluids, Noradrenaline should be started. A low dose steroid should be started if hypotension remains refractory to treatment. Contrary to the previous guidelines *new studies do not recommended tight glycemic control in septicemia.*

Very high cost and disappointing results have lead to withdrawn of activated protein C (Drotrectogin alfa) for the treatment of even severe sepsis. Other modalities like fibronectin or monoclonal antibodies have also shown the disappointing results.

PULMONARY EDEMA

Pulmonary edema is defined as abnormal accumulation of fluid in interstitial and alveolar spaces of lungs. Pulmonary edema is divided into:
- Hemodynamic type.
- Increased permeability type.

HEMODYNAMIC TYPE

The most common cause of hemodynamic pulmonary edema is left heart failure (cardiogenic edema). Pulmonary edema develops when pulmonary artery occlusion pressure (previously called as pulmonary capillary wedge pressure), i.e. left atrial pressure rises to more than 25 mm Hg (or 30 cm H_2O).

Other causes of hemodynamic pulmonary edema are:
- Excess volume (reperfusion type)
- Sudden expansion of collapsed lung (re-expansion type)
- Decreased oncotic pressure like in hypo-albuminemia
- Neurogenic.

Treatment of Cardiogenic Edema
- Propped up position.
- Oxygen inhalation.
- Morphine:
  – Relieves the anxiety of patient.
  – Reduces central sympathetic outflow.
  – Shifts fluid from pulmonary to systemic circulation.
- Remove fluids from lungs by diuretics (furosemide)
- Reduction of preload by nitroglycerine infusion (venodilator)
- Reduction of afterload by sodium nitroprusside infusion (arteriolar dilatation).
- Improve cardiac output by:
  – Cardiac glycosides.
  – Dopamine.
  – Dobutamine.
- Rotating tourniquets: Not used now-a-days.
- *Treatment of underlying cause:* Most commonly it is due to myocardial ischemia therefore treat ischemia and control arrhythmias.
- If oxygenation is not improved by these measures, patient should be taken up for mechanical ventilation with PEEP.

INCREASED PERMEABILITY TYPE (NON-CARDIOGENIC)—ADULT RESPIRATORY DISTRESS SYNDROME

The basic pathology is increased capillary permeability leading to pulmonary edema followed by epithelial cell damage. This type of increased capillary permeability pulmonary edema constitutes a syndrome called as *adult respiratory distress syndrome (ARDS).*

The overall mortality in ARDS is 30–40% and is due to multiorgan failure. Risk factors for increased mortality in ARDS include old age, *low PaO$_2$/FiO$_2$ ratio,* septic shock, *high sequential organ failure assessment (SOFA) score,* and associated comorbidities like renal or liver disease.

Diagnosis of ARDS

American–European definition which had classified ARDS on the spectrum of acute lung injury had significant limitations and confusion therefore a simplified *Berlin definition of ARDS is followed in current practice* which has simply divided ARDS severity into three stages:

Mild: PaO_2/FiO_2 ≤300 mm Hg with PEEP or CPAP ≥5 cm H_2O

Moderate: PaO_2/FiO_2 ≤200 mm Hg with PEEP ≥5 cm H_2O

Severe: PaO_2/FiO_2 ≤100 mm Hg with PEEP ≥5 cm H_2O

Other criteria of Berlin definition to diagnose ARDS are:

- Onset of respiratory symptoms within 1 week of a known clinical insult.
- Bilateral opacities on X-ray chest which are not nodules, effusions, or lung collapse.
- Respiratory failure not explained by cardiac failure or fluid overload (ruled out by echocardiography).
  Low PAOP (PCWP) {< 18 mm Hg} essentially rules out cardiogenic pulmonary edema however is not the part of Berlin definition.
  Low pO_2, decreased functional residual capacity (FRC) and decreased static compliance of lungs are the hallmark of ARDS while pCO_2 may be low (if patient is hyperventilating to compensate for low pO_2), normal or high.

Causes of ARDS

- *Sepsis*: Sepsis is the most common cause of ARDS.
- *Lung infection*: Pneumonitis.
- Pulmonary aspiration of gastric contents.
- Polytrauma (shock lung syndrome).
- Toxins, inhalation of smoke, fumes, carbon dioxide/monoxide.
- Oxygen toxicity.
- Air, fat or amniotic fluid embolism.
- Blood transfusion (mismatch transfusion reaction).
- Pancreatitis, peritonitis.
- Drowning
- Anaphylactic reaction.
- Radiation pneumonitis.
- Acid inhalation.
- Thoracic trauma.
- Burns.

Management of ARDS

- Supplement oxygen if patient is able to maintain pO_2 >60 mm Hg, pCO_2 <50 mm Hg and respiratory rate <35/min. If not then add CPAP/BIPAP with CPAP/BIPAP device. If the patient does not maintain oxygen saturation with NIPPV then intubate and start mechanical ventilation.
- Mechanical ventilation:
  - Select control/assist control mode
  - *Use low tidal volume of 6 mL/kg. Low tidal volumes have not only seen to decrease the morbidity, ventilator days and ICU stay but have also found to decrease the overall mortality significantly (9%).*
  - Initial respiratory rate should be the rate which maintains baseline minute ventilation of patient (but, of course, not be >35 breath/min). The aim should be to maintain normal pCO_2.
  - *Keep plateau airway pressure (P_{plt}) <30 cm H_2O*
  - Inspiratory flow rate should be above the patient demand (usually 80 L/min)
  - FiO_2: 1.0 to start with and then keep on decreasing with a target of <0.5
  - PEEP of 5–12 cm H_2O is invariably required. Higher PEEP is not advisable as it does not offer any additional advantage rather increases the risk of barotrauma and hypotension.
  - Muscle relaxants should be used to paralyze the patient if absolutely necessary. Inadvertent use of muscle relaxants can cause muscular weakness and difficulty in weaning.
- Bronchodilators (if there is reflex spasm), antibiotics (if there is associated evidence of infection) and mucolytics to clear secretions.
- *Steroids: The use of steroids still remains controversial in ARDS;* some studies have shown the improvement in morbidity and mortality while others have shown the conflicting results.
- *Prone position*: The prone position leads to better drainage of secretions and improves oxygenation by eliminating the effects of gravity on ventilation perfusion mismatch however studies has found no difference in morbidly and mortality in patients ventilated in supine vs. prone position therefore *the routine*

use of prone position is not recommended for the treatment of ARDS.

- *Recruitment maneuvers*: Recruitment maneuvers mean using high inspiratory pressures to improve oxygenation. These maneuvers can significantly increase the risk of barotrauma and improves oxygenation only transiently without improving mortality *therefore, are not recommended routinely.*
- *Inhaled nitric oxide*: As ARDS is associated with pulmonary hypertension, inhaled nitric oxide appears to be beneficial by causing selective pulmonary vasodilatation (It does not produce systemic vasodilatation because it is rapidly metabolized by hemoglobin in pulmonary vasculature); however, studies showed no long-term difference in overall prognosis of the patients received nitric oxide. Therefore, *inhaled nitric oxide is not recommended for routine use in ARDS.*
- Treat the underlying cause.

Management of Refractory ARDS

If, in spite of the above said measures pO_2 remains <60 mm Hg, pO_2/FiO_2 ratio <100 and airway pressure more than 30 cm H_2O *rescue therapy* should be instituted which includes:

- *Extracorporeal membrane oxygenation (ECMO)*: In this technique patient's venous blood is withdrawn through a large bore cannula, circulated through an external oxygenation device (artificial lung) for oxygenation and then returned back to patient through another venous cannula. The aim of ECMO is not only to provide external oxygenation but also to give rest to diseased lung and time to clinician to treat the cause. *The major complication of ECMO is bleeding* due to the use of anticoagulants (anticoagulants are given so that blood does not clot in ECMO circuits).
- In current day practice, the use of recruitment maneuvers, prone position, inhaled nitric oxide and muscle relaxants are reserved for refractory ARDS.

CHRONIC OBSTRUCTIVE PULMONARY DISEASE

The management of chronic obstructive pulmonary disease (COPD) patient is very tricky. The important considerations in management of COPD patient includes:

- *These patients survive on hypoxic drive therefore during oxygen supplementation it is necessary to keep the low flows (1–2 liter/min),* otherwise hypoxic drive may be lost and the patient can go in apnea.
- Once put on ventilator *COPD patients are most difficult to be weaned therefore maintaining oxygenation by noninvasive positive pressure ventilation (NIPPV) with CPAP/BIPAP should be the prime goal.* Early institution of NIPPV has found to significantly decrease the need of mechanical ventilation. Some intesivists have suggested that removal of CO_2 by extracorporeal CO_2 elimination techniques should be done before putting the patient on mechanical ventilation.
- These patients should be put on ventilator based on *clinical judgment* rather than by blood gas reports. It is very common to see the patient of COPD comfortable at very low pO_2 and very high pCO_2.
- Ventilator setting includes small tidal volume, *low breath rate (6–8/min) and longer expiratory time to allow maximum exhalation.*
- These patients have decreased body resistance; therefore, prone for infection necessitating the need for asepsis during any procedure.

CARBON MONOXIDE POISONING

Usually defined as carboxyhemoglobin >20% in blood. The affinity of carbon monoxide (CO) to bind to hemoglobin is 240 times than oxygen; it bind to hemoglobin replacing oxygen from there producing *anemic hypoxia*. Moreover, CO shifts the O_2 dissociation curve to left further decreasing the oxygen supply to tissues. Levels >30% are associated with neurologic impairment and acidosis.

Treatment

Half-life of CO at atmospheric air is 214 minutes which can be reduced to 1 hour if 100% oxygen is used and can further be reduced to 20 minutes with hyperbaric oxygen (2.8 atm.). Based on this fact, many clinicians reserve hyperbaric oxygen only for severe cases; however, number of studies have proven better prognosis after hyperbaric therapy than normobaric oxygen therapy.

ACID-BASE MANAGEMENT

Acid-base disturbances may be respiratory or metabolic based on arterial pH, partial pressure of CO_2 (pCO_2) and bicarbonate levels (HCO_3^-).

Blood Gas Sample

Arterial sample is taken either from radial artery or femoral artery (radial preferred). Sample must be taken in heparinized syringe (glass syringe preferred over plastic syringe because oxygen can diffuse through plastic), all air (even minute droplet) should be removed from syringe and sample to be sent in ice if immediate analysis is not possible.

Interpretation of Normal Blood Gas

pH	: 7.35–7.45
pCO_2	: 35–45 mm Hg
HCO_3^-	: 24–26 mEq/L
Base deficit	: –3 to + 3
$SpO2$ (oxygen saturation)	: 96 to 98%
(A – a) DO_2 (alveolar to arterial difference)	: 3 to 5 mm Hg

The normal pH is maintained by the normal 20 : 1 ratio of bicarbonate to carbon dioxide as described by Henderson–Hasselbalch equation which is:

$$pH = pK + \log \frac{HCO_3^-}{0.03 \times pCO_2}$$

So, if this ratio is maintained at 20 : 1 the pH may be normal in spite of acid-base imbalances or in other words, it can be said that acid-base abnormalities have been compensated.

To compensate or maintain normal ratio any increase in pCO_2 is associated with increase in bicarbonate (bicarbonate retention by kidney) and any decrease in pCO_2 is associated with decrease in bicarbonate (excess excretion of bicarbonate by kidneys).

Diagnostic Approach for Establishing the Acid Base Abnormality

The acid-base disturbances may be respiratory acidosis, respiratory alkalosis, metabolic acidosis and metabolic alkalosis.

The problem in interpretation arise when more than one abnormality coexist at a time e.g. respiratory acidosis in COPD patients may be associated with metabolic acidosis due to decreased cardiac output (cor pulmonale) and renal flow.

The acid-base disturbances may be acute (non-compensated) or chronic (compensated).

The diagnostic approach is first see the pH. It may be normal, increased or decreased. Then see pCO_2 it may be again normal, increased or decreased. Now see the bicarbonate level this may be unchanged, decreased or increased. Now interpret as shown in **Flow chart 40.1**.

RESPIRATORY ACIDOSIS

Definition

It is defined as increase in pCO_2 sufficient enough to decrease the pH to less than 7.35.

Causes

- Hypoventilation which may be because of overdosage of drugs and anesthetics.
- Disorders of neuromuscular junction effecting muscles of respiration.
- Central depression of CNS.
- Lung diseases like COPD, etc.
- Excessive CO_2 production, e.g. malignant hyperthermia.

Respiratory acidosis may be associated with metabolic alkalosis if there are decreased body stores of chloride and potassium.

Treatment

- Mechanical ventilation; if pCO_2 is high (>50 mm Hg).
- Acidosis should be treated slowly.
- Treatment of the underlying cause.

RESPIRATORY ALKALOSIS

It is defined as decrease in pCO_2 sufficient to increase the pH to more than 7.45.

Causes

- *Hyperventilation*: This is the usual cause during general anesthesia (with hand ventilation there is always a tendency to hyperventilate).
- Iatrogenic.
- Pregnancy.
- Salicylate poisoning.
- Hypoxia.
- CNS trauma.

Treatment

- Adjustment of ventilator setting (decrease the frequency) and increasing the rebreathing (i.e. exhaled gases containing CO_2).

Flow chart 40.1: Diagnostic approach for acid-base abnormality

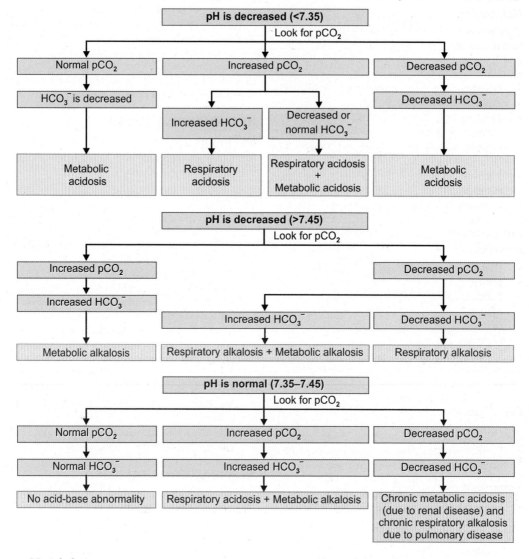

- CO_2 inhalation.
- Treat the underlying cause.

METABOLIC ACIDOSIS

Defined as decrease in pH <7.35.

Causes

- Renal failure.
- Circulatory failure (shock) leading to accumulation of lactic acid.
- Hepatic failure.

- Diarrhea with loss of bicarbonate.
- Cyanide poisoning.

Anion Gap

Also called as unmeasured anion concentration. Normally anion gap is constituted by sulfates, phosphates, organic acids and plasma proteins. *Anion gap is mainly constituted by plasma albumin.*

Anion gap = Sodium concentration – (chloride + bicarbonate concentration).

Normal anion gap = 8–16 mM/L (average 12 mM/L).

Conditions Associated with Normal Anion Gap

Conditions primarily associated with bicarbonate loss is accompanied by equivalent rise in chloride and hence a normal anion gap. These conditions are:

- Diarrhea.
- Enterostomies.
- Renal tubular necrosis, obstructive uropathies, chronic pyelonephritis. In these conditions kidney primarily loses bicarbonate but chloride is retained.
- Administration of hydrogen or ammonium chloride.
- Carbonic anhydrase inhibitors.

Conditions Associated with Increased Anion Gap

- Diabetic ketoacidosis.
- Ketoacidosis associated with starvation.
- Lactic acidosis: This is the *most common cause* of metabolic acidosis in anaesthesia and is due to tissue hypoxia.
- Salicylate poisoning.
- Methanol and ethylene glycol poisoning.
- Renal failure, leading to decreased excretion of acid, phosphates and sulfates.

Conditions Associated with Decreased Anion Gap

- Hypoalbuminemia.
- Multiple myeloma.

Treatment of Metabolic Acidosis

- *Sodium bicarbonate:*
  Dose can be calculated by formula:
  Sodium bicarbonate (mEq) = 0.3 × body weight × base deficit.
  Half of the calculated dose is to be given immediately and the remaining dose only after getting the next blood gas analysis report. *It is mandatory to have adequate ventilation before giving sodium bicarbonate* because sodium bicarbonate produces carbon dioxide on metabolism (1 mEq produces 180 mL of CO_2) and can worsen the acidosis. Another problem with sodium bicarbonate is its hypertonicity (6 times more than plasma) which can result in hypernatremia and hyperosmolarity.

Other buffers:
  - *Carbicarb* (sodium bicarbonate + sodium carbonate): It is a non CO_2 generating alternative to sodium bicarbonate but clinical studies are lacking.
  - *THAM:* Non-sodium containing compound.
- Treat the underlying cause.

METABOLIC ALKALOSIS

Defined as pH >7.45.

Causes

- Vomiting.
- Ryle's tube aspiration (loss of HCl).
- Diuretics.
- Hypovolemia.
- Diarrhea with loss of chloride.
- Iatrogenic.

Treatment

- Treat the underlying cause.
- IV infusion of ammonium chloride or 0.1 N hydrochloric acid (not more than 0.2 mEq/kg/hr).
  For summary of findings of acid base disturbances see **Table 40.2**.

■ **Table 40.2:** Summary of findings of acid base disturbances

Abnormality	pH	pCO₂	HCO₃⁻
Respiratory acidosis			
Acute (noncompensated)	↓↓	↑↑↑	↑
Chronic (compensated)	↓	↑↑↑	↑↑
Respiratory Alkalosis			
Acute (noncompensated)	↑↑	↓↓↓	↓
Chronic (compensated)	↑ or normal	↓↓↓	↓↓

Abnormality	pH	pCO₂	HCO₃⁻
Metabolic acidosis			
Acute (noncompensated)	↓↓↓	↓	↓↓↓
Chronic (compensated)	↓	↓↓	↓↓↓
Metabolic alkalosis			
Acute (noncompensated)	↑↑↑	↑↑	↑↑↑
Chronic (compensated)	↑↑	↑↑	↑↑↑

Abbreviations: ↑↑↑, marked increase; ↓↓↓, marked decrease; ↑↑, moderate increase; ↓↓, moderate decrease; ↑, mild increase; ↓, mild decrease.

KEY POINTS

- Oxygen therapy is helpful in improving oxygen saturation in all types of hypoxia except histotoxic hypoxia.
- Ventilatory breath may be volume controlled or pressure controlled.
- The chief advantage of volume controlled ventilation is decreased chances of hypoventilation and chief disadvantage is increased chances of barotrauma.
- The chief advantage of pressure controlled ventilation is less chances of barotrauma while main disadvantage is increased possibility of hypoventilation.
- Pressure regulated volume control (PRVC) can be considered as mode of choice for ventilation in current day critical care practice.
- Ideal PEEP is the PEEP which maintain oxygen saturation >90% without decreasing the cardiac output significantly. Usually, it is between 5–12 cm H_2O.
- Leakage is the major problem during NIPPV.
- It is possible to wean patient in any mode of ventilation except control mode ventilation.
- The most common source of nosocomial infections in ICU are urinary tract infections.
- Majority of nosocomial infections in ICU are caused by gram-negative organisms.
- Positing head at 30 degrees proves to be simplest and most cost effective method to decrease ventilator associated pneumonia.
- Current guidelines for hemorrhagic shock are in favor of hypotensive resuscitation which means maintaining SBP between 80–100 mm Hg and MAP between 60–65 mm Hg.
- Correction of coagulopathy called as hemostatic resuscitation is of utmost importance in hemorrhagic shock.
- The concept of hypotensive and hemostatic resuscitation is called as balanced resuscitation.
- Modified shock index (MSI), ratio of heart rate to mean blood pressure (MAP) is considered as better predictor of outcome in shock then shock index.
- Mixed venous oxygen saturation is overall the best guide to assess tissue perfusion while urine output is considered as best clinical guide to assess tissue perfusion.
- Stroke volume variation is considered as most reliable to assess fluid status and titrate fluid therapy.
- Crystalloids are preferred over colloids for shock and Ringer is the most preferred crystalloid.
- Phenylephrine is the vasopressor of choice for neurogenic shock, ephedrine for spinal shock and nor-epinephrine for septicemic shock.
- Metabolic acidosis due to shock should be treated by fluids and vasopressors not by soda bicarbonate unless severe (pH <7.15).
- Enteral route is always preferred over parenteral route for nutrition.
- Subclavian is vein of choice for parenteral nutrition.
- Out of the total energy required 60–70% should be provided by carbohydrates (dextrose) and 30–40% by fats. Amino acids are given as supplement, never as a substrate for source of energy.
- Sepsis is the leading cause of death in ICU.
- New studies do not recommended tight glycemic control in septicemia.
- Low pO_2, decreased functional residual capacity (FRC) and decreased static compliance of lungs are the hallmark of ARDS while pCO_2 may be low, normal or high.
- Low tidal volume (6 mL/kg), airway plateau pressure < 30 cm H_2O and low FiO_2 (<0.5) are the key in the management of ARDS.
- Extracorporeal membrane oxygenation (ECMO) should be instituted early for refractory ARDS.
- In current day practice the use of recruitment measures, prone position, inhaled nitric oxide and muscle relaxants are reserved for refractory ARDS.
- For COPD patients it is necessary to keep the low flows (1–2 L/min) of oxygen to preserve hypoxic drive.
- Maintaining oxygenation by non-invasive positive pressure ventilation (NIPPV) with CPAP/BIPAP should be the prime goal in COPD patients.
- Ventilator setting for COPD patients includes small tidal volume, low breath rate (6–8/min.) and longer expiratory time to allow maximum exhalation.
- Lactic acidosis is the most common cause of metabolic acidosis in anesthesia and is due to tissue hypoxia.
- Soda bicarbonate should be used to treat only severe acidosis (pH <7.15).

CHAPTER 41

Cardiopulmonary and Cerebral Resuscitation

- Cardiopulmonary resuscitation (CPR) nowaday is called as cardiopulmonary and cerebral resuscitation (CPCR).
- Cardiac arrest is defined as "inability of heart to produce effective cardiac output, impairing tissue perfusion".
- Cardiac arrest may be of cardiac origin or non cardiac; in adults is usually of cardiac origin and in children it is usually of respiratory origin.
- Cardiac arrest may be witnessed (monitored) or unwitnessed (unmonitored). It may be inside hospital (IHCA) or outside hospital (OHCA). *Unwitnessed cardiac arrest in adults should be considered due to ventricular fibrillation until proved otherwise and in children should be considered due to asystole until proved otherwise.*
- *Rhythms in cardiac arrest*: The following three rhythms are seen in cardiac arrest:
  1. *Ventricular fibrillation (and pulseless ventricular tachycardia)*: More common in adults
  2. *Asystole*: More common in children.
  3. Pulseless electrical activity (PEA)

MANAGEMENT OF CPCR

Management guidelines are based on the *recent recommendation (2015)* by American Heart Association (AHA) and Emergency Cardiovascular Care (ECC) with International Liaison Committee on Resuscitation (ILCOR).

AHA and ECC have given 4 link chain of survival:
1. Early recognition and activation of emergency medical services.
2. Immediate CPR (every minute delay decreases prognosis by 7–10%).
3. Early shock (CPR + shock within 5 minutes has survival rate of 49–75%).
4. Early advanced life support.

Management of CPR is done under three heads:
1. Basic life support (BLS)
2. Advanced cardiovascular life support (ACLS)
3. Post cardiac arrest care.

Whether the CPR is provided by BLS or ACLS the primary focus is the management of airway, breathing, circulation and early defibrillation. *The standard age long sequence of A (Airway) → B (Breathing) → C (Circulation) was changed to C → A → B in 2010 CPR guidelines*, which means the rescuer will first give 30 compressions in approximately 18 seconds before proceeding to airway and breathing. The reasons for this change are:
  i. There is enough oxygen present in blood which just needs to be pushed to vital structures like heart and brain with cardiac compressions.
  ii. Studies have shown that it takes around 18–20 seconds to assemble equipment for airway management, during which time the rescuer can start compressions while assistants can prepare equipment for airway management.

BASIC LIFE SUPPORT (TABLE 41.1 AND FLOW CHART 41.1)

Basic life support (BLS) as the name suggests can be employed with minimal or no instruments therefore is more suitable for outside hospital CPR provided by lay rescuers and paramedics or as an

■ **Table 41.1:** Differences between BLS and ACLS

Parameter	Basic life support	Advanced cardiovascular life support
Airway management	Manual	With equipment
Breathing	Bag and mask/ mouth to mouth	Advanced methods like endotracheal tube, LMA, combitube or tracheostomy tube
Circulation	Cardiac massage	Cardiac massage
Defibrillation	Automatic external defibrillator	Manual defibrillator
Drugs	–	+

immediate step to start CPR in in-hospital cardiac arrests till advance life support arrives.

Basic life support includes:
- Airway management by manual methods.
- Rescue breathing by bag and mask or mouth to mouth. *Mouth to mouth is recommended only for trained personal.*
- Circulation by cardiac massage.
- *Defibrillation by automatic external defibrillator (AED)*: AED are the devices which automatically detect the rhythm and give shock if rhythm is shockable. Since AED can be used by lay rescuer, they are the part of basic life support. As AED are meant for public use they are now better known as public assess defibrillators (PAD); like west they should ideally be present at all public locations like airports, railway stations, bus stations, etc.

ADVANCED CARDIOVASCULAR LIFE SUPPORT (ACLS)

ALS is usually employed in continuation of BLS however sometimes in monitored in-hospital arrest (particularly in ICU) CPR can directly be started with ALS.

Advanced life support includes:
1. Airway management by equipment like Guedel's airway, laryngeal mask airway or endotracheal tube.
2. Breathing by advanced methods, i.e. endotracheal tube, laryngeal mask, combitube or tracheostomy.
3. Circulation by cardiac massage.

4. *Defibrillation by manual defibrillators*: In manual defibrillators, rescuer has to detect rhythm, select energy and give shock therefore, can be used only by medical personnel and hence is a part of advance life support.
5. *Drugs*: can be used only in hospital set up by medical personal therefore are the parts of ALS.

AIRWAY MANAGEMENT

Interestingly, as per the newer studies epiglottis, rather than tongue fall, has been found to be the more important cause of airway obstruction in unconscious patient. However, tongue falling back on posterior pharyngeal still plays a very important role in airway obstruction.

This tongue/epiglottis fall can be managed by:
- *Manually:* This includes:
  - Open mouth and clear airways (if something is clearly visible in oral cavity).
  - Tilt head backwards (i.e. neck extension) and chin lift.
  - Jaw thrust, i.e. mandible is pulled forward.
    - In patients with suspected cervical spine fracture head tilt and chin lift should be avoided and airway should be managed only by jaw thrust however *if airway is not manageable by jaw thrust alone then head tilt and chin lift can be given* because life takes the priority over cervical spine.
- *Airway insertion*: Most commonly used in Guedel airway. Others are Safar, nasopharyngeal and laryngeal mask airway (LMA)
- *Endotracheal tube*: It is the most definitive method to maintain airway.

Management of Airway Obstruction due to Foreign Body

- *Infant chest thrust:* 4 blows given on sternum with thrust by heel of hand between the shoulders.
- *Back blows:* 4 blows on the middle of back. Back blows are also performed for infants if sternal thrusts do not work.
- *Heimlich maneuver:* Manual thrust with the patient standing, rescuer behind the patient and compressing the abdomen 6–10 times.

Flow chart 41.1: Algorithm showing basic life support (BLS)

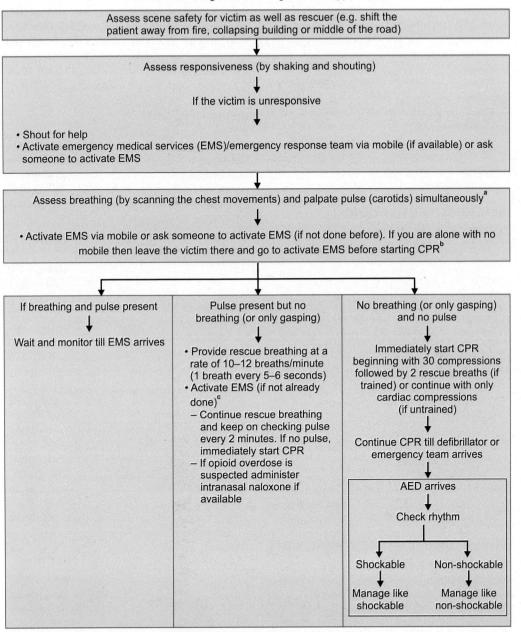

a. Breathing and pulse check should not take more than 10 seconds.
b. In an adult victim, the cause of cardiac arrest should be considered ventricular fibrillation until proved otherwise therefore arranging defibrillator before starting CPR is must.
c. Note that new guidelines allow activation of EMS at any step.

This method is used for adults and older children.

- *Chest thrust (manual compression over lower sternum):* Employed in very obese or pregnant patient where abdominal compression is not possible.
- *Finger sweep method:* Possible in unconscious patients only.
- *Cricothyroidotomy:* As a life saving procedure to secure airway.

Airway obstruction due to other causes like laryngeal edema, acute epiglottitis and laryngo-tracheobronchitis where intubation is not possible, may require tracheostomy.

BREATHING (VENTILATION)

Breathing can be accomplished by:

- *Mouth to mouth/mouth to nose:* Rescue breath by mouth to mouth or mouth to nose is reserved only for trained rescuers (medical as well as non-medical). It is neither expected nor warranted for untrained lay rescuer; *for untrained lay rescuer CPR means "hands only" i.e. only cardiac massage.*
- *Bag and mask:* The major disadvantage of bag and mask ventilation are:
  - Exhausting.
  - Increased dead space.
  - Increased chances of aspiration.
- Ventilation by advanced methods:
  - *Endotracheal tube: Intubation is the most definitive and best method for ventilation.*
  - Laryngeal mask airway.
  - Combitube.
  - Tracheostomy-other than endotracheal intubation, the only other definitive method of ventilation is tracheostomy.

AIRWAY AND BREATHING FOR PATIENTS WITH CERVICAL SPINE

For patients with cervical spine fractures intubation should be performed with neck in neutral position and only after stabilization. Neck stabilization can be done manually and with hard cervical collars. As intubation often requires removal of cervical collar *manual stabilization is always preferred over collar stabilization.*

Studies have shown more harm than benefit with cervical collars therefore routine application of cervical collars by first aid providers is not recommended. If cervical spine injury is suspected then ensure that patient remains still as far as possible (*for detailed management of patients with cervical spine see Chapter 5, page nos. 55 and 56*).

CIRCULATION

This is accomplished by *cardiac massage.*

Method (Fig. 41.1)

It is done with patient in supine position however in very rare cases, where supine position is not possible it can be done in prone position too. The rescuer stand (or bend on knee if the victim is on floor) on side (usually right side), lock one hand over other and provide compression over the lower third of sternum (2 fingers above xiphoid process). The victim must lie on hard surface and rescuer should exert pressure through shoulders (elbow should remain straight).

The force generated during massage should be able to depress sternum by *2 inches* (5 cm) *but not more than 2.4 inches* (6 cm) to avoid complications due to excessive pressure.

During cardiac massage compression relaxation (chest to recoil) should be equal. To allow full

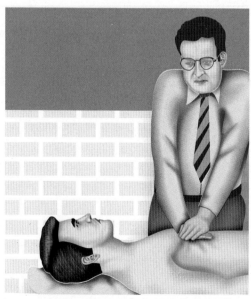

Fig. 41.1: Cardiac massage (note the extension at elbow, pressure exerted from shoulder). Patient should lie flat on hard surface

recoil the rescuer must not lean (a very common practice) on patient chest between compressions.

The rate of compression should be *100–120 compressions/minute but not more than 120* because studies have shown that at compression rate more than 120/min, compression depth decreases significantly. No intervention (intubation, pulse check) should stop cardiac massage for >10 seconds.

Physiological Considerations of Cardiac Massage

Heart compressed between sternum and spine results in ejection of blood from heart *(cardiac pump theory)* however another convincing theory is *thoracic pump theory* which states that cardiac compression raises intrathoracic pressure forcing blood out of chest and dynamic venous compression preventing backward flow, heart acting only as a passive conduit.

Effective cardiac output generated by successful massage is only 30% of normal therefore all efforts should be directed to establish spontaneous circulation.

COMPRESSION (C) TO VENTILATION (V) RATIO

Without advanced airway (i.e. ventilation with mouth to mouth or bag and mask), *the ratio should be 30:2* (30 compressions followed by 2 breaths) irrespective of number of resuscitators. *With advanced airway* (intubation, LMA) *compression will be continued at a rate of 100–120 compressions/ minute and breathing at a rate of 10 breaths/ minute (1 breath after every 6 second) without any synchronization, i.e. no pause for ventilation.* The aim is uninterrupted compressions.

If there are 2 rescuers they should rotate with each other after 2 minutes (or 5 cycles of 30:2) to avoid fatigue of one person providing compression.

MONITORING OF CPR

- *Capnography:* Capnography is the simplest and highly reliable method to see the effectiveness of CPR. *Successful cardiac massage should be able to produce ETCO₂ of at least 20 mm Hg.* If ETCO₂ is less than 10 mm Hg then cardiac massage should be considered grossly abnormal. ETCO₂ becoming normal

(40 mm Hg) is the earliest indicator of return of normal circulation.

In the current day CPR *Capnography is considered essential* not only to confirm the position of endotracheal tube but also to assess the performance of CPR.

- *Diastolic blood pressure (intra-arterial):* Diastolic blood pressure <20 mm Hg indicates grossly abnormal CPR.
- *Venous oxygen saturation:* CPR should be considered ineffective if it is not able to produce oxygen saturation of at least 30% in venous blood (normal is 75%).
- *Audiovisual feedback devices:* These devices provide real-time monitoring and feedback of quality of CPR however currently they are used only during training sessions.

MANAGEMENT OF ARRHYTHMIAS SEEN DURING CARDIAC ARREST

One of the most important parts of ACLS is arrhythmia management.

Arrhythmias seen during cardiac arrest have been divided into *shockable rhythms* (which include ventricular fibrillation, pulseless ventricular tachycardia and polymorphic ventricular tachycardia i.e. torsade pointes) and *nonshockable rhythms* (which include asystole and pulseless electrical activity).

Management of Shockable Rhythms (Flow Chart 41.2)

(Ventricular fibrillation, pulseless ventricular tachycardia and polymorphic ventricular tachycardia).

Defibrillation

Defibrillation is done for ventricular fibrillation, pulseless ventricular tachycardia and polymorphic ventricular tachycardia. Defibrillators have been classified as monophasic (delivers current of one polarity only) and biphasic (delivers current of two polarities). Although studies have not proven clear cut superiority of biphasic defibrillators still majority of defibrillators manufactured today are biphasic. A defibrillator may be manual or automatic (AED).

Defibrillation should be done as soon as the defibrillator is ready. Ideally, in monitored patients defibrillation should be done within 3 minutes.

Position of defibrillation paddles: The ideal position would be like that the heart is sandwiched between paddles, i.e. one is placed anteriorly at the precordial region and second posteriorly however this is not possible because the patient lies supine therefore one paddle (sternal paddle) is placed right infraclavicular and second (apex paddle) over precordium. Paddle should be applied with pressure equivalent to 10 kg. Defibrillation pads in patients with intra- cardiac devices (ICD) should be away from ICD device.

Paddle size:
- For adults: 13 cm.
- For children: 8 cm.
- For infants: 4.5 cm.

Latest recommendations for energy selection and shock protocol:
- *With monophasic defibrillators all shocks should be of 360 Joules (J). With biphasic defibrillators, the shock energy should be 150–200 J (if exponential waveform is used)* or 120 J *(if rectilinear waveform is used). The clinician should go by the manufacturer's recommendation.*
- Immediately after giving shock give 5 cycles of 30:2 (without advanced airway) or 2 minutes of CPR (with advanced airway) before checking rhythm. The rationale for this recommendation is that it actually takes around 2 minutes for heart to generate cardiac output even if rhythm becomes sinus therefore CPR during these 2 minutes is required to maintain coronary and cerebral perfusion. Or in simple words it can be said that *end point to stop CPR is the return of spontaneous circulation (ROSC)* assessed by palpating carotids, not the rhythm even if it is sinus.

MANAGEMENT OF NONSHOCKABLE RHYTHMS (FLOW CHART 41.3)

(Asystole, pulseless electrical activity)

Pulseless Electrical Activity (PEA)

PEA used to be called as electromechanical dissociation (EMD). As the name suggests, PEA is

Flow chart 41.2: Algorithm showing shockable rhythms

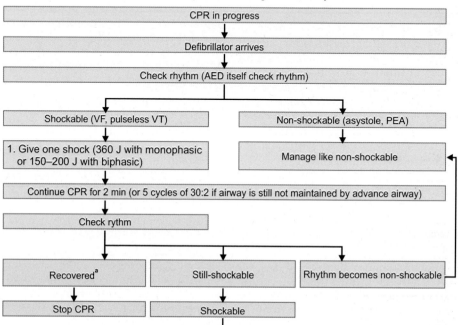

Contd...

Contd...

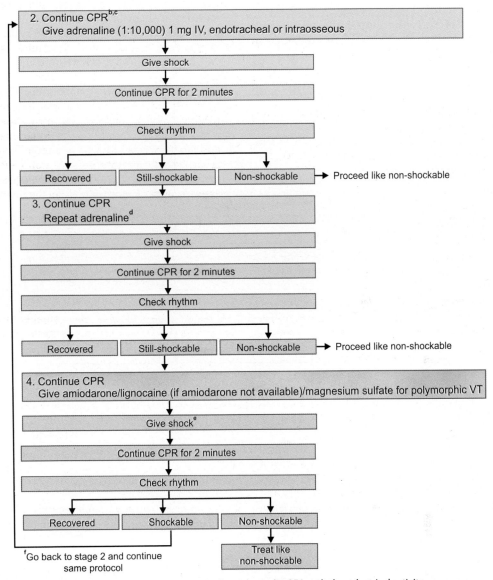

Abbreviations: VF, ventricular fibrillation; VT, ventricular tachycardia; PEA, pulseless electrical activity
a. Recovered means return of spontaneous circulation (ROSC) as judged by palpation of carotid pulse or return of normal end tidal CO_2
b. CPR should be resumed immediately after defibrillation (gap should not be more than 10 seconds)
c. Consider intubation and putting I/V line at this stage. Defibrillation takes the priority; intubation and IV access should not delay defibrillation if ventilation can be achieved by bag and mask. In fact, there have been many instances where patient recovers with first shock avoiding the intubation.
d. Vasopressin, which was given after 1st dose of adrenaline has been, removed from 2015 CPR guidelines.
e. Defibrillation should be attempted 2 minutes after epinephrine and amiodarone injection.
f. Consider termination of efforts if no response for 20 minutes

Flow chart 41.3: Algorithm showing management of nonshockable rhythms

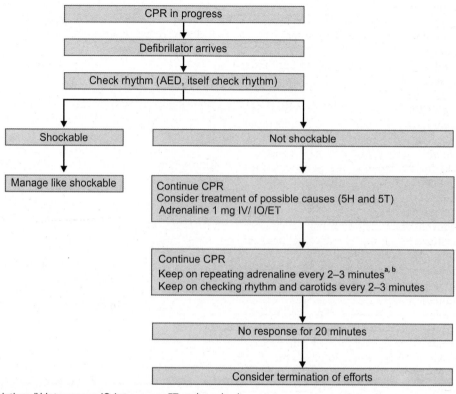

Abbreviations: IV, intravenous; IO, intraosseus; ET, endotracheal
a. Vasopressin, which was given after 1st dose of adrenaline has been removed from 2015 CPR guidelines.
b. Atropine has already been removed in 2010 guidelines.

the condition in which peripheral pulses are not palpable but heart shows some electrical activity on ECG other than ventricular tachycardia and ventricular fibrillation. Most common electrical activity seen is idioventricular rhythm or bradya-systole.

Causes

The causes of PEA have been divided into 5H and 5 T.

5H

  i. *Hypovolemia*: *Hypovolemia (shock) is the most common cause of PEA*
 ii. Hypokalemia/hyperkalemia
iii. Hypothermia
 iv. Hypoxia
  v. Hydrogen ion (acidosis)

5T

  i. Tension Pneumothorax
 ii. Tamponade (cardiac)
iii. Thrombosis (coronary, pulmonary)
 iv. Tablets (drug overdoses)/toxins (accidental)
  v. Trauma

Asystole

Asystole is the terminal event of all arrhythmias. The prognosis of asystole is very poor as compared to PEA and ventricular fibrillation.

NEWER TECHNIQUES/VARIATIONS IN CPR

• *Impedance threshold device (ITD) and chest compression devices (CCD)*: The routine use of ITD and CCD is not recommended.

- *Extracorporeal CPR (ECPR)*: It means initiation of extracorporeal circulation and oxygenation. ECPR provides circulation and oxygenation till the cause of cardiac arrest is reversed.
- *Simultaneous abdominal compression*: Limits caudal movement of diaphragm and limits dissipation of intrathoracic pressure however is hardly used.
- *Cough CPR*: It is applicable to a conscious patient having VF. If a patient coughs during VF, increase in intrathoracic pressure can maintain cerebral perfusion (i.e. consciousness) for 90 seconds therefore ask these patients to cough every 1–3 sec till he/she is defibrillated.
- *Delayed ventilation*: Studies have shown improved survival and neurologic recovery in witnessed cardiac arrest with shockable rhythm if continuous 200 compressions with interposed shocks are given without providing ventilation; oxygen is delivered by passive insufflation. This study obviously endorses the role of "hands only" CPR for untrained lay rescuers.
- *Steroids and vasopressin*: The routine use of steroids and vasopressin is not recommended in present day CPR, nonetheless they can be considered for special circumstances along with adrenaline where standard CPR is failing to revive the patient.
- *Intravenous lipid emulsion (ILE)*: Not only for local anesthetic toxicity, ILE is now recommended empirically for cardiac arrest caused by other drugs and not responding to standard CPR.
- *Empiric naloxone*: Administration of IM or Intranasal (IN) Naloxone is recommended empirically to patients having suspected opioid poisoning (no breathing, pulses present) by health care as well as trained lay rescuers.

POSTCARDIAC ARREST CARE

Postcardiac arrest care is required for the patients who had survived the cardiac arrest. It includes:

- *Optimization of circulation*: The aim should be to maintain systolic blood pressure >90 mm Hg and mean arterial pressure > 65 mm Hg.
- *Optimization of ventilation*: Hyperoxia can produce complications including ARDS therefore use minimum FiO_2 which maintains target SPO_2 between 94 and 98%.
- *Targeted temperature management (TTM)*: Induced hypothermia after cardiac arrest is now called as TTM. As hypothermia is the only recommended method for brain protection TTM is applied to the patients who had survived the cardiac arrest but are comatose. *TTM means maintaining core body temperature for 32–36° for 24 hours.*
- *Moderate glycemic control*: Both hypoglycemia and hyperglycemia are unacceptable therefore moderate blood sugar (144–180 mg/dL or 8–10 mmol) should be maintained in post-resuscitation period.
- *Early percutaneous coronary intervention (PCI)*: Emergency (preferably within 90 minute) coronary angiography/angioplasty is recommended for all patients with ST elevation myocardial infarction (STEMI) and for hemodynamically unstable MI without ST elevation (Non-STEMI). However, if the center is not equipped to do PCI then patient should be transferred to PCI center preferably within 3–6 hours after medical management.
- *Early prognostication of neurologic outcome*: Prognostication is recommended *72 hours after return of spontaneous circulation* for those who have not been given TTM. For those who have received TTM prognostication should be done *72 hours after the completion of TTM.*
- All patients who progress to brain death should be considered potential organ donors and their relatives must be counseled for organ donations.
- Lignocaine or Amiodarone infusion is recommended to prevent the recurrence of VT.

PEDIATRIC CPR (EXCLUDING NEWBORN)

Age classification (From CPR point of view)
- *Neonate*: First 4 weeks after birth.
- *Infant*: 4 weeks to 1 year.
- *Child*: 1 year till puberty
- *Adult*: Beyond puberty.

Differences from Adults

- *Difference in BLS algorithm*:
  - *For single rescuer*:
    After assessing consciousness activate EMS via mobile however if activation

via mobile is not possible then assess breathing and circulation and if absent then *give 5 cycles of CPR (30:2) before going to activate EMS* (contrary to adults where activation of EMS is done before starting CPR). The reason for this difference in algorithm sequence is that the cause of cardiac arrest in children should be considered asystole until proved otherwise therefore rescuer is not in that hurry to get AED.

– *For 2 rescuers*:

Activation of EMS and CPR can go hand in hand; one person can activate EMS while second can continue with CPR.

For witnessed cardiac arrest if the cause is ventricular fibrillation or pulseless VT then algorithm sequence remains same as that of adult.

Cardiac arrest in children is usually asphyxial (respiratory) therefore there lies the great value of rescue breaths however untrained layman can continue with "hands only CPR".

- Ratio of compression to breathing: Ratio of compression to ventilation *without advanced airway is 30:2 for one rescuer and 15:2 for 2 rescuers* (While for adults it is 30:2 irrespective of rescuers). With advanced airway in place compression and breathing rate remain same for all ages, i.e. 100–120 compressions and 10 breaths/minute without any synchronization.
- If there is only respiratory arrest (no cardiac arrest, pulses are palpable) then give breath at a rate of 12–20/min (Adults 10–12/min).
- *Pulse check*:
  – *Infants*: Brachial/Femoral.
  – *Children*: Carotid.
  – *Adult*: Carotid/Femoral.
- Cuffed endotracheal tubes can be used in pediatric patients; nonetheless a leak must be maintained around the cuff (inflated or not inflated) at a pressure of more than 15–20 cm H_2O.
- Heart rate <60/min with signs of poor perfusion (pallor/cyanosis) is the indication to start chest compressions in pediatric age group.
- Advanced cardiac life support protocol for pediatric patient remains same with some notable difference like:

– Energy selection for shock (manual) is 2 J/kg for first shock and 4 J/kg subsequently. If AED is used it automatically select energy and do attenuation accordingly. *Pediatric AED are only recommended for children < 8 years (or <25 kg). Children > 8 years (> 25 kg) should be defibrillated with adult defibrillators.* For infants, manual defibrillators should be preferred over AED

– Endotracheal concentration of adrenaline for adults is 1:10,000 while for pediatric age group it is 1: 1000.

- *Targeted temperature management*:

For comatose children resuscitated after outside hospital cardiac arrest normothermia (36°C to 37.5°C) for 5 days or hypothermia (32°C to 34°C) for 2 days followed by normothermia for 3 days is recommended. For in-hospital cardiac arrests maintaining normothermia for 5 days is advocated.

- Systolic blood pressure should be maintained above the fifth percentile for age in post cardiac arrest care.
- Maintain normoxia—both hypoxia and hyperoxia are detrimental.

NEWBORN CPR

The detailed discussion of newborn CPR is beyond the scope of this book however some of the notable points are:

- Rate of ventilation (breathing) is 40–60 breaths/min (if only ventilation is given).
- Indication of chest compression is HR (heart rate) < 60/min in spite of adequate ventilation with 100% oxygen for 30 seconds.
- The primary measure for successful ventilation is increase in heart rate.
- 2 thumbs with encircled chest is preferred method for compression over only 2 thumb technique.
- Compression ventilation ratio is 3:1 (90 compressions with 30 breaths) and synchronized.
- Reassessment to be made every 30 sec and continue compression till HR >60/min.
- Adrenaline indicated if HR <60/min.
- Preterm babies should receive FiO_2 of 21–30%.
- Stop resuscitation if no signs of life after 10 minutes.

CPR IN PREGNANCY

- Studies have shown that lateral tilt compromises the quality of CPR therefore *lateral lilt has been eliminated from new CPR guidelines and aortocaval compression should be achieved by uterine displacement.*
- Sodium bicarbonate administration is advocated early.
- Early insertion of endotracheal tube is recommended to prevent aspiration. During mask ventilation cricoid pressure should be applied continuously till the patient is intubated.
- Pregnant patients are more prone for hypoxia therefore use of high FiO_2 is recommended.
- *Emergency LSCS (cesarean section) should be considered if fetus >25 week and LSCS can be performed within 4 minutes of maternal arrest.*

OPEN CHEST MASSAGE

Indications are:
- *Cardiac tamponade.*
- Penetrating blunt trauma.
- Air embolism.
- Arrest during intrathoracic procedures.
- Chest deformities.

COMPLICATIONS OF CPR

- Rib fracture.
- Pneumothorax.
- Pneumopericardium.
- Pneumomediastinum.
- Injury to diaphragm.
- Gastric injury.
- Lung injury.
- Injury to major vessels particularly by fractured rib.
- Injury to abdominal organs: Liver, spleen and stomach.

OUTCOME OF CPR

Outcome depends on the cause, time of initiation of CPR and duration for which CPR is performed. *Survival is better, if basic life support (BLS) is initiated within 4 minutes of arrest, ALS within 8 minutes and CPR time is less than 30 minutes.*

Fortunately most common cause of cardiac arrest is ventricular fibrillation which if detected in time can have 50 to 60% success rate. Average survival rate of in-hospital arrest is 8 to 21%.

IMPORTANT CONSIDERATIONS IN CPR

Intravascular Access

Any peripheral or central vein can be chosen for IV access. Subclavian is the most preferred central vein in emergency situations. In case of non-availability of intravascular access other routes which can be utilized are intraosseous and endotracheal.

Intraosseous (IO)

As per the current guidelines *intraosseous route is recommended for all ages* (previously employed only for children < 6 years), *anything can be given* (even blood transfusion) *and is preferred over endotracheal route.* A 16 or 18 G needle is inserted over anterior surface of tibia 2–3 cm below the tibial tuberosity. The drug/fluid is injected directly in medullary cavity.

Endotracheal (ET)

Rates of absorption of drug from endotracheal route are almost similar to intravenous route. Drugs which can be delivered by ET route are:
- Adrenaline
- Atropine
- Lignocaine (Xylocard)
- Naloxone.

The *dose by endotracheal route is 2.5 times of intravenous dose* and the drug should be diluted with 10 mL of saline in adults and 5 mL in children.

Fluid During CPR

Glucose containing solutions should not be used as hyperglycemia increases cerebral edema. Ringer lactate should be avoided as calcium present in ringer lactate can cause neuronal injury. Therefore, *fluid of choice during CPR is normal saline.*

Intracardiac Adrenaline

This route offer no advantage rather injection in myocardium can cause significant myocardial injury therefore *adrenaline by intracardiac route is contraindicated in present day CPR.*

Calcium

Calcium as a routine is contraindicated in CPR because excess calcium worsens cellular death. Calcium is only recommended if cardiac arrest is due to hypocalcemia, hyperkalemia and over dosage of calcium channel blockers.

Use of Sodium Bicarbonate

Use of sodium bicarbonate without proven acidosis on blood gas analysis do more harm than benefit due to the following reasons:

- Sodium bicarbonate on metabolism produces carbon dioxide which can change cerebral pH and can worsen the neuronal injury.
- Excess CO_2 increases the intracranial tension.
- Diffusion of CO_2 into cell can worsen intracellular acidosis (paradoxical acidosis).
- Sodium bicarbonate is hypertonic therefore can increase plasma osmolarity significantly.

Therefore, it can be very well concluded that routine use of sodium bicarbonate is *not recommended*; it should be given only if there is proven acidosis (pH <7.15) in blood gas analysis.

Dose: $0.3 \times$ body weight $\times$ base deficit.

Cerebral Protection

Cerebral hypoxia and brain damage is a constant fear in medical practice. Although theoretically there is conventional notion that irreversible brain damage occurs if there is significant hypoxia for >6 minutes however there are enough evidences that irreversible brain damage has not occurred even after complete hypoxia of 20 minutes (that is why patient can be declared dead only after resuscitation of 20 minutes).

The only recommended modality for global cerebral ischemia seen in CPR is targeted temperature management. It can be achieved by cold IV saline infusion, covering the patient with cold blankets or at least putting ice on carotids. Other agents like Barbiturates (Thiopentone), Propofol or calcium channel blockers (Nicardipine, Nimodipine) are useful for focal ischemia however their role in global ischemia is not proven.

Brain Death

Brain death is the irreversible cessation of all brain functions.

Criteria

- Rule out all reversible causes of coma (hypothermia, drug intoxication, metabolic encephalopathy, shock etc.)
- Absent cerebral functions: No motor activity (even decorticate or decerebrate activity should be absent), no cerebral responsiveness.

- Absent brainstem reflexes (cough, pupillary, corneal, pharyngeal, laryngeal and carinal)
- Clinical test
    - No spontaneous respiration even if pCO_2 increases to 60 mm Hg
    - No spontaneous respiration and cough reflex on carinal stimulation
    - No increase in heart rate in response to 2 mg atropine
- Highly desirable (but not necessary)
    - Flat (isoelectric) EEG
    - Absent evoked responses
    - Radiological evidence of absent cerebral perfusion.

Declaration should be done by two doctors; one among those should be the neurologist.

SUMMARY OF CHANGES AS PER 2015 GUIDELINES IN COMPARISON TO 2010

See **Table 41.2**.

DRUGS FOR CPR

Adrenaline (Epinephrine)

It stimulates both α and β receptors (both $\beta1$ and $\beta2$). It increases stroke volume, heart rate and cardiac output. It increases the systolic while decreases the diastolic blood pressure. Vasoconstriction seen in cerebral, pulmonary and coronary blood vessels is far less as compared to vasoconstriction seen in other vascular beds like skin or splanchnic leading to *diversion of blood flow from non critical to vital structures like brain and heart* (a very beneficial effect of adrenaline in CPR).

Pharmacokinetics

Available as 1 mL injection containing 1 mg of adrenaline in 1 : 1,000 concentration. It can be given by IV, IO (Intraosseous), endotracheal route (ET), I/M and subcutaneous (S/C).

Concentration and Dose

See **Table 41.3**.

Amiodarone

Amiodarone is *considered as drug of choice for ventricular tachycardia. It can be used for ventricular as well as supraventricular tachycardia.* First dose is 300 mg IV and subsequent doses are 150 mg.

■ **Table 41.2:** Comparison between 2010 and 2015 guidelines

S. no.	Factor	2015	2010
1.	Chest compression	Not more than 2. 4 inches (6 cm)	At least 2 inches (5 cm), no upper limit
2.	Compression rate	100–120 but not more than 120	100/min
3.	Breath rate	10/minute	8–10/minute
4.	Vasopressin	No vasopressin	Vasopressin after 1st or 2nd dose of adrenaline
5.	Activation of emergency medical services (EMS)	Flexibility at multiple stages of CPR	Activation at 2nd step after assessing responsiveness
6.	Assessment of breathing and pulse	Simultaneously	Separately
7.	Targeted temperature management	32–36° C for 24 hours	32–34° C for 12 hours
8.	Extracorporeal circulation (ECC)	Employed early	Less liberal approach towards ECC
9.	Prognosis	To be assessed only after 72 hours	No specific time was mentioned
10.	Organ donation	More emphasis	Comparatively less emphasis

■ **Table 41.3:** Concentration of adrenaline

Dose	Concentration
1. CPR: 1 mg to be repeated every 3–5 minutes	IV/IO/ET—1: 10,000 If premixed 1: 10000 is not available then dilute 1 amp. (1: 1000) with 10 mL of saline
	ET in children—1: 1,000
2. Anaphylaxis: 0.5–1 mg to be repeated every 3–5 minutes	IM (and S/C)—1: 1000 IV/IO/ET—1: 10,000
3. With local anesthetics	1: 2,00,000
4. For producing local ischemia	1 : 1,00,000

■ **Table 41.4:** Summary of cardiopulmonary and cerebral resuscitation (CPCR)

	Newborn	Infant	Child	Adult	Comments
Age criteria		0–1 year	1 year- puberty	Above puberty	
Pulse check	Heart (auscultation)	Brachial/femoral	Carotid	Carotid/femoral	
Compression area	Lower 1/3 of sternum	Midsternum (line below intersection of intermammary line)	Midsternum (line below intersection of intermammary line)	Lower 1/3 sternum (2 finger above xiphisternum)	
Compression method	2 thumb with encircled chest	2–3 fingers	Heel of one hand	Heel of two hand one locked over other	Compression in newborn and infant should be started if HR <60/min
Sternal depth	1 inch	1.5 inch (4 cm) {1/3 of AP diameter of chest}	2 inch (5 cm) {1/3 of AP diameter of chest}	2 inch (5 cm)	Compression depth should not exceed >2.4 inch (6 cm)

Contd...

Contd...

	Newborn	Infant	Child	Adult	Comments
Compression rate	90/min	100–120/min	100–120/min	100–120/min	Rate should not be >120/min
Ventilation rate • If compression is also provided simultaneously	30/min	10/min	10/min	10/min	
• If only ventilation is needed	40–60/min	12–20/min	12–20/min	10–12/min	
Compression ventilation ratio: • Without advanced airway in place (i.e. ventilation with bag and mask)	3:1 with pause for ventilation [90 compression with 30 breaths]	30:2-for single resuscitator, 15:2-for two resuscitators	30:2-for single resuscitator, 15:2-for two resuscitators	30:2 irrespective of no. of resuscitators	Previously it was 15:2 for adults before intubation
• With advanced airway in place (i.e. endotracheal tube, LMA, combitube, tracheostomy tube)	– same –	100 compression/min and 10 breath/min without any synchronization (i.e. no pause for ventilation)	100 compression and 10 breath/min without synchronization	100 compression 10 breath/min without any synchronization	

Xylocard

Xylocard is preservative free Lignocaine used for the treatment of ventricular tachyarrhythmia. The dose is 1.5–2 mg/kg followed by infusion at a rate of 1–4 mg/min.

For summary of cardiopulmonary and cerebral resuscitation (CPCR) see **Table 41.4**.

KEY POINTS

- Unwitnessed cardiac arrest in adults should be considered due to ventricular fibrillation until proved otherwise and in children should be considered due to asystole until proved otherwise.
- The standard sequence of CPR, i.e. A (airway) → B (breathing) → C (circulation) was changed to C → A → B in 2010 CPR guidelines.
- Epiglottis, rather than tongue fall, has been found to be the more important cause of airway obstruction in unconscious patient.
- In patients with suspected cervical spine fracture if airway is not manageable by jaw thrust alone then head tilt and chin lift can be given.
- For patients with cervical spine fractures intubation should be performed with neck in neutral position and only after stabilization. Manual stabilization is preferred over collar stabilization.
- Rescue breath by mouth to mouth is reserved only for trained rescuers.
- For untrained lay rescuer CPR means "hands only" i.e. only cardiac massage.
- Intubation is the most definitive and best method for ventilation.
- Cardiac massage should be able to depress sternum by 2 inches (5 cm) but not more than 2.4 inches (6 cm).
- During CPR rescuer must not lean on patient chest between compressions.
- The rate of cardiac compression should be 100–120 compressions/minute but not more than 120.

Contd...

Contd...

- Without advanced airway the ratio of compression to breathing for adults should be 30:2 irrespective of number of resuscitators while for children this ratio is 30: 2 for single rescuer and 15:2 for two rescuers.
- With advanced airway compression is continued at a rate of 100–120 compressions/minute and breathing at a rate of 10 breaths/minute without any synchronization.
- In the current day CPR Capnography is considered essential.
- Successful cardiac massage should be able to produce $ETCO_2$ of at least 20 mm Hg.
- Ventricular fibrillation, pulseless ventricular tachycardia and polymorphic ventricular tachycardia are shockable rhythms while pulseless electrical activity and asystole are considered as nonshockable rhythms.
- Shock energy should be 360J with monophasic defibrillators and 150–200 with biphasic defibrillators.
- Immediately after giving shock give 5 cycles of 30:2 or 2 minutes of CPR before checking the rhythm.
- The end point to stop CPR is the return of spontaneous circulation (ROSC) assessed by palpating carotids.
- Vasopressin, which was given after 1st dose of adrenaline, has been removed from 2015 CPR guidelines.
- Defibrillation should be attempted 2 minutes after epinephrine and Amiodarone injection.
- Consider termination of CPR efforts if no response for 20 minutes.
- Hypovolemia (shock) is the most common cause of pulseless electrical activity (PEA).
- Targeted temperature management is the only recommended method for brain protection.
- Targeted temperature management means maintaining core body temperature between 32–36° for 24 hours.
- Prognostication is recommended after 72 hours.
- In unwitnessed cardiac arrest in children 5 cycles of CPR are given before activating EMS.
- During CPR in pregnancy aortocaval compression should be prevented by uterine displacement, not by lateral tilt.
- Emergency cesarean section should be considered if fetus >25 week and cesarean section can be performed within 4 minutes of maternal arrest.
- Intraosseous route is recommended for all ages, anything can be given and is preferred over endotracheal route.
- Fluid of choice during CPR is normal saline.
- Adrenaline by intra-cardiac route is contraindicated in present day CPR.
- The routine empiric use of sodium bicarbonate is not recommended.
- The intravenous/intraosseous/endotracheal tube (IV/IO/ET) concentration of adrenaline during CPR is 1: 10,000.
- Amiodarone is considered as drug of choice for ventricular tachycardia.

Conversion of Pressure

SI unit is kPa

1 atmosphere = 760 mm Hg = 1.033 kg/cm^2 = 1.013 bar = 14.7 PSI (pounds per square inch) = 101.32 kPa

1 kPa = 7.5 mm Hg

1 mm Hg = 1 torr = 1.3 cm H$_2$O = 13 mm H$_2$O

Units used in India are PSI and Kg/cm^2 (1 kg/cm^2 = 14.1 PSI)

For example: In a full oxygen cylinder the pressure is 2000 PSI which will be 141 kg/cm^2 or 139 bar or 14000 kPa or 1,06,000 mm Hg.

Drugs Metabolized by Plasma Cholinesterase (Pseudocholinesterase)

- Suxamethonium
- Mivacurium
- Ester-linked local anesthetics (except cocaine)

Drugs Metabolized by RBC Esterase

- Remifentanil
- Esmolol

Methemoglobinemia is seen with

- Prilocaone
- Benzocaine
- Nitroglycerine
- Impurities in nitrous oxide cylinder

Agents Producing Convulsions

- Methohexitone
- Enflurane
- Sevoflurane
- Atracurium/cisatracurium
- Local anesthetic toxicity

Antanalgesics

- Thiopentone (at sub-anesthetic doses)
- Promethazine

Bag and Mask Ventilation is Contraindicated in

- Full stomach
- Pregnancy
- Intestinal obstruction
- Conditions increasing intra-abdominal pressure like obesity, abdominal tumor and ascites
- Conditions impairing the tone of lower esophageal sphincter like hiatus hernia and neuromuscular diseases
- Conditions delaying gastric emptying like diabetes mellitus and opioids
- Neonatal emergencies
  - Diaphragmatic hernia
  - Tracheoesophgeal fistula
  - Meconium aspiration syndrome
  - Pyloric stenosis

Index